IMMUNOLOGY

Other Books by the Authors

Biochemistry: A Problems Approach by Wood, Wilson, Benbow, and Hood
Molecular Biology of Eucaryotic Cells by Hood, Wilson, and Wood
Essential Concepts in Immunology by Weissman, Hood, and Wood

IMMUNOLOGY

Leroy E. Hood
California Institute of Technology

Irving L. Weissman
Stanford University

William B. Wood
University of Colorado, Boulder

The Benjamin/Cummings Publishing Company, Inc.
Menlo Park, California • Reading, Massachusetts
London • Amsterdam • Don Mills, Ontario • Sydney

Front cover photo: Lymphocytes and macrophages. [Courtesy of J. Orenstein and E. Shelton.]

Sponsoring editor: Mary Forkner
Production editor: Margaret Moore
Editor: Jim Hall
Cover designer: Paul Quin
Artist: Georgeann Waggaman

The Benjamin/Cummings Publishing Company, Inc.
2727 Sand Hill Road
Menlo Park, California 94025

Preface

Scope and Purposes of the Book

Although the study of immunology began in the 19th century, it remained largely a descriptive science until the early 1960s. During the last 15 years, however, the tools of modern biochemistry, genetics, and molecular biology have transformed immunology into a discipline with a dual nature. Aspects such as the structures of antibody molecules and genes are understood at the molecular level, whereas others, including much of cellular immunology, are still in a descriptive stage. In this book we attempt to describe both aspects clearly and, where possible, to integrate phenomenology with the detailed molecular picture that is emerging.

In this text, we have organized the subject matter of immunology into five chapters. Chapter 1, "The Immune System," deals with structural and functional aspects of the immune system from the perspective of cellular and developmental biology. Chapter 2, "Immunopathology," analyzes medically significant disorders of the immune system with a view toward further understanding of basic immunological principles. An appendix to this chapter discusses methods for measuring antigen–antibody interactions and their uses as tools in solving both fundamental and clinical problems. Chapter 3, "Antibodies," considers the structures and functions of antibody molecules as well as the organization, regulation, and evolution of antibody genes. Chapter 4, "Molecular Recognition at Cell Surfaces," represents a departure from standard immunology texts; it is an attempt to integrate current knowledge of cell-surface macromolecules and their organization, prevertebrate cell–cell recognition systems, cell-surface receptors of the immune system, and the vertebrate major histocompatibility complex, with the goal of understanding how external signals may trigger intracellular events in the immune response. Chapter 5, "Cancer Biology and Immunology," considers basic aspects of cancer and cancer therapy that relate to immunology.

Using the Book

Each chapter is comprised of four sections: Essential Concepts, References, Problems, and Answers. The Essential Concepts are the text sections; they present the most important general principles of each subject first, followed by more detailed information in sub-paragraphs.

The References offer short "where to begin" sections that cite readable introductory materials, followed by references to longer reviews and specific journal articles. We have included seminal articles from the classical literature as well as the most up-to-date references.

The Problems sections, we believe, contain much of the teaching value of the book. They provide from 11 to 27 problems each, of increasing difficulty. New concepts and techniques often are presented in the introductions to problems. Many problems have been drawn from the contemporary literature, so that the reader is exposed to data analysis in many areas of modern immunology. All information required to work these problems is contained in the book.

The Answers sections provide readers with detailed feedback on their efforts to obtain solutions, often by describing the analytical process originally used to interpret data in the literature.

In using these materials for courses in immunology at California Institute of Technology and Stanford University, we cover the Essential Concepts of Chapter 1 slowly, at the rate of 1 to 3 per lecture. Subsequent chapters then are covered more rapidly. For courses that emphasize immunoglobulin structure early, there is a natural break following Essential Concept 1-3, where Essential Concepts 3-1 through 3-6 may be inserted.

Audience

We have written *Immunology* with three audiences in mind: undergraduate and graduate students taking a first course in immunology; doctoral students in the health professions doing course work in immunology; and physicians wishing a text suitable for self-instruction with which to review modern immunology. The organization of the text allows its use at several levels, from a quick scan of the Essential Concepts and their opening statements as a review of principles in contemporary immunology, to detailed study of all the text and accompanying problems as a comprehensive introduction to the subject.

The immune system is complex, and immunologists have employed a complex terminology to describe it. We have taken pains to minimize the considerable problem that this terminology can pose for the nonimmunologist, by defining all terms clearly as they are introduced and by avoiding jargon and unnecessary abbreviations.

For all readers, we feel that the emphasis on problem solving can be a particularly valuable feature of the book. In order to gain an active working knowledge of immunology, we have found it essential for students to confront actual experimental data and solve concrete problems in addition to reading, listening to lectures, and learning factual material. Consequently, we have included simple as well as challenging problems with detailed answers in each chapter of the book. Students in the immunology courses we have taught often report that they have learned more from solving these problems than from any other aspect of the course.

Acknowledgments

Many people have contributed to the creation of this book. We are indebted to Jonathan Howard for extensive criticism and helpful suggestions on Chapter 1, and to Mert Bernfield, Barbara Birshtein, Mike Cecka, Henry Claman, Robert Fox, Jonathan Fuhrman, Henry Huang, Minnie McMillan, Carol Nottenberg, Bob Sanders, and Stewart Sell for reading and criticizing portions of the text. We are also indebted to Alfred Dorfman, Gerald Edelman, Sylvia Friedberg, George Gutman, Elias Lazarides, Jan Orenstein, Robert Rouse, Willem van Ewijk, and Roger Warnke for making photomicrographs available, and to Jonathan Fuhrman for contributing many of the problems. We thank the students and teaching assistants in our Caltech and Stanford immunology courses for their patience with early versions of the text and for their helpful suggestions. We are indebted to Jim Hall for creating the hospitable and productive environment of the Aspen Writing Center, and to Don King and the staff at the Given Institute of Pathology in Aspen for their generosity in allowing us to use their library facilities and participate in stimulating discussions with visitors at the Institute. Georgeann Waggaman skillfully transformed our crude drawings into finished artwork; Jim Hall and Mary Forkner provided invaluable editorial help; Claire Wolf and members of the Caltech Biology Division typing pool contributed expert secretarial assistance. Finally, we appreciate the support and understanding of our families during the writing of this book.

L. E. Hood, I. Weissman, W. B. Wood

Contents

5 CANCER BIOLOGY AND IMMUNOLOGY   401

Essential Concepts

1 THE IMMUNE SYSTEM

Vertebrates possess a surveillance mechanism, called the immune system, that protects them from disease-causing (pathogenic) microorganisms, such as bacteria and viruses, and from cancer cells. The immune system specifically recognizes and selectively eliminates foreign invaders. Immunology, the study of the immune system, has contributed significantly to modern medicine in areas such as blood transfusion, vaccination, organ transplantation, and the treatment of allergy, autoimmune disease, and cancer. Immunology also has made vital contributions to cell biology by advancing our understanding of differentiation, cell-cell cooperation, and the triggering of proliferation and differentiation by cell-surface receptors. This chapter considers the cell biology of the vertebrate immune response.

The immune system is highly complex and not yet understood completely. Much of the information in this chapter has been obtained recently. In addition, much of it is based on experiments with one organism, the mouse, or with artificial *in vitro* systems, which may prove inapplicable to humans and other mammals. Although most of the conclusions presented seem likely to be proven correct, a number of them are currently tentative and may be modified as additional evidence accumulates.

Essential Concepts 1–1 through 1–3 present an overview of the immune system and its response to foreign invaders. The remaining essential concepts deal with current knowledge of the development, anatomy, and function of the system in more detail.

Essential Concepts

1–1 Two systems of immunity protect vertebrates

A. Immune protection in vertebrates is provided by a dual system that maintains two basic defenses against foreign invaders. Both systems respond specifically to most foreign substances, although one response generally is favored. The *cellular* immune response is particularly effective against fungi, parasites, intracellular viral infections, cancer cells, and foreign tissue. The *humoral* immune response defends primarily against the extracellular phases of bacterial and viral infections.

Cellular immunity resides in cells of the lymphoid system. Humoral (circulating) immunity resides ultimately in the *serum,* which is the fluid residue of blood after cells and fibrinogen have been removed by clotting and centrifugation. Thus the two systems of immunity are distinct but provide overlapping protection.

B.   The duality of the immune system results from two populations of morphologically indistinguishable lymphoid cells, called *lymphocytes.* Each lymphocyte in these two populations is poised to recognize and respond to one or a few closely related foreign substances.

1.   One class of lymphocytes, the *T cells,* mediates the cellular immune response. When the organism is invaded by a foreign substance, the T cells that recognize it are activated and initiate a reaction that includes binding to and eliminating the substance (Figure 1–1).

2.   The other class of lymphocytes, the *B cells,* initiates the humoral immune response. Individual B cells, when activated by recognition of a foreign invader, differentiate to plasma cells which secrete *antibodies,* proteins that bind specifically to the foreign substance and initiate a variety of elimination responses (Figure 1–1).

C.   In addition to lymphocytes, the immune system depends upon several other kinds of accessory cells (Figure 1–2). Their functions include accumulation of foreign substances in the body for presentation

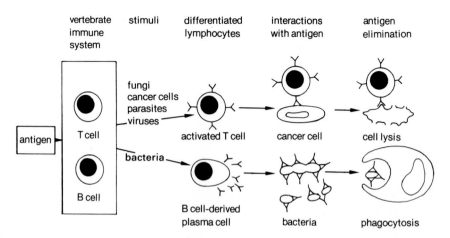

Figure 1–1 Differentiation, interaction, and elimination events that may occur upon stimulating T and B cells of the immune system.

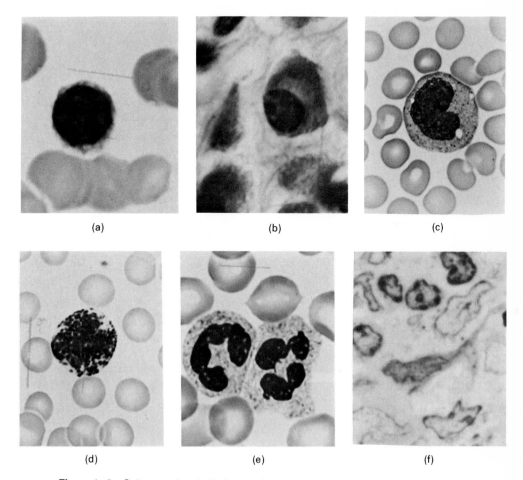

(a)   (b)   (c)

(d)   (e)   (f)

Figure 1–2   Cells associated with the vertebrate immune response: (a) blood lymphocyte (B or T), (b) plasma cell, (c) blood monocyte, (d) basophile, (e) polymorphonuclear leukocytes, (f) dendritic reticular cell. [Photomicrographs (a)–(e) courtesy of R. Rouse; (f) courtesy of G. Levine.]

to lymphocytes, scavenging of foreign invaders attacked by the immune system, and mediation of physiological changes that accompany the immune response.

D.   The dual system of T- and B-cell immunity appears to be restricted to vertebrates. Specific cellular and humoral immune responses are found in bony fishes and even in the lowest vertebrates. The extent to which cellular and humoral immunity occur in invertebrates is still unclear, although efficient cellular scavenging mechanisms, transplant rejection, and potent inducible antibacterial substances have been demonstrated in several subvertebrate species.

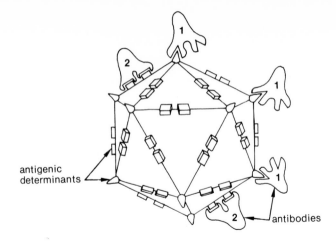

Figure 1–3 A virus interacting with antibodies specific to two types of antigenic determinants.

1-2 The immune system recognizes foreign entities by their molecular features

A. The essence of the immune system is its capacity to recognize surface features of macromolecules that are not normal constituents of the organism. The components of the organism that carry out this specific recognition are protein molecules called antibodies; the foreign entities that they recognize are termed *antigens*. That portion of the antigen to which an antibody binds is called an *antigenic determinant* (Figure 1-3). Antibodies recognize and bind antigens by molecular complementarity, which permits multiple noncovalent interactions of the same types that confer specificity on enzyme–substrate binding. An antigen complementary to a specific antibody is called a *cognate* antigen.

B. An antigen that elicits a response from the immune system is referred to as an *immunogen*. Macromolecules such as foreign proteins, nucleic acids, and carbohydrates usually are effective immunogens; molecules with molecular weights of less than 5000 usually are not. However, many small nonimmunogenic molecules, termed *haptens*, can stimulate an immune response if covalently attached to a large *carrier* molecule. For example, the 2,4-dinitrophenyl group rarely is immunogenic unless attached to a carrier protein such as serum albumin (Figure 1-4).

Animals that have an appropriate number of activated specific T cells or an appropriate concentration of specific antibody in their blood are *immune* to the cognate antigens.

C. Antibodies belong to a class of proteins called *immunoglobulins*. The basic unit of immunoglobulin structure is a complex of four polypeptides, two identical "light" (low molecular weight) chains and two identical "heavy" (high molecular weight) chains, linked together by disulfide bonds (Figure 1-5).

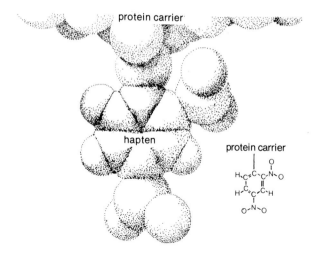

Figure 1–4 Three-dimensional representation of a simple hapten, the dinitrophenyl group, attached to a hypothetical protein carrier. The structural formula of the dinitrophenyl group is shown at right. [Adapted from G. Edelman, *Sci. Am.* **223,** 34 (1970). Copyright © 1970 by Scientific American, Inc. All rights reserved.]

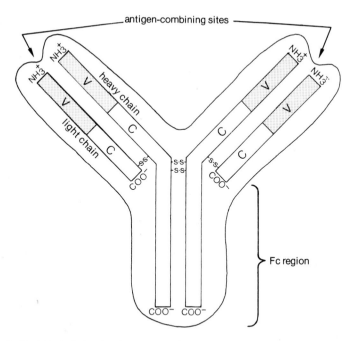

Figure 1–5 A two-dimensional representation of the antibody molecule. The heavy and light chains are joined by disulfide bridges. The N-terminal (NH$_3^+$) and C-terminal (COO$^-$) ends and the variable (V) and constant (C) regions of each chain are oriented as shown. The envelope around the immunoglobulin molecule approximates its three-dimensional shape. The antigen-combining sites are located between the V regions of the light and heavy chains.

The carboxyl-terminal (C-terminal) portions of the light and heavy chains, termed the *constant* regions, are nearly identical for antibodies of the same class. The stem of an immunoglobulin molecule, formed by the C-terminal halves of the two heavy chains, is called the *Fc* region. The amino-terminal (N-terminal) portions of the light and heavy chains differ substantially in amino acid sequence between individual species of antibody. These *variable* regions of the light and heavy chains combine to form the antigen-binding sites of an antibody molecule, as shown in Figure 1–5. The *valence* of an antibody is the number of identical antigen-binding sites per molecule. The *affinity* of an antibody-combining site is a measure of the strength of its binding to an antigenic determinant. The term *avidity* is used to describe the net strength of interaction of a *multivalent* antibody with a *multideterminant* antigen.

1.   The variable and constant regions, respectively, are responsible for the two functions of an antibody: the *antigen-recognition function* and the *effector function*. Circulating antibodies have a variety of characteristic effector functions that are involved in the elimination of foreign antigens.

2.   Immunoglobulins in mammalian serum can be divided into five classes on the basis of amino acid sequence differences in the constant regions of their heavy chains. These classes, designated IgM, IgG, IgA, IgD, and IgE, correspond to antibodies with different effector functions.

3.   The antigen-binding sites of individual antibodies are unique combinations of light-chain and heavy-chain variable regions, and consequently exhibit unique protein structures. If a specific antibody from one animal is injected as an immunogen into a suitable second animal, the injected antibody will elicit production of host antibodies. Some of these antibodies will be specific for the unique determinants of the variable regions of the injected antibody. Such antigenic determinants are known collectively as the *idiotype* of the immunizing antibody. Every species of antibody will exhibit unique idiotypic determinants, some of which are determined by its antigen-binding site and some of which are determined by structural features outside the binding site.

The structures and molecular functions of antibody molecules are discussed in more detail in Chapter 3.

1–3   Each lymphocyte is predetermined to express a homogeneous set of membrane-bound receptors with a single specificity for antigen

A.   The general mechanism by which a vertebrate can mount an immune response specific to any of a nearly infinite variety of antigens was explained in the 1950's by the clonal selection theory of antibody formation, a set of postulates put forward by Jerne, Burnet, Lederberg, and Talmage. Subsequent research has substantiated these postulates, which are stated in their modern form in Sections B through E and are diagramed in Figure 1–6.

B.   The cell surfaces of lymphocytes carry membrane-bound antibodies or antibody-like molecules that function as antigen receptors. The receptors of B cells are known to be antibodies, which are present on the membrane in a quantity of about 10^5 molecules per cell. The receptors of T cells appear to have similar properties, but their molecular nature is still unknown. Binding of an antigen to a receptor initiates a humoral or a cellular immune response, depending upon whether a B-cell or a T-cell receptor is stimulated.

Each lymphocyte carries only one kind of specific receptor, and therefore will respond to only a few closely related antigenic determi-

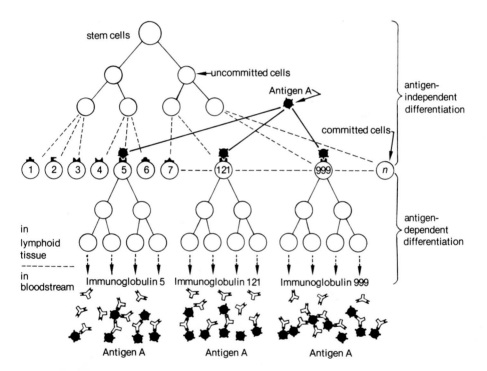

Figure 1–6   The clonal selection theory of antibody formation. Stem cell progeny undergo an antigen-independent differentiation that ultimately commits each of 10^5 to 10^8 clones to the synthesis of its own molecular species of antibody (numbers). These antibodies are displayed as receptors on the cell surfaces. A particular antigen (A) usually interacts with several clones to initiate the antigen-dependent stage of differentiation, which leads to proliferation of clones of antibody-producing cells with complementary receptors and to the synthesis of specific antibody molecules. [Adapted from G. Edelman, Sci. Am. **223**, 34 (1970). Copyright © 1970 by Scientific American, Inc. All rights reserved.]

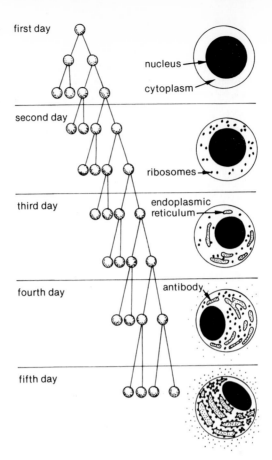

first day

nucleus

cytoplasm

second day

ribosomes

third day

endoplasmic
reticulum

fourth day

antibody

fifth day

Figure 1–7 Successive stages in the development of mature plasma cells after triggering by antigen. This process takes about five days and eight cell generations. The mature plasma cell has an extensive endoplasmic reticulum whose internal cavities are filled with antibody molecules. [Adapted from G. J. V. Nossal, *Sci. Am.* **211,** 109 (1964). Copyright © 1964 by Scientific American, Inc. All rights reserved.]

nants. However, a mammal contains 10^8 to 10^{12} lymphocytes, which collectively possess the capacity to respond to an enormous variety of antigens. This lymphocyte population is thought to consist of 10^5 to 10^8 clones of cells with different receptor specificities. Therefore, the sizes of these clones are thought to range from about 1 to about 10^7 cells. However, the number of lymphocytes in the population that potentially can react with a typical antigen is much larger, because such an antigen displays many determinants, and because a given determinant can be recognized by more than one kind of receptor.

C. Lymphocytes that bind an antigen may be triggered to proliferate and differentiate. They form clones of progeny lymphocytes, each of which displays surface receptors of the same idiotype as its parent cell. In the process of proliferation, some progeny differentiate into *effector cells,* the functional end products of the immune response (Figure 1–7). The B lymphocyte effector cells are *plasma cells* (Figure 1–2b), which secrete humoral antibodies of the same idiotype and antigen-recognition specificity as their cell-surface receptors (Figure 1-7). T lymphocytes give rise to several types of effector cells with different functions. One of these types is the *cytotoxic* or *killer T cell* (T_C cell), which eliminates foreign cells directly. Other types of effector T cells are responsible for delayed hypersensitivity (T_D cells), for helping B-cell differentiation and proliferation (T_H cells), for amplifying killer T-cell differentiation and proliferation (T_A cells), and for suppressing immune responses (T_S cells).

D.   The clonal selection process explains the phenomenon known as *immunologic memory*. For example, when a mammal first encounters an antigen, its so-called primary immune response exhibits the kinetics shown in Figure 1-8. However, if the mammal encounters the same antigen after an interval of a few days, or at any later time during its life, its specific response is both more rapid and of greater magnitude. The initial encounter causes specific B- and T-cell clones to proliferate and differentiate. The progeny lymphocytes include not only effector cells, but also expanded clones of *memory cells*, which retain the capacity to produce further progeny cells of both the effector and memory types upon subsequent stimulation by the original antigen. Whereas the lifetime of an effector cell is measured in days, the memory cells produced in a primary response can remain in the lymphocyte population for decades. Thus if the same antigen is encountered again, its cognate

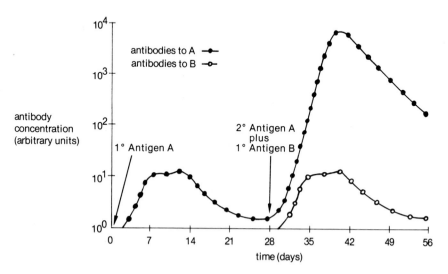

Figure 1-8 Kinetics of the appearance of immunoglobulins in the serum following primary (1°) and secondary (2°) immunizations at days 0 and 28, respectively. The secondary immunization includes a control antigen to demonstrate the specificity of immunological memory. The secondary response is both faster and greater than the primary response.

memory cells rapidly produce large numbers of effector cells to give the rapid increases in specific humoral antibodies and effector T cells characteristic of a secondary response.

E.   The clonal selection process also must account for the phenomenon of *tolerance*, a mechanism that prevents organisms from mounting immune responses to the antigenic determinants of their own macromolecules. Tolerance is created by a process that eliminates or suppresses all clones of lymphocytes that could respond to normal constituents of the organism.

1-4   Precursor lymphocytes differentiate along one of two pathways to produce functionally distinct T and B cells

A.   In mammals the primordial lymphocyte precursors arise in the blood islands of the yolk sac and then migrate successively to the embryonic liver and bone marrow. Throughout the remainder of the organism's lifetime the bone marrow produces blood-forming (hematopoietic) stem cells, which have lymphocyte precursors among their progeny.

All of the cells in the hematolymphoid system (Figure 1–9) follow analogous maturation pathways. They derive from a common stem cell, which gives rise to cells that somehow are precommitted to entering a particular tissue microenvironment. Interaction of the microenvironment with the precommitted cell induces further proliferation and differentiation to committed cells equipped with surface receptors for specific stimuli. Committed cells, when triggered by a specific stimulus, undergo terminal differentiation to effector cells with various functions. All the committed and effector cells shown in Figure 1–9, except erythrocytes, are involved in host defense mechanisms. In this section we shall discuss only the maturation of the lymphocyte series. These cells mature through one of two developmental pathways into immunologically competent T and B cells.

B.   Maturation of both T and B cells is believed to include an antigen-independent phase and an antigen-driven phase (Figure 1–6). Each phase may involve several steps, each of which yields cells at a defined maturational stage that is characterized by a distinct set of cell-surface antigens. These sets of antigens may be used as *differentiation markers.* The differentiation steps that occur in the fetus or in organs that do not accumulate and process foreign antigens currently are thought to be antigen-independent. Lymphocytes that differentiate in these environments become *immunocompetent;* that is, they acquire antigen-specific cell-surface receptors and the cellular machinery to respond to antigen stimulation. These cells are called *virgin lymphocytes.* Antigen-driven differentiation of these lymphocytes results eventually in the generation of memory cells and effector cells. However, there

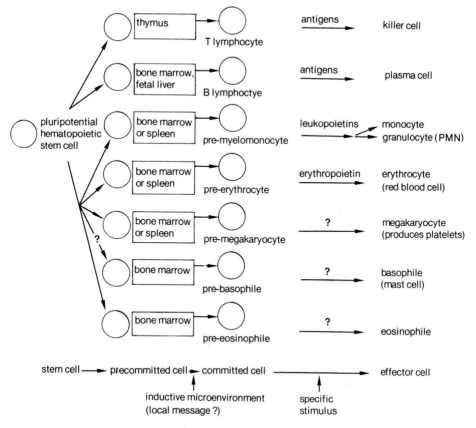

Figure 1–9 Differentiation pathways in the mammalian hematolymphoid system. Branch points between the pluripotential hematopoietic stem cell and precommitted cells indicate probable intermediate precursor cells.

is considerable evidence that the latter two cell types derive not directly from virgin lymphocytes, but rather from an intermediate class of immunocompetent cells, which provisionally have been termed *mature lymphocytes*. It is not yet clear whether the steps that lead from virgin to mature lymphocytes are antigen-driven, but the differentiation of mature lymphocytes to effector cells definitely requires stimulation by a specific antigen. Thus the term "mature" will be used to designate immunocompetent lymphocytes that already may or may not have undergone some antigen-dependent differentiation.

C.   Maturation of the T-cell lineage involves at least four distinct events: embryological establishment of the maturational microenvironment in the thymus, seeding of the thymic microenvironment by precommitted hematopoietic T-cell precursors, intrathymic proliferation and differentiation, and migration of T cells to T-cell domains in peripheral lymphoid tissues. In the process of maturation the T cells must be equipped with cell-surface molecules for specific recognition of other cells, for specific recognition of antigens, and eventually for the execution of T-cell effector functions.

1. The thymus, along with other internal organs, originates embryologically with the movement of cells from one embryonic germ layer, the endoderm, into another layer, the mesoderm (mesenchyme). The third and fourth pouches of the anterior endoderm penetrate the surrounding mesenchyme to initiate formation of the thymus and parathyroids (Figure 1–10). The thymus rudiment detaches itself and migrates down into the chest cavity.

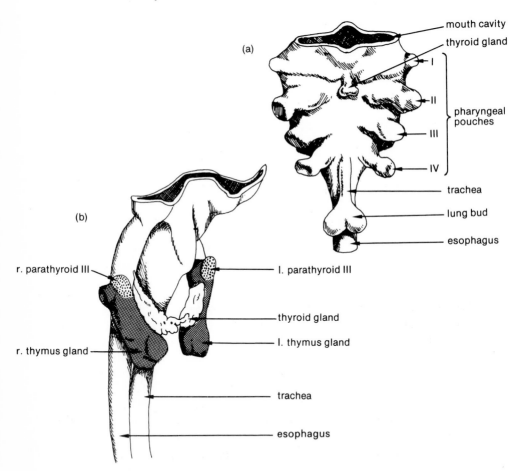

Figure 1–10 Embryological development of the thymus. (a) The third and fourth endodermal pharyngeal pouches migrate laterally into surrounding mesenchyme, and then split. The portions that remain in the neck (b) form the parathyroids, while the portions that migrate down into the chest cavity form the thymic lobes. [Adapted from G. L. Weller, *Contrib. Embryol. Carneg. Inst.* **24,** 93 (1933).]

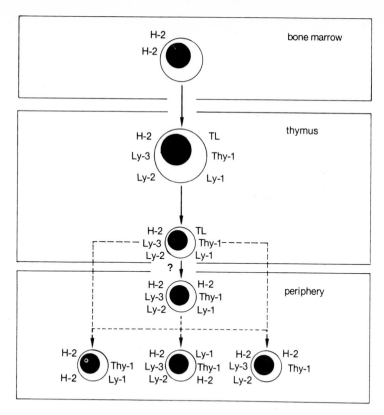

Figure 1–11 Differentiation of mouse T cells with acquisition of differentiation antigens. Dashed lines indicate possible alternative routes of differentiation. TL, Ly-1, Ly-2,3, Ly-1,2,3, and Thy 1 are T-cell differentiation antigens found on the cell surface. H-2 antigens are found on cell surfaces in most tissues of the mouse. Boxes indicate distinct anatomical compartments.

2. For a brief interval just after its downward migration, the thymic rudiment collects T-cell precursors from the blood. These cells rapidly are induced to express some cell-surface molecules characteristic of thymus cells (thymocytes), and other molecules that are common to all T cells. In mice some of the differentiation molecules have been detected serologically and are designated TL, Thy-1, and Ly-1, Ly-2, and Ly-3.

The expression of TL is closely linked genetically to that of several other cell-membrane molecules. The TL antigen is expressed on ≥95% of normal thymocytes and is present on most thymic leukemia (TL) cell lines. Most if not all peripheral T cells are TL-negative. Thy-1 is a membrane glycoprotein found on thymocytes, peripheral T cells and effector T cells, but not on B cells or other hematolymphoid cells. Ly-1, Ly-2, and Ly-3 antigens *all* are expressed on ≥95% of thymocytes and on nearly 50% of peripheral T cells; these cells are designated Ly-1,2,3 (Figure 1-11). The other 50% of peripheral T cells carry either the Ly-1 antigen alone, or the Ly-2 and Ly-3 antigens together (designated Ly-1 and Ly-2, 3 respectively). No other cells express these antigens.

Throughout life the hematopoietic tissues of the bone marrow provide a low level of thymic precursors, and also can provide a reservoir for massive thymic regeneration if necessary. Precommitment of these marrow cells to the T lineage does not involve expression of thymus cell-surface markers. Nevertheless, these cells have gained the ability to home specifically to the thymus, and the ability to be triggered specifically by the thymic microenvironment or by an extracted thymic hormone to express thymus cell-surface markers.

3. Soon after hematopoietic precursors appear in the thymus these cells organize into a layer 2 to 10 cells thick and become large, dividing cells (Figure 1–12), which give rise to all thymic

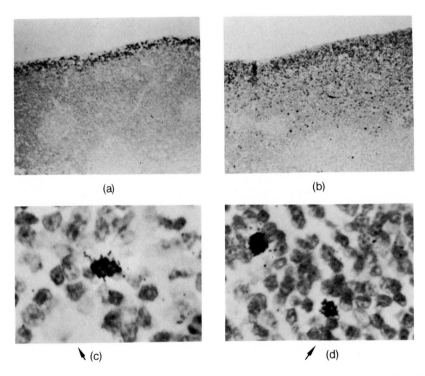

(a)   (b)

(c)   (d)

Figure 1–12 Radioautographs of thymus cells. A radioactive DNA precursor, tritiated thymidine, was applied to the thymus surface at time zero. Within an hour the layer of dividing thymus cells beneath the surface had incorporated this label into their DNA (a). One day later these labeled cells had migrated from the thymus surface to deeper areas of the cortex and to the medulla (b). By the second or third day, labeled cells were found in the lymph nodes (c) and the spleen (d). [Adapted from I. Weissman, *J. Exp. Med.* **126,** 291 (1967) and **137,** 504 (1973). © 1973 by The Rockefeller University Press.]

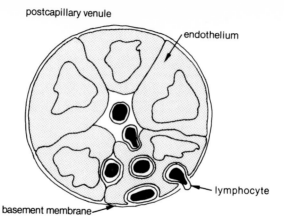

postcapillary venule

endothelium

lymphocyte

basement membrane

Figure 1-13 Diagrammatic cross-section of a lymph node postcapillary venule. Small dark cells are lymphocytes adhering to and migrating across the specialized endothelial walls of these vessels. [Redrawn from J. L. Gowans, *Hosp. Pract.* **3(3),** 34 (1968).]

lymphocytes and eventually to peripheral T cells. Under steady-state conditions this population of large dividing cells represents 5% of thymus cells. It gives rise to most (85–90%) of the deep cortical small thymocytes, as well as to a minor (3–5%) population of medium-size medullary thymocytes. The small thymocytes leave the thymus and are replaced by new cells every 3 to 5 days, so that in the mouse, for example, there is a daily turnover of 50 million to 100 million cells in the thymus. The fate of this rapidly turning-over population is not completely understood. Many cells migrate from the thymus, but many must die there or in the periphery, because the peripheral T-cell pool is not replaced at a comparable rate. Most peripheral T cells are long-lived, and only a few thymus cell migrants are allowed entry to this pool of more mature cells.

While in the thymus, T cells may become immunocompetent. A small proportion of competent cells remains in the thymus as medullary thymocytes. The population that migrates from the thymus contains competent T cells, although it is not clear what proportion of the population they comprise.

Although the thymus decreases considerably in size after puberty, in response to release of steroid hormones, it remains functional throughout life.

4. Thymus-cell migrants, equipped with the capacity for specific lymphoid homing, enter predetermined T-cell domains after traversing specialized small veins (postcapillary venules) in peripheral lymphoid tissues (Figure 1-13). These T cells possess surface receptors for antigens, although it is not known whether they can respond to antigenic stimulation by differentiation to effector cells. Most recently arrived thymus-cell migrants appear to be short-lived.

5. It has been proposed that these virgin T cells are triggered by cognate antigen to mature to long-lived, circulating peripheral T cells, and that only these mature cells respond to further antigenic stimulation by differentiating terminally to effector cells.

In mice, the first peripheral T cells that appear in development are Ly-1,2,3. As the animal ages, Ly-1 and Ly-2,3 cells appear. These latter cells differentiate to effector T cells. It has been proposed that Ly-1,2,3 thymic cells give rise to Ly-1,2,3 T cells, which in turn give rise to the mature Ly-1 and Ly-2,3 subsets (Figure 1–11). However, the existence of this sequence so far has not been proven by direct lineage analyses.

In summary, antigen-independent maturation of T cells in the thymus gives rise to a diverse population of short-lived antigen-specific T cells. Those cells that meet a cognate antigen in the periphery appear to complete their maturation sequence and gain the property of longevity.

D.   Maturation of B cells involves antigen-independent induction by a microenvironment as well as peripheral differentiation to mature subpopulations of immunocompetent cells. In the process, B cells, like T cells, acquire specific homing and cell-recognition properties, antigen-specific cell-surface receptor antibodies, and eventually B-cell effector functions.

1.   In mammals, precommitment of hematopoietic cells to the B-cell lineage and microenvironmental induction to virgin B cells occur in the liver and perhaps the spleen during fetal life, and in the bone marrow during adult life. Very little is known about early events in B-cell maturation, except that they include the expression of stage-specific B lineage cell-surface molecules, which have been detected as serological markers. One of these molecules is a membrane-bound IgM immunoglobulin.

In all vertebrate species tested, subclasses of B cells express one or both of two receptors for immunologically significant molecules: one for the Fc region of IgG immunoglobulins (Figure 1–5), and the other for the activated form of a serum complement component (C3b; Essential Concept 1–10C). The functional significance of these receptors is still unknown, but they provide useful markers for the identification of B cells in humans (Figure 1–14), and may represent stage-specific differentiation markers.

In mice, cell-surface markers specific for cells in the B lineage include the antigens Ly-4 and Pc-1. Ly-4 is found on B cells but not on plasma cells. Pc-1 is found only on plasma cells.

2.   Following their generation in bone marrow, the antigen-specific virgin B cells migrate to peripheral B-cell domains. In general, these cells are believed to be short-lived. Like virgin T cells,

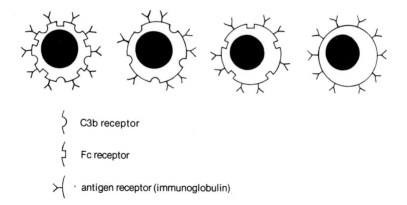

> C3b receptor

> Fc receptor

> · antigen receptor (immunoglobulin)

Figure 1–14 A diagram of four classes of B cells with differing combinations of B-cell-specific surface receptors. It is not known whether these B cells result from distinct pathways of differentiation or whether they represent different stages along a single differentiation pathway.

they probably require stimulation by a cognate antigen to undergo further differentiation to mature, long-lived, recirculating B cells, which respond to further antigenic stimulation by proliferating and terminally differentiating to memory B cells and antibody-secreting plasma cells.

3.   In birds, development of the B-cell but not the T-cell system is prevented by exposing the embryo to the male hormone testosterone. The *bursa of Fabricius,* a lymphoid pouch that connects with the intestinal lumen, fails to develop in these birds, and B cells and plasma cells do not appear. It seems likely that the lack of a bursa and the failure of B-cell system development are linked. Many immunologists believe that the bursa is the site for generation of virgin B cells in birds; in fact, this belief gave rise to the designation "B" for bursal cells. However, there is still no definitive proof that B-cell maturation in birds occurs solely in the bursa and not in hematopoietic tissues, as in mammals.

E.   The analysis of T- and B-cell differentiation sequences is difficult and still incomplete. Several animal and human lymphoid cancers appear to be of either T-cell or B-cell origin. Many of these cancer cell lines express different specific differentiation markers, as if frozen at various stages of maturation. Therefore, these tumor cell lines may prove extremely useful for further elucidating lymphocyte differentiation pathways.

F.   The ontogenic maturation time of the lymphoid system relative to birth differs from one species to another. As measured by the onset of immune responsiveness as well as by the appearance of peripheral

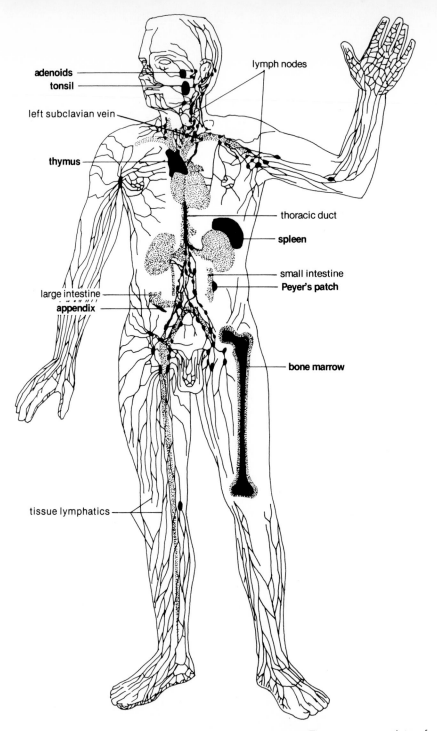

adenoids

tonsil

left subclavian vein

thymus

lymph nodes

thoracic duct

spleen

small intestine

Peyer's patch

large intestine

appendix

bone marrow

tissue lymphatics

Figure 1–15 A diagram of the human lymphoid system. The system consists of circulating lymphocytes and the lymphatic organs, which include the tree of lymphatic vessels and the lymph nodes stationed along them, the bone marrow (in the long bones, only one of which is illustrated), the thymus, the spleen, the adenoids, the tonsils, the Peyer's patches of the small intestine, and the appendix. The lymphatic vessels collect the lymphocytes and antibody molecules from the tissues and lymph nodes and return them to the bloodstream at the subclavian veins. [Adapted from N. K. Jerne, *Sci. Am.* **229,** 52 (1973). Copyright © 1973 by Scientific American, Inc. All rights reserved.]

T and B cells, mice and birds develop their immune systems just before and after birth, whereas sheep and humans develop functional immune systems early in gestation, well before birth. However, in all species the immediate postnatal period is marked by dramatic differentiative changes in the immune system, reflecting the sudden exposure to a host of environmental antigens.

1-5   Lymphocytes encounter and respond to antigens in specialized lymphoid organs

A.   Lymphocytes are carried throughout most of the tissues and organs of higher vertebrates by two circulatory networks, the blood and lymphatic systems. Lymphocytes make up 20–80% of the nucleated cells in the blood, and over 99% of the nucleated cells in the lymphatic fluid (lymph). However, lymphocytes contact and respond to immunizing antigens in specialized lymphoid organs that provide accessory cells and tissue architecture appropriate for antigen processing and presentation. The lymphoid system (Figure 1–15) has three principal functions: (1) to concentrate antigens from all parts of the body into a few lymphoid organs; (2) to circulate the lymphocyte population through these organs, so that every antigen is exposed to the organism's repertoire of antigen-specific lymphocytes in a short period of time; and (3) to carry the products of the immune response, antigen-specific effector T cells and humoral antibodies, to the bloodstream and the tissues.

B.   Antigens are collected and processed by different lymphoid organs (Figure 1–15), depending upon their route of entry into the body. Processing in all these organs involves white blood cells called *phagocytes* (*phago*, eating; *cyte*, cell), which take up antigens from the circulating fluid for presentation to lymphocytes. The large phagocytes found in lymphoid organs are called *macrophages* (Figure 1–2c).

   1.   Antigens that enter the intercellular spaces of any tissue are swept into the lymphatic system by lymph, the interstitial fluid that bathes the tissues. The lymphatic system is an extensively branched and widely dispersed network of thin-walled vessels with one-way valves and interspersed filtering organs called *lymph nodes*. The typical lymph node (Figure 1–16) is a bean-shaped organ that consists of an outer layer, the *cortex*, and an inner core called the *medulla*. A fibrous tissue network (reticulum) throughout the node supports macrophages and extensively branched *dendritic reticular cells;* the reticulum and its adherent cells trap antigens and provide passageways and niches for lymphocytes and their progeny (Figure 1–17).
      The lymphatic vessels originate in the interstitial spaces of the tissues. Interstitial fluid is pulled into and pumped through

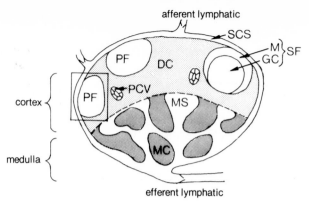

Figure 1–16 The general structure of a lymph node. The cortical subcapsular sinus (SCS) lies beneath the capsule of the node and communicates extensively with the sinuses of the medulla. The subcapsular sinus drains the extracellular space via afferent lymphatics, and is lined with phagocytic cells. The primary follicle (PF), lying directly under the SCS in the cortex, is an ovoid accumulation of small lymphocytes lying in a meshwork of dendritic reticular cells. The secondary follicle (SF) is composed of the mantle (M), the components of which are similar to those of the primary follicle, and the germinal center (GC), which contains small and large lymphocytes, many large blast cells with abundant cytoplasm, "tingible body" macrophages (containing phagocytized cell debris), and dendritic reticular cells. The diffuse cortex (DC) includes many small lymphocytes, macrophages, and post-capillary venules (PCV). The medullary sinus (MS) is lined by phagocytic cells. This sinus constitutes the route of emigration of itinerant T and B lymphocytes, as well as blast cells after antigen stimulation. The medullary cords (MC) are close-packed, interconnected spaces containing cords of cells, particularly plasma cells and large lymphoblasts.

the lymphatics by osmotic pressure and muscular contraction. The fluid is transported through *afferent lymphatic* vessels to lymph nodes. It enters a node through a series of cavities (*sinusoids*) that are lined with macrophages, percolates through the tissue of the lymph node, and exits via an *efferent lymphatic* vessel. Several efferent lymphatics come together and fuse into larger lymphatic ducts, which in turn empty into the venous sytem. The interstitial lymphatic fluid is replaced by diffusion

Figure 1–17 Microscopic anatomy of a lymph node. (a) Scanning electron micrograph (SEM) of the subcapsular sinus; the flattened bodies with long branching processes are part of the reticulum, and the adherent cells with multiple globular protrusions are macrophages. Notice the large intercellular spaces in the sinus. (b) SEM of the medullary sinus; again a flattened reticulum with adherent macrophages is evident. The smaller round cells with or without filamentous protrusions are lymphocytes, and a biconcave red blood cell is seen at the right. (c) An electron microscopic view of a cross-section of the medulla. The clear space is the medullary sinus with a few large pale macrophages and many small dark lymphocytes. The highly cellular portions are medullary cords, containing lymphoblasts and plasma cells. (d) SEM view of the diffuse cortex, where a fine meshwork of reticulum surrounds many lymphocytes. (e) Light microscopic view of a standard histological section of a lymph node from a thymus-deprived mouse. The only region containing large numbers of small, dark, round lymphocytes is the primary follicle. (f) SEM view of a primary follicle; dendritic reticular cells with long lacy processes surround densely-packed small lymphocytes. [Electron micrographs (a)–(d) and (f) courtesy of W. van Ewijk; photomicrograph (e) by I. Weissman.]

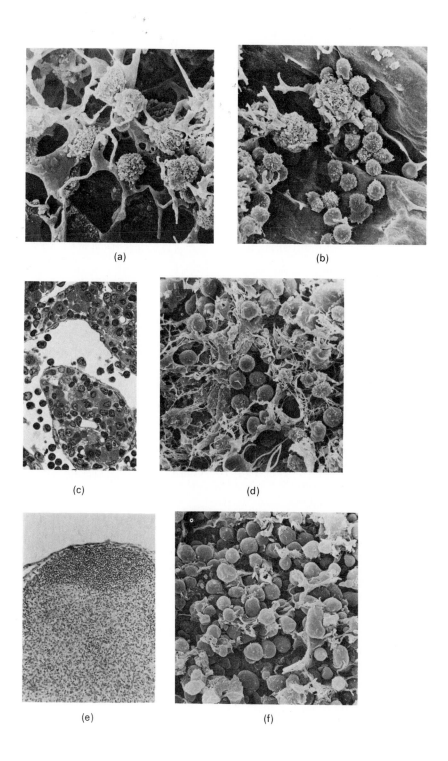

(a)

(b)

(c)

(d)

(e)

(f)

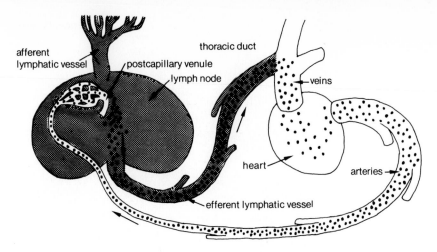

Figure 1–18 The pathway of lymphocyte recirculation. Blood lymphocytes enter lymph nodes, adhere to the walls of specialized postcapillary venules, and migrate to the lymph node diffuse cortex. Many lymphocytes then migrate to T- or B-cell domains and percolate through lymphoid fields to medullary lymphatic sinuses and then to efferent lymphatics, which in turn collect into major lymphatic ducts in the thorax that empty into the neck veins leading to the heart. [Redrawn from J. L. Gowans, *Hosp. Pract.* **3(3),** 34 (1968).]

of water, ions, and selected proteins through the walls of blood capillaries in the tissues, to complete the lymphatic circulation.

2. Antigens that enter the body via the upper respiratory and gastrointestinal tracts are filtered through local lymph nodes as well as several specialized lymphoid organs: the tonsils, adenoids, Peyers patches, and appendix (Figure 1–15).

3. Antigens that enter the bloodstream are filtered out by macrophages that line sinusoidal blood vessels in the spleen, liver, and lungs. However, only the spleen is capable of mounting an immune response to blood-borne antigens. The spleen is differentiated into two types of tissue, called *lymphoid white pulp* and *erythroid red pulp*. The white pulp, which surrounds small splenic arteries (arterioles) from their origins as arterial branches to their termini, is analogous in structure and function to the cortex of the lymph node. The red pulp is involved in scavenging old red blood cells (*erythrocytes*), and is a reserve site for hematopoiesis.

C. Recirculating lymphocytes pass from the blood through the lymphoid system and back to the blood. On the way they percolate through lymphoid organs where they may contact processed antigens (Figure 1–18).

1. In the resting lymph node the cortex is divided into discrete B-cell domains, called the *primary follicles,* and an adjacent T-cell domain, the *diffuse cortex* (Figure 1–19). Lymphocytes enter the

(a)

(b)

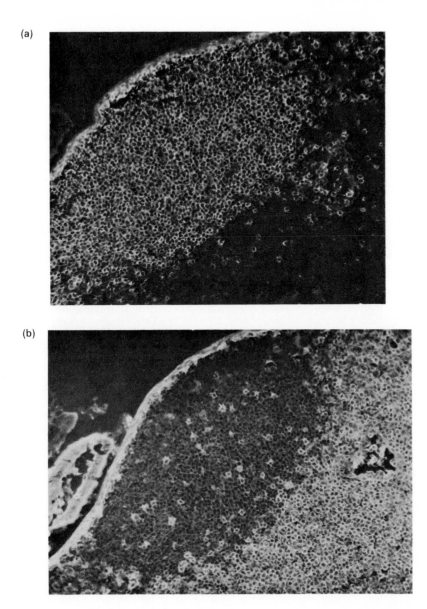

Figure 1–19 Localization of T and B cells in a lymph node. A lymph node was frozen rapidly, and sections of the node were stained with antibodies coupled to a fluorescent tracer. Photomicrographs were taken to locate bound fluorescent antibodies.(a) Anti-B-cell fluorescent antibodies were used to stain the cortex of a node containing a primary follicle (top left) and its adjacent diffuse cortex (bottom right) containing a postcapillary venule (PCV). B cells predominate in the primary follicle; they are found also in the lumen and wall of the PCV, presumably just having entered via the bloodstream. (b) A serial section adjacent to the one in (a), stained with anti-T-cell fluorescent antibodies. T cells predominate in the diffuse cortex and also are found in the PCV. [Photomicrographs by G. A. Gutman and I. Weissman.]

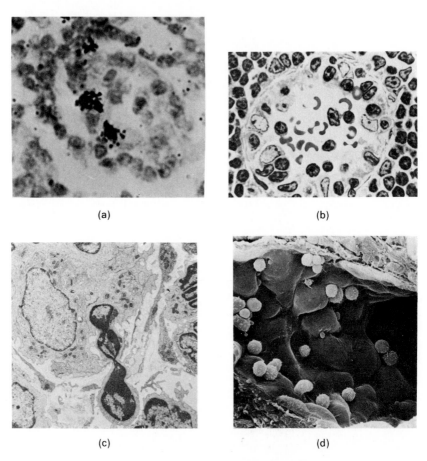

(a)

(b)

(c)

(d)

Figure 1–20   Microscopic views of lymphocytes traversing postcapillary venules. (a) An autoradiograph of labeled lymphocytes in the walls of a postcapillary venule within minutes after their injection into the bloodstream [G. A. Gutman and I. Weissman, *Transplantation* **16,** 621 (1973)]. (b) A thin section of a postcapillary venule under high power, showing lymphocytes in different stages of passage with several red blood cells in the vessel lumen. [Photomicrograph courtesy of G. Levine.] (c) An electron microscopic view of a lymphocyte (lower right) squeezing through a narrow passageway in a postcapillary venule. Lymphocyte nuclei stain densely, while endothelial nuclei stain lightly with a dark rim just inside the nuclear membrane. [Electron micrograph courtesy of G. Levine and G. A. Gutman.] (d) A scanning electron microscopic view of several lymphocytes in contact with the inner surface of postcapillary venule endothelial cells. [Electron micrograph courtesy of W. van Ewijk.]

lymph node from the bloodstream via arterioles and capillaries to reach postcapillary venules in the diffuse cortex. Both T and B cells, but not other blood cells, adhere specifically to large, specialized endothelial cells in the venule walls, and then traverse these walls to enter the node. Upon entry, B cells migrate to the follicles and T cells remain in the diffuse cortex, suggesting that each type of cell recognizes and responds to a different cortical microenvironment (Figure 1-20).

In resting lymph nodes, the medulla serves primarily as a collecting point for sinusoids that lead to the efferent lymphatic vessels. After traversing their specific cortical domains, recirculating B and T cells enter these sinusoids, and then are transported via the main lymphatic ducts back into the venous system for recirculation. The lymphocyte fields of the lymph nodes thus contain slowly moving masses of B and T cells, most of which are on their way from blood to lymph and back to blood.

2. The specialized lymphoid organs attached to the respiratory and gastrointestinal tracts—in mammals the adenoids, tonsils, Peyers patches, and appendix (Figure 1-15)—also have both specialized postcapillary venules, which serve as lymphocyte entry sites, and specific B-cell and T-cell domains. Birds lack tonsils and appendix, and have only a single Peyers patch. However, birds possess the bursa of Fabricius, anterior to the cloaca. It is unclear whether this organ is a major site of immune response to gastrointestinal antigens, a major site of B-cell maturation, or both.

3. Most lymphocytes enter and leave the spleen directly via the bloodstream. The lymphoid white pulp of the spleen (Figure 1-21) takes the form of a bumpy sheath that surrounds entering arterioles. It is separated from the red pulp by the marginal zone, which receives blood from a specialized venule called the marginal sinus. This sinus arises at the termination of the arteriole and curves back to envelop the white pulp. The bumps on the sheath are primary follicles, that is, B-cell domains, whereas the sheath itself consists of T-cell domains (Figures 1-22 and 1-23). Circulating B and T cells, but no other blood cells, enter the white pulp by traversing the walls of the marginal sinus, and then migrate to their respective domains. Lymphocytes then may cross the border from white pulp through the marginal zone via so-called bridging channels to the red pulp, where they are taken up by veins that leave the spleen. However, some lymphocytes appear to flow into splenic efferent lymphatics, which transport them via the lymphatic ducts back to the venous system

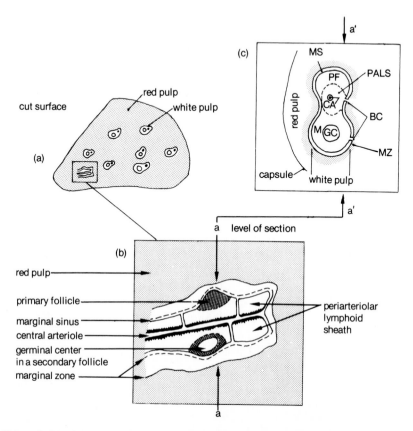

Figure 1–21   General structure of a spleen. (a) A cross-section of the spleen. (b) Enlarge-ment of an area of white pulp. (c) Cross-section of an area of white pulp. *White pulp:* The central arteriole (CA), a branch of a trabecular artery, has branches that empty into the marginal zone (MZ), marginal sinus (MS), and red pulp. The periarteriolar lymphoid sheath (PALS) is an accumulation of small lymphocytes surrounding the central arteriole. The primary follicles (PF), mantle (M), and germinal center (GC) are similar to those described for the lymph node (Figure 1–16). *Marginal area:* The marginal sinus (MS) separates the white pulp from the marginal zone (MZ) and red pulp. The marginal areas, including the sinuses, receive much of the blood entering the spleen. These areas are major sites of entry of T and B cells. Bridging channels (BC) appear to interrupt the marginal area and form connections between the white and red pulp. *Red pulp:* In addition to hematopoietic cells (in the mouse), plasma cells appear in this site and are particularly prominent after antigenic stimulation.

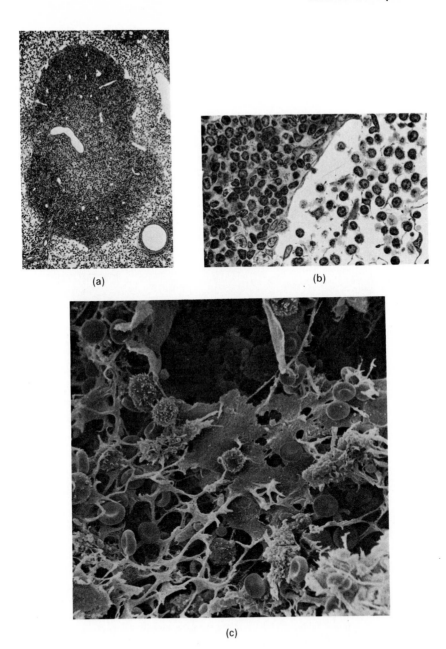

(a)

(b)

(c)

Figure 1–22 Microscopic anatomy of the spleen. (a) A light micrograph of a section of the spleen. The structures have the same relationship to each other as diagramed in Figure 1–21c. (b) An electron microscopic view of a primary follicle (upper left) and the marginal zone (lower right). One cell appears to be traversing the boundary. (c) A scanning electron microscopic view of the marginal zone. The dendritic reticulum and its adherent macrophages surround the space containing lymphocytes and red blood cells. [Electron micrographs courtesy of W. van Ewijk.]

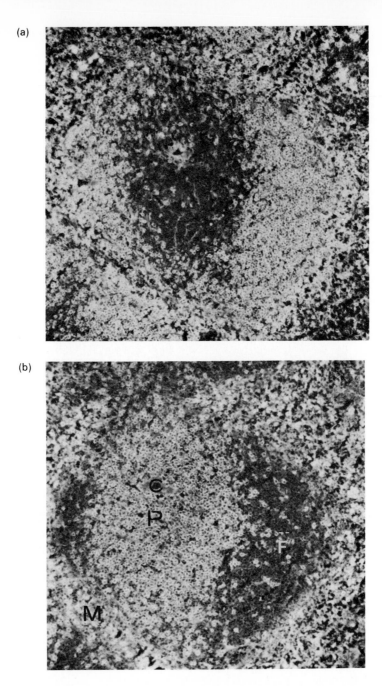

Figure 1–23 Localization of T and B cells in the spleen. Photomicrographs are of sections stained as in Figure 1–19. (a) Anti-B-cell stain of a spleen. The central arteriole (C) is immediately surrounded by a fluorescent-negative periarteriolar lymphoid sheath (P). B cells predominate in the eccentric folicles (F) and are interspersed around the marginal zone (M). (b) Anti-T-cell stain of serial section: T cells predominate in the periarteriolar lymphoid sheath and are interspersed around the marginal zone. [Micrographs by G. A. Gutman and I. Weissman.]

(Figure 1–23). In rodents, recirculating T and B cells take about 6 hours to traverse the lymphoid fields of the spleen, and somewhat longer to traverse the fields of the lymph nodes. On the average, lymphocytes have a total recirculation time of about 24 hours.

D.   The products of an immune response in any lymphoid tissue are effector T cells and humoral antibodies produced by plasma cells. These products, which must be distributed to the bloodstream and the tissues to play their defensive roles, are transported via efferent lymphatic vessels and lymphatic ducts into the venous system. Of the five classes of humoral antibodies (Essential Concept 1–2c), IgG can traverse blood-vessel walls and enter the interstitial spaces of tissues most efficiently. Typically about 50% of an organism's IgG antibodies are found in the interstitial fluid and 50% in the bloodstream. The remaining classes of circulating antibodies, IgA, IgD, IgE, and IgM, are confined primarily to the bloodstream or to specific local sites.

Effector T cells in the bloodstream collect rapidly on blood-vessel walls near a site where cognate antigens have invaded the tissues. The T cells then migrate through the vessel walls into the tissues, where they initiate inflammatory and elimination responses to the invading agent.

1–6   Antigen binding to lymphocyte surface receptors triggers an immune response

A.   Antigen-triggered lymphocyte proliferation and differentiation occurs in lymphoid organs. Antigen that enters a lymph node via the afferent lymphatics is taken up by macrophages in the afferent sinusoids, the diffuse cortex, and the medulla, within minutes after infection or injection. Most of this antigen becomes incorporated into special vacuoles, called *phagosomes,* in the cytoplasm of macrophages. The vacuoles fuse with *lysosomes,* vesicles that contain hydrolytic enzymes, to form *phagolysosomes.* The enzymes degrade most of the antigen to nonantigenic components. However, the macrophage cell surface retains or receives a small amount of highly immunogenic material for presentation to antigen-specific lymphocytes.

Nonmacrophage-associated antigen begins to collect within primary follicles at about 24–48 hours after injection. This antigen is retained on the web of dendritic reticular cell processes in close proximity to most B cells in the follicle.

B.   B and T cells entering a lymph node are small cells with dense nuclei surrounded by a thin layer of cytoplasm that contains few mitochondria, no polysomes, and little endoplasmic reticulum. Binding of a cognate antigen to the surface receptors of either type of lymphocyte triggers a general activation (Figure 1–7): the cell enlarges; the nucleolus swells; polysomes and microtubules form; and rates of macromolecular synthesis increase markedly. This process is called *blast transformation* (Figure 1–24). The activated cells proliferate and differentiate, with concomitant changes in the morphology of the lymph node.

During the first 24–48 hours following antigenic stimulation of the organism, antigen-specific lymphocyte clones are retained in those lymphoid organs that contain the antigen. During this period these clones are largely depleted from the recirculating lymphocyte population.

1.   Small T cells that enter the lymph node through postcapillary venules encounter processed antigen and transform to large lymphocytes in the diffuse cortex, which is the T-cell domain (Figure 1–19). These cells initiate DNA synthesis, divide (beginning about 30–40 hours after injection of antigen), and give rise to clones of memory and effector T cells.

2.   Small B cells with appropriate receptor specificities also react with processed antigen. The wave of T-cell division in the diffuse cortex is followed closely by transformation of small B cells to large B cells in the follicle. These cells also initiate DNA synthesis, divide, and give rise to memory and effector cells of the B-cell lineage.

3.   Some T cells migrate into the follicle, where a focus of dividing T and B cells as well as active macrophages builds up to form a *germinal center,* which compresses the follicle into a crescent around it. Follicles with germinal centers, known as

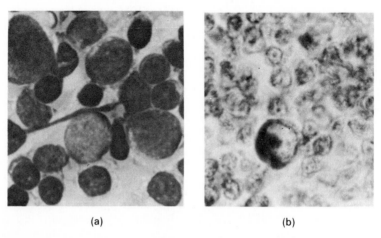

(a)   (b)

Figure 1–24   Antigen-induced activation of T cells. (a) The appearance of a T cell (lymphoblast) activated *in vitro* and surrounded by resting T cells. (b) The appearance of an activated T cell in the tissue. The peculiar morphology of this cell is emphasized by using a dye (pyronin Y), which stains RNA intensely. [Photographs courtesy of R. Rouse.]

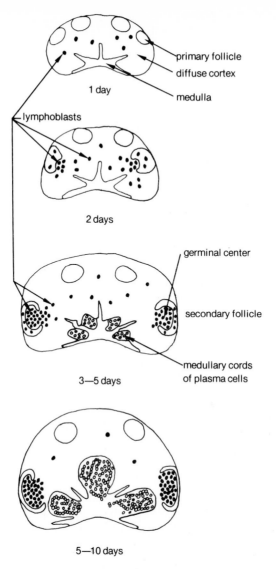

primary follicle

diffuse cortex

1 day

medulla

lymphoblasts

2 days

germinal center

secondary follicle

medullary cords
of plasma cells

3—5 days

5—10 days

Figure 1–25 Morphological changes in a lymph node after stimulation with a thymus-dependent antigen. The diagram depicts the time course of antigen-dependent changes in multi-cellular structures, and emphasizes changes in size and shape of the separate lymphoid compartments, largely caused by selective proliferation and altered movement patterns of lymphocyte subclasses. Analogous changes occur in antigen-activated spleen.

secondary follicles (Figure 1–25), appear 4–5 days after antigen injection, and may remain for several days. At the same time plasma cells begin to settle between the sinusoids of the medulla, to form medullary cords. Other activated B-cell progeny, as well as most activated T cells and their progeny, percolate through the lymph node and spread to other lymphoid tissues and the bloodstream via the efferent lymphatics and the major lymphatic ducts. Thus most memory and effector T cells and memory B cells eventually reenter the general circulation following antigenic stimulation, whereas most effector B cells (plasma cells) are retained in the lymph node.

4.   Following antigenic stimulation of a lymph node (Figure 1–26) activated B and T cells release soluble factors that cause local vessel dilation, which allows leakage (transudation) of plasma fluids into the lymph node. Other factors may attract macrophages and other blood phagocytes into the node. The resulting accumulation of cells and fluid may plug some of the medullary sinusoids that lead to efferent lymphatics. The combination of specific cellular proliferation, increased fluid in the tissues (edema), increased numbers of nonlymphoid cells, and retention of normally recirculating lymphocytes causes the lymph node to enlarge rapidly, causing the typical "swollen glands" of infection. The nodes return to their original size only as the response to infection abates.

C.   The mechanism by which antigen binding to surface receptors activates cells is not yet understood. Presumably only receptors that bind antigen with some threshold avidity can initiate activation. Although there will be low-avidity interactions between any given antigen and many lymphocyte receptors, only one in 10^4 to 10^5 cells will bind strongly enough to trigger a primary immune response. Even in a secondary response following clonal expansion of the antigen-specific cells, a maximum of about 1% of the lymphocyte population has the capacity to bind the antigen, and very few of these cells are likely to traverse the site of antigen deposition and be stimulated. Consequently it is difficult to study the triggering event directly with antigens. However, progress is being made in studies of two presumably closely related processes: the response of cell membranes to binding of surface molecules in general, and the action of substances called *mitogens*, which induce many kinds of cells to divide by interacting with their surfaces.

Figure 1–26 Microscopic views of antigen and germinal centers in antigen-draining $\longrightarrow$
lymph nodes. (a) Labeled antigen detected by autoradiography inside a phagolysosome (pl) of a macrophage. [Courtesy of J. J. Miller III.] (b) An autoradiogram of labeled antigen adhering to the processes of follicular dendritic reticular cells. [Courtesy of J. J. Miller III and G. J. V. Nossal.] (c) The distribution of antigen within a primary follicle 1–2 days after immunization, shown by immunofluorescence. [Courtesy of J. J. Miller III.] (d) The appearance of germinal centers in a hyperimmune lymph node. [Courtesy of R. Warnke.] (e) Immunofluorescence of antigen bound to follicular dendritic reticular cells which have been compressed into a crescent by the development of a germinal center. [Courtesy of J. J. Miller III.] (f) Immunofluorescence identification of T cells in the upper pole of a germinal center. [Photomicrograph by G. A. Gutman and I. Weissman.]

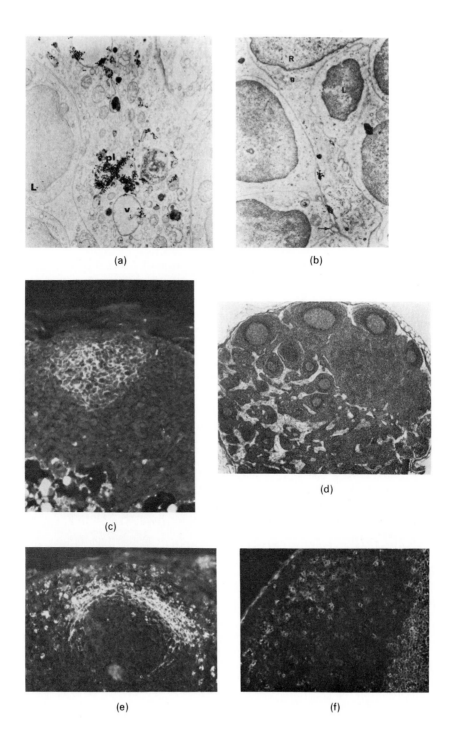

(a)

(b)

(c)

(d)

(e)

(f)

1. Cross-linking and rearrangement of cell-surface antibody receptor molecules could be the event that triggers changes in the nucleus. Since receptor proteins in the cell membrane are mobile, they can be cross-linked by specific reagents, such as divalent ligands (or antibodies), to form areas of two-dimensional precipitation that have been called *patches*. These patches coalesce into a polar *cap*, most of which is shed from or ingested by the cell (Figure 1–27). Different receptors can usually be capped independently, which suggests that normally they are not physically associated. Cap formation is an energy-requiring process that involves contractile microfilament activity. The microfilaments may play a role in transmitting the binding signal from the membrane to the nucleus; this process will be discussed further in Chapter 4.

2. The preceding notions on receptor cross-linking as a trigger for cellular differentiation gain support from the observation that

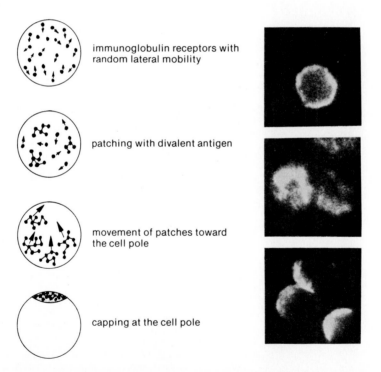

immunoglobulin receptors with random lateral mobility

patching with divalent antigen

movement of patches toward the cell pole

capping at the cell pole

Figure 1–27 Diagrams illustrating how a multivalent antigen causes mobile immunoglobulins to cluster in discrete *patches* that migrate toward one end of the cell and *cap* together at a single pole in the cell membrane of a small lymphocyte. [Photomicrographs courtesy of G. E. Edelman.]

a number of general mitogens also bind to cell-surface molecules and induce capping. Certain mitogenic agents will stimulate a large fraction of the lymphocyte population to proliferate and differentiate. These agents include the mitogenic *lectins,* plant proteins that bind specifically to various carbohydrate groups; lipopolysaccharides, which are large polymers found in the cell walls of gram-negative bacteria; and a few chemical reagents such as periodate. Mitogenic stimulation requires that the mitogen bind to cell-surface molecules in the proper conformation. Stimulation also requires that this binding signal somehow be transduced to the cell interior, there to initiate the sequence of metabolic events that precede proliferation and differentiation. These events include changes in cyclic nucleotide levels, in lipid turnover rates, in transport of ions and small molecules, and in nucleic acid metabolism. The binding events occur in seconds to minutes, whereas the metabolic changes take minutes to hours. If mitogen is removed prior to the metabolic changes, proliferation and differentiation do not occur.

3.   Although mitogens interact with specific carbohydrate groups that are about equally represented on the glycoproteins of T- and B-cell surfaces, they affect the two cell types differently. The lectins phytohemagglutinin and concanavalin A stimulate differentiation of T cells only, whereas pokeweed mitogen stimulates differentiation of both B and T cells. Lipopolysaccharides from gram-negative bacteria are selectively mitogenic for B cells in rodents. Mitogenic activation by T-cell-specific or B-cell-specific substances often leads to differentiation of the activated cells to effector cells. This activation is polyclonal; that is, all members of the population can become activated regardless of their antigenic specificity.

4.   The foregoing observations have led to three hypotheses currently under consideration to explain B-cell activation by antigen binding (Figure 1–28).

   (i)   B cells require one signal only, from a multideterminant antigen that cross-links cell-surface *receptor immunoglobulins.*

   (ii)   B cells require one signal only, from mitogenic groups on the antigen that interact with *mitogen receptors* on the cell surface. In this model the antigen-specific receptor immunoglobulins play an important but passive role in triggering, by binding a cognate antigen and thereby focusing its mitogenic signal onto the cell surface. Whereas the antigen receptors vary from one B cell to the next, mitogen receptors could be common to all B cells at a particular stage of maturation.

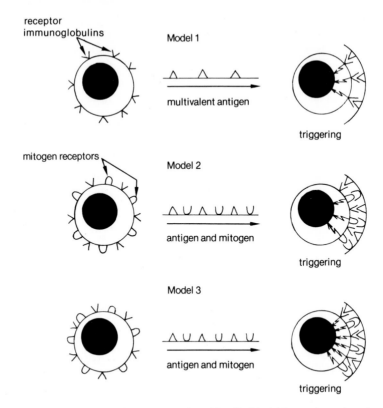

Figure 1–28   Three models for the triggering of B cells. Model 1 postulates that triggering occurs via bound or cross-linked receptor immunoglobulins. Model 2 suggests that triggering occurs via bound or cross-linked mitogen receptors. Model 3 postulates that triggering requires signals from both receptor immunoglobulins and mitogen receptors.

(iii)   B cells require two signals to be triggered, one through their antigen-specific receptor immunoglobulins, and the other through mitogen receptors. Either signal alone would be insufficient to stimulate the cell to differentiate and divide.

It is not yet known which if any of these hypotheses is correct.

1-7   The magnitude and duration of any specific immune response are regulated by several feedback mechanisms

A.   Antigenic stimulation causes several categories of cells to proliferate and differentiate, resulting in the generation of several specific and nonspecific effector mechanisms. Uncontrolled continuation of an immune response could lead to pathological lymphoid proliferation, excessive antibody production, and even anti-self reactions. Five major mechanisms are known to control the magnitude and duration of immune responses. Recognition of the latter two of these mechanisms constituted an important advance in understanding cellular interactions in the immune system. The five mechanisms are described in the following paragraphs; misregulation and its pathological consequences will be considered further in Chapters 2 and 5.

1. Effector cells have a lifespan of only a few days, and new effector cells appear only via antigenic stimulation.

2. Antigen is removed as a result of effector cell functions.

3. Antigen bound to macrophages and reticular cells may become coated with antibodies of high avidity, so that the antigen no longer can stimulate lymphocytes. This process creates a negative-feedback loop that prevents production of a large number of like antibody molecules.

4. Antigenic stimulation of specific T-cell clones may induce specific suppressor T cells, which somehow function to inhibit antigen triggering of other lymphocytes.

5. The idiotypic determinants of the antibodies produced in an immune response are themselves potential immunogens to which the organism is not tolerant. If their concentration reaches immunogenic levels, the organism may mount an anti-idiotypic immune response, which may inhibit the lymphocytes that express these idiotypes. Thus anti-antibodies may be important elements in controlling the magnitude of an immune response.

The anti-idiotypic response is the key element in an hypothesis put forward by Jerne, called the *network theory of immunological regulation*. The theory postulates that in the course of an anti-idiotypic response, the idiotype-specific lymphocytes that proliferate will bear their own new idiotypic determinants, which in turn will stimulate new immune responses (Figure 1–29). Continuation of this process leads to a network of receptor–antireceptor interactions throughout the lymphoid system.

Recent experiments indicate that at least some antibody responses are followed by anti-idiotypic responses from both T cells and B cells. Thus there must exist T-cell receptors and B-cell receptors that recognize self idiotypic determinants. It is not yet known if all subclasses of T and B cells bear anti-idiotypic receptors or whether all manifestations of T-cell and B-cell immunity are activated by idiotypic determinants.

Jerne points out that the set of idiotypic internal antigens may include "internal images" of all the external antigens to which an organism can respond. Consequently anti-idiotypic responses may play an important role during ontogeny in the

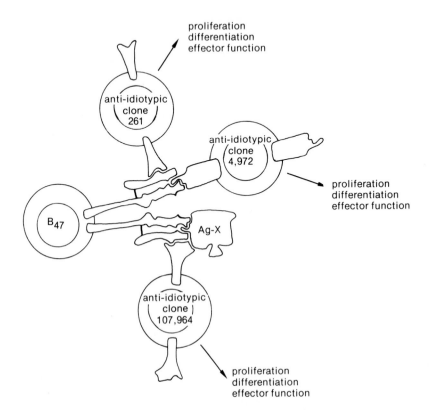

Figure 1–29 In this model, B-cell clone 47 is the predominant clone reacting to an antigenic determinant on antigen X. Having expanded to the point that its antigen-binding receptors reach an immunogenic level, B clone 47 stimulates three separate lymphocyte clones, each of which possesses surface receptors that recognize idiotypic determinants on the immunoglobulins expressed by B clone 47 and its progeny cells. Anti-idiotype clone 4,972 recognizes idiotypic determinants within the antibody combining site, whereas clone 261 recognizes L-chain idiotypic determinants outside the combining site, and clone 107,964 recognizes L-chain idiotypic determinants in combination with determinants on antigen X. Each of these anti-idiotype clones could be in the T-cell or B-cell series, and the cells or their products could express helper or suppressor functions, leading respectively to idiotype specific augmentation (positive feedback) or inhibition (negative feedback) of this immune response. In turn, as each anti-idiotype expands to the point that its antigen-specific receptors reach immunogenic levels, anti-(anti-idiotypic) responses of a positive and negative type could be induced.

generation of expanded responding clones of diverse immuno-specific lymphocytes. If this view is correct, the definitions of antigen-independent and antigen-dependent phases of lymphocyte maturation will have to be changed to take into account the role of idiotypic internal antigens.

1–8 The antibodies produced in a humoral immune response are heterogeneous in specificity and may include all immunoglobulin classes

A.   An individual B cell activated by a cognate antigen proliferates and differentiates to form plasma cells that begin to synthesize identical antibodies with a single specificity at the rate of 3,000 to 30,000 molecules per cell per second. However, an organism's total response to the simplest antigens almost always is heterogeneous with respect to antibody specificity. This heterogeneity is due to two factors: most antigens have multiple antigenic determinants that trigger the activation of different B cells, and even a single antigenic determinant generally activates several different B cells that display receptor immunoglobulins with similar but not identical specificities (Figure 1–30). Consequently the serum of any vertebrate contains an extremely heterogeneous collection of immunoglobulin molecules whose specificities reflect the organism's past antigenic history.

B.   The B-cell response to a single antigen may produce antibody molecules of all five known classes of immunoglobulins: IgA, IgD,

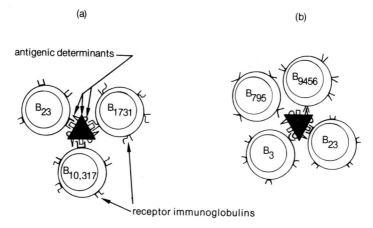

Figure 1–30 Two sources of heterogeneity in an antibody response to an antigen. (a) The same antigenic determinant triggers B cells with functionally related but different receptor immunoglobulins. (b) Different antigenic determinants on the same antigen trigger B cells with different receptors.

IgE, IgG, and IgM. The immunoglobulins of the five classes differ in the structures of their heavy-chain constant regions, although antibody molecules of two different classes may exhibit identical antigen-binding specificities and idiotypes, and therefore probably possess identical variable regions. The molecular basis for this apparent paradox is discussed in Chapter 3. Antibodies of the five classes mediate different physiological effector functions (Table 1–1). They are present in normal human serum at very different concentrations, and they differ significantly in normal serum half-life (Table 1–1). In addition, the five classes are produced in different relative amounts in primary and secondary immune responses (Figure 1–31).

1.   IgM, the first antibody produced in response to an immunogen, is a pentamer of the basic antibody structural unit. IgM is particularly effective against invading microorganisms. Although the affinity of each IgM active site for a cognate antigenic determinant may be low, the overall avidity of the IgM pentamer for a complex antigen is very high, due to the presence of repeating determinants on most complex cell-membrane antigens. Because of its pentameric structure, IgM is about 1000 times more effective on a molar basis at agglutinating cells by cross-linking than are monomeric divalent antibodies. In addition, IgM bound to an antigenic target cell stimulates its ingestion by macrophages, and its destruction by complement fixation.

IgM is principally an antibody of the blood. Because of its

Table 1–1

Physiological properties of the five immunoglobulin classes in humans

Class	Mean adult serum level (mg/ml)	Serum half-life (days)	Physiological functions
IgM	1.0	5	Complement fixation; early immune response; stimulation of ingestion by macrophages
IgG	12	25	Complement fixation; placental transfer; stimulation of ingestion by macrophages
IgA	1.8	6	Localized protection in external secretions
IgD	0.03	2.8	Function unknown
IgE	0.0003	2	Stimulation of mast cells; possibly parasite expulsion

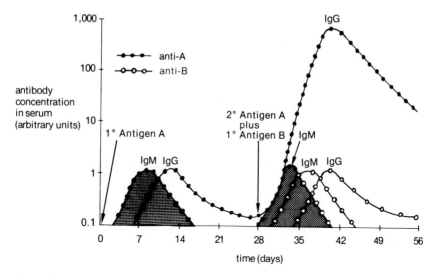

Figure 1-31 Kinetics of IgM and IgG appearance in the serum following primary and secondary immunizations. The secondary response to Antigen A demonstrates that the IgM response is slightly more rapid and intense than the primary IgG response. However, most of the secondary response is of the IgG class.

large size it enters the interstitial fluid slowly, if at all. It does not cross the placenta to enter the fetal circulation. IgM also is displayed as a monomer on the surfaces of B cells, where it may act as a receptor immunoglobulin.

2. IgG is a monomeric antibody produced later in the immune response than IgM. Low doses of antigen stimulate IgM production only; higher doses are required to stimulate IgG appearance. IgG is the most prevalent antibody in the blood, and is a major antibody in tissue spaces. The prevalence of IgG in the bloodstream makes it a major trigger of complement fixation, although on a molar basis it is many times less effective than IgM at this function. IgG also activates macrophage ingestion of antigenic particles by coating them with antibody. IgG is the only class of antibody that can cross the placenta to provide immunity for a developing fetus.

The average affinity for antigen of the IgG antibodies produced in a primary response increases with time after immunization. This phenomenon, known as affinity maturation, is thought to occur because decreasing levels of antigen lead to progressively more selective triggering of B cell receptors with higher affinity for antigen.

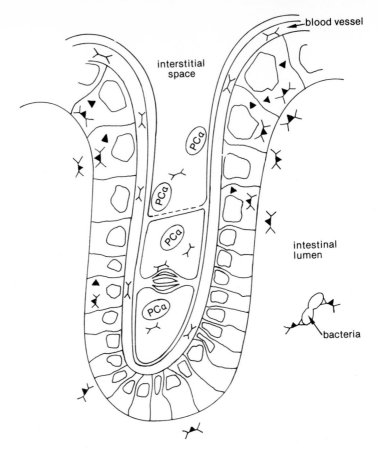

Figure 1–32 Representation of intestinal villus with epithelial cells producing secretory component (▲), which facilitates the transport of dimeric IgA (>—<) from the interstitial spaces into the intestinal lumen. PC_α indicates IgA producing plasma cells in the interstitial space of the villus.

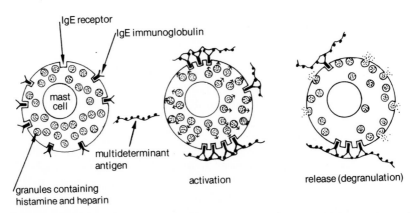

Figure 1–33 Activation of a mast cell by multivalent antigen bound to passively acquired IgE. Activation leads to the exocytosis of granules containing heparin and histamine, and to their release into the extracellular fluid.

3. IgA, also produced later in an immune response than IgM, can exist as a monomer, dimer, or trimer of the basic immunoglobulin structural unit. IgA antibodies are thought to act as a protective barrier against microorganisms at several potential points of entry. Some epithelial cells produce a polypeptide called *secretory component* (Sc), which complexes to the Fc region of IgA antibodies and specifically mediates their transport from interstitial spaces to the epithelial surface (Figure 1–32).

B-cell precursors of IgA-secreting plasma cells are found in highest frequency in lymphoid organs that drain the gastrointestinal tract. Upon antigenic stimulation, progeny of these lymphocytes are released via efferent lymphatics and collecting ducts to the blood. Most of these cells home preferentially to the gastrointestinal tract, where they come to rest in the tissue spaces just under the epithelial mucosal cells, and there differentiate to IgA-secreting plasma cells.

Similar precursor lymphocytes home to the mammary gland, where they differentiate into IgA-secreting plasma cells just under the epithelial glandular cells. IgA is a major immunoglobulin in milk and colostrum, where it may function to protect the gastrointestinal tracts of nursing infants. IgA also is found in saliva, tears, and sweat.

4. IgD, a monomeric antibody, normally is present in only minute concentrations in the blood. It also is present as a cell-surface receptor on a majority of circulating B cells, but its functions are still unknown.

5. IgE, a monomeric, heat-labile antibody, also is normally present in the blood in only minute concentrations. IgE antibodies bind tightly via their Fc regions to *mast* cells in connective tissue and blood basophiles. Interaction of bound IgE with a cognate antigen can trigger the mast cell to *degranulate,* that is, to release the contents of its intracellular vacuoles, which contain *histamine* and a sulfated polysaccharide called *heparin* (Figure 1–33). Since monovalent haptens will not trigger this release, it is likely that either conformational change or intermolecular cross-linking of the IgE antibodies is required. Triggering involves the cyclic nucleotide system, as in other cellular responses to stimulation of a surface receptor. The release of histamine and heparin results in local vessel dilation and smooth muscle contraction.

C.   A given plasma cell secretes antibody of only one class. The class that a plasma cell secretes generally is the same as the class of receptor immunoglobulin displayed by its B-cell precursor. Mature B cells and memory B cells that display the various classes of immunoglobulins as receptors are designated by the corresponding Greek letters:

for example, B_μ cells carry monomeric IgM molecules as receptors, B_γ cells carry IgG molecules as receptors, and so on. Plasma cells are designated in the same manner, as PC_μ, PC_γ, and so on.

Some B cells clearly are class-restricted: for example, all PC_α cells are derived from antigen-activated B_α lymphocytes. However, there are several intriguing and still unexplained observations connected with the class relationships of plasma cells and their B-cell precursors.

1.   There are differences in the secondary or memory responses of different immunoglobulin classes. Restimulation of a host with an antigen results in an IgM response only slightly higher than the primary IgM response, with a slightly shorter lag period between antigen injection and appearance of antibody (Figure 1–31). Since all PC_μ cells are derived from B_μ cells, and since B_μ cells are the first B cells that appear during ontogeny, it is possible that all IgM antibody formation results from stimulation of virgin B cells, and that no B_μ memory cells are produced in a primary response.

In contrast, a secondary IgG response appears more rapidly and is orders of magnitude higher than the primary IgG response to the same antigen (Figure 1–31). PC_γ cells derive mainly from B_γ precursors with some contribution from $B_{\mu+\delta}$ precursors. A primary immune response usually triggers a large clonal expansion of B_γ memory cells, but B_γ cells still represent only a small fraction of circulating B cells.

The behavior of IgA is intermediate between that of IgM and IgG; although IgA is produced in much higher concentrations during a secondary response than during a primary response, it never approaches the levels reached by IgG in secondary responses.

2.   There are quantitative discrepancies between the relative numbers of class-specific B cells and the relative amounts of the corresponding antibodies produced in an immune response. As mentioned in the preceding section, B_γ cells represent a minority of circulating B cells, yet IgG is the major class of antibody produced in an immune response. Conversely, IgD is a common receptor immunoglobulin on B-cell surfaces, and yet only minute concentrations of IgD antibodies are found in the blood. B_δ cells appear after B_μ cells during ontogeny and are distributed differently than B_μ cells in the body. B_δ cells are relatively infrequent in the spleen, but they represent the major class of B cells in thoracic duct lymph. It is unknown whether IgD can be the sole class of receptor immunoglobulin on a B cell; most B_δ cells also exhibit IgG or IgM receptors. PC_δ cells

are extremely rare; therefore the consequences of B_δ cell activation are unclear.

3. Some B cells display two classes of receptor immunoglobulin molecules with identical idiotypes. For example, many B_γ cells carry either IgM ($B_{\gamma+\mu}$) or IgD ($B_{\gamma+\delta}$) in addition to IgG receptors, and $B_{\mu+\delta}$ cells are common. These observations, as well as the finding that some plasma-cell tumors secrete antibodies of two classes with identical idiotype, have raised the possibility that in the course of their differentiation B cells may switch from production of one immunoglobulin class to another, without changing the idiotype or specificity of the antigen-recognizing portion of the molecule. This phenomenon and its possible molecular mechanism are discussed in Essential Concept 3–8.

4. It is not yet known whether all classes of B cells arise as virgin B cells by antigen-independent differentiation pathways, or whether some classes arise following antigenic stimulation of a precursor class. At present, three possible models for B-cell class differentiation are under active investigation by immunologists (Figure 1–34).

The first model postulates that B-cell precursors become class-restricted prior to expression of their cell surface receptors, that is, that class differentiation is antigen-independent. Class differentiation may result in the expression of only the new class (as in Figure 1–34a) or of both the old and the new class. If this model is correct, the lymphocyte population in a mature organism should include virgin B cells, memory B cells, and plasma cells representing each of the five classes.

The second model postulates that B_μ cells arise by antigen-independent maturation (Figure 1–34b) and that B_α, B_γ, and perhaps B_ε cells are derived from them by either an antigen-dependent or an antigen-independent process. According to the antigen-dependent version of this model, initial stimulation of B_μ cells by cognate antigens causes proliferation and differentiation to produce mature B_α, B_γ, and B_ε cells in addition to PC_μ cells. Some of these mature cells also may express μ receptors, but only a single notation is used for simplicity in Figure 1–34. Continued antigenic stimulation triggers the mature B_α, B_γ, and B_ε cells to proliferate and differentiate into the corresponding classes of memory cells and plasma cells.

The third model postulates that class switch occurs at the memory-cell or plasma-cell stage of differentiation rather than at the mature cell stage (Figure 1–34c).

None of these models accounts for the high proportion of

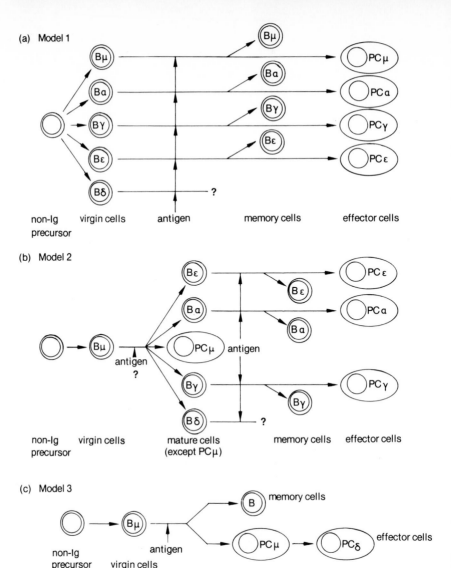

Figure 1–34 Three models for B-cell differentiation (see text).

B_δ cells in the lymphocyte population, and none explains the existence of cells that carry two receptor classes of immunoglobulin, except as cells in transition from one class to another.

1-9 Humoral antibodies initiate several effector mechanisms for eliminating foreign cells and macromolecules

A. The biological activity of some foreign invaders is neutralized by simple combination with antibody of any class. For example, the binding of antibodies to toxins or destructive foreign enzymes, such

as snake venom esterases, inhibits the interaction of these macromolecules with target ligands or substrates. Binding of antibody to surface
components of viruses can prevent their attachment to target cells.
Thus the humoral antibody response is effective in combating the
extracellular phase of a viral infection.

B.   Prior to an antibody response, the phagocytic cells of the
blood—monocytes, macrophages, and polymorphonuclear leukocytes
(PMN's; Figure 1–2f)—bind and ingest foreign substances. However,
the rate of binding and phagocytosis increases by an order of magnitude
if the foreign substance is coated with IgG antibodies. This process
of preparing foreign particles for ingestion by phagocytes is called
opsonization, and the specifically bound antibodies are called *opsonins*
(Figure 1–35). Phagocytic cells bear multiple low-affinity receptors for
the constant regions of IgG molecules. A particle coated with many
IgG molecules binds with high avidity to these receptors and triggers
phagocytosis (Figure 1–36).

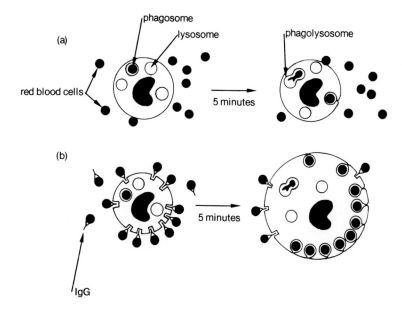

Figure 1–35   Macrophage phagocytosis of red blood cells (RBC) in the absence (a) or
presence (b) of antibodies. Antibody (IgG) bound to RBC's allows macrophages with receptors for the Fc portion of the IgG molecules to bind them to the macrophage surface.
Because each RBC is coated with many antibodies, the macrophage–Fc bond to any one
RBC is multivalent. Bound RBC's are engulfed by membrane–Fc interactions that continue
over the entire RBC surface, until macrophage membranes meet and fuse. The resulting
intracellular vesicle that contains the RBC is called a phagosome. This vesicle fuses with a
lysosome, and lysosome enzymes digest the RBC. Opsonizing antibody increases the
number of RBC's bound to the macrophage membrane, but does not increase the rate of
phagocytosis (per RBC) and digestion.

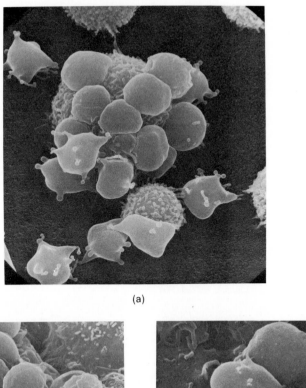

(a)

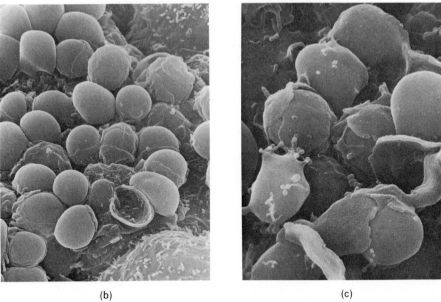

(b)   (c)

Figure 1–36 Scanning electron micrographs showing phagocytosis of red blood cells. (a) Several distorted antibody-coated RBC's bound to a few macrophages. One RBC has a leaflet of macrophage membrane extending over its lower pole. (b) A later stage in phagocytosis; several leaflets extend over each RBC, and one region of a macrophage membrane cup has been exposed by removal of a RBC. (c) Several enveloped RBC's, one with only a triangle of red cell membrane uncovered, and one empty macrophage membrane cup. [Photomicrographs courtesy of J. Orenstein and E. Shelton.]

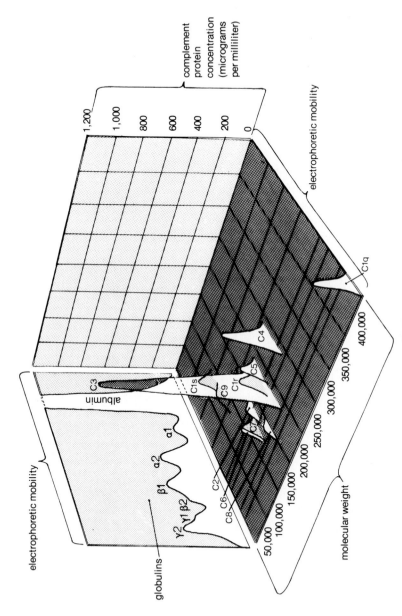

Figure 1-37 Human complement proteins characterized by molecular weights, electrophoretic mobilities at pH 8.6, and concentrations in the blood serum. For purposes of comparison, the mobilities and concentrations of globulins (α, β, and γ) and albumin are shown as well. [From M. Mayer, "The Complement System," *Sci. Am.* **229**, 54 (1973). Copyright © 1973 by Scientific American, Inc. All rights reserved.]

1.   Cells in the monocyte lineage may interact with IgG-coated foreign cells to cause contact lysis rather than phagocytosis. This process, called antibody-dependent cell-mediated cytotoxicity (ADCC), is independent of the complement system (defined in the following section). The effector cells for this process, called killer (K) cells, are distinct from the cytotoxic killer T cells. Although a subclass of B cells also may act as K cells, it is clear that most K cells are nonphagocytic members of the monocyte–macrophage lineage, and do not bear surface markers characteristic of either T- or B-cell lineages. Thus cells of the monocyte–macrophage lineage are important both in initiating and effecting immune responses.

2.   Another recently recognized type of killer cell is active against the transformed cells of virus-induced leukemias. This so-called natural killer (NK) cell is present in highest concentrations in bone marrow, and does not bear T-cell or B-cell differentiation markers. Its relationship to the K cell of the monocyte-macrophage lineage is unknown, although both NK and K cells possess Fc receptors.

C.   IgM and most subclasses of IgG antibodies activate the *complement system* when they bind to foreign antigens. The complement system is a set of eleven proteins that constitute about 10% of the globulins in the normal serum of man and other vertebrates (Figure 1–37). Complement proteins are distinct from immunoglobulins, and their concentrations are not affected by immunization. The complement system is triggered by antigen-antibody complexes to initiate a cascade of proteolytic cleavage and protein-binding reactions, with at least three important consequences for host defense (Figure 1–38). First, if the antigen–antibody complex is on the surface of a foreign cell, activated complement components attack the cell membrane to cause lysis and cell death. The utilization of complement components in this process is called *complement fixation.* Second, a cleavage product of complement component C3 binds to foreign particles that have complexed with antibodies. The attached C3 fragment (C3b) interacts with C3b-specific receptors on phagocytic cells to promote the process of immune adherence, which is similar to opsonization. Third, release of other cleavage products results in the development of a local, acute inflammatory reaction that walls off the area and attracts large numbers of phagocytic polymorphonuclear leukocytes (PMN's).

1.   The complex sequence of events in complement activation is diagramed in Figure 1–39. Complement fixation is initiated by the binding of one IgM or several IgG molecules—perhaps as few as two in close proximity—to an antigen on a foreign cell surface. This binding exposes a complement-binding site on

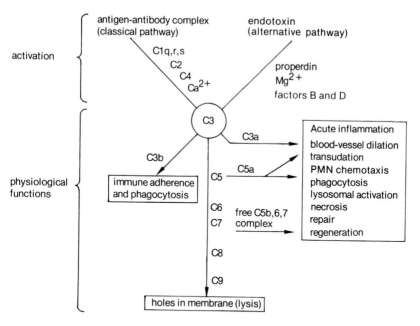

Figure 1–38 Activation pathways and physiological functions of complement components.

the Fc region of the antibody molecule. Complement component C1, a heat-labile complex of three proteins, binds to the antigen–antibody complex via its C1q subcomponent, a molecule with multivalent binding sites specific for IgM and IgG Fc regions. In the presence of Ca^{2+}, the binding activates C1s, another subcomponent with proteolytic activity, to cleave C4. The larger of the two C4 fragments, in association with C1, then specifically cleaves C2. The larger fragments from C4 and C2 combine on the membrane to form a specific protease that cleaves C3. The two resulting fragments of C3 have distinct activities. C3a (molecular weight ~7000) causes local blood-vessel dilation and also may attract polymorphonuclear leukocytes. C3b attaches over the entire cell membrane, promotes opsonization, and combines with the C4–C2 complex to initiate cleavage of C5. The smaller of the resulting C5 fragments (molecular weight ~15,000) is vasoactive like C3a, and may attract polymorphonuclear leukocytes. The larger C5 fragment binds to the cell membrane and combines with C6 and C7 to form a trimolecular complex, C5,6,7, which in turn can bind C8 and C9. In addition, free forms of the C5,6,7 complex are strong chemotactic attractants for polymorphonuclear leukocytes.

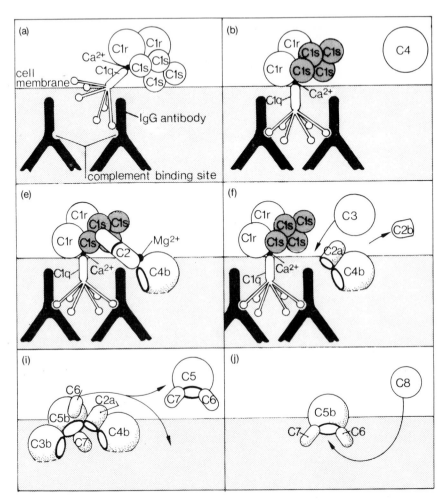

Figure 1–39 Diagrammatic representation of the sequence of events in complement activation on a cell membrane. (a) When two IgG molecules bind to adjacent sites on a foreign cell, they can activate complement factor C1. C1 consists of three subunits, C1q, C1s, and C1r, which are held together by a calcium ion. (b) C1 is inactive until it binds antibody through the C1q subunit. Then C1s, a serine esterase, becomes activated (shading). (c) C4 is cleaved into two parts, C4a and C4b. (d) C4b binds to the cell surface nearby. (e) C2 is split by the activated C1s. (f) the C2a fragment combines with C4b to form a proteolytic enzyme that splits C3. (g) The C3b fragment binds to the surface. (h) If C3b is

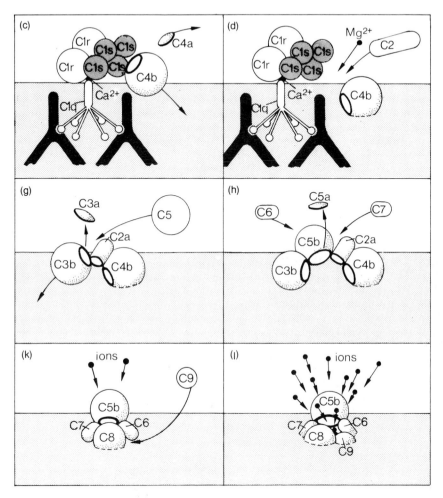

near C4b,2a complex, they bind together and cleave C5. (i) C5b then binds to C6 and C7. (j) The C5b,6,7 complex can act as an inflammatory mediator, or it can bind to the surface at a new site where it complexes with C8. (k) These components form a small hole in the membrane through which a few ions can pass. (1) The addition of C9 greatly enlarges the hole and speeds up the flow of water and ions, leading to osmotic lysis. The C3a, C5a and C5b,6,7 fragments mediate various aspects of the inflammatory response (see text). [From M. Mayer, "The Complement System," *Sci. Am.* **229**, 54 (1973). Copyright © 1973 by Scientific American, Inc. All rights reserved.]

Upon binding of C8 and C9, the cell membrane develops characteristic circular lesions (Figure 1–40) that permit cell contents to leak out. Since no concomitant covalent changes in the membrane constituents have been detected, the lesions probably do not result from direct enzymatic attack. Instead, they may arise by incorporation of C8 and C9 into the membrane to form a cylindrical channel with a hydrophobic outer surface and a hydrophilic central pore, by analogy with the action of some cyclic peptide antibiotics such as gramicidin (Figure 1–40).

2.   An alternative pathway of complement activation is important in host defense against gram-negative bacteria that inhabit the gastrointestinal tract. Lipopolysaccharides (endotoxins) from the cell walls of these organisms combine directly with a serum factor called *properdin,* which then, in the presence of Mg^{2+} and two serum cofactors designated D and B, cleaves C3 as in the "classical" pathway. This alternative pathway bypasses the need for antibody, C1, C4, or C2, and thus allows the complement system to be activated acutely in response to some infections (Figure 1–38).

3.   At least three complement components, C2, C4, and alternative pathway cofactor B, are coded for or regulated by genes in the chromosomal region known as the *major histocompatibility*

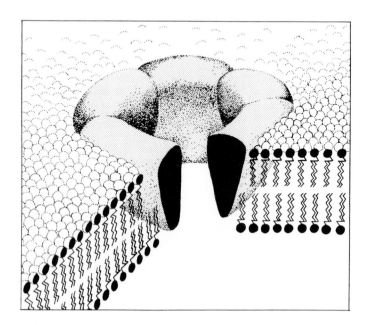

Figure 1–40   A hypothetical model of a cell-membrane pore created by complement action. [From M. Mayer, "The Complement System," *Sci. Am.* **229,** 54 (1973). Copyright © 1973 by Scientific American, Inc. All rights reserved.]

complex (MHC), which is important in several aspects of host defense.

D.   Inflammation, a common host response to injury, can be induced by antigen–antibody reactions that activate the complement system. The four cardinal signs of inflammation are *heat* (calor), *redness* (rubor), *swelling* (tumor), and *pain* (dolor).

1.   *Acute* inflammatory responses, induced by antibodies or other agents, involve a rapid set of events at the site of injury (Figure 1–41a). Local vessel dilation (which causes redness and heat) allows influx of plasma proteins and phagocytic cells into the tissue spaces (to cause swelling). Local release or activation of other vessel-active enzymes, and increased tissue pressure, trigger local nerve endings (to cause pain).

If the acute response rids the host of the agents that induce inflammation, repair and regeneration ensue. If not, the continued influx of polymorphonuclear leukocytes and serum products leads to cell death and, in some cases, to the formation of an abcess—a swelling bounded by fibrin from clotted blood and cells involved in phagocytosis and repair, with a central cavity of live and dead polymorphonuclear leukocytes, tissue debris, and the injurious or infectious agents. The center of an abcess is said to be purulent, and the liquid it contains is commonly known as pus.

2.   Continuing acute inflammatory responses may become chronic inflammatory responses, with the same four cardinal signs, but different cellular and soluble-protein participants. Chronic inflammatory responses are characterized by an infiltration of lymphocytes and cells of the monocyte–macrophage

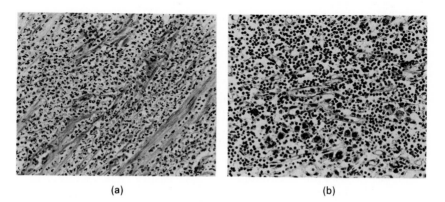

(a)   (b)

Figure 1–41 Photomicrographs of (a) acute and (b) chronic inflammation. Polymorphonuclear leukocytes predominate in acute inflammation, whereas lymphocytes and macrophages predominate in chronic inflammation. [Photomicrographs by R. Rouse and I. Weissman.]

lineage (Figure 1–41b). These responses may be induced by immunological injury initiated by effector T cells.

3. Both acute (antibody-induced) and chronic (T-cell induced) inflammation may occur in the skin. These responses are called *immediate* and *delayed hypersensitivity*, respectively. Immediate hypersensitivity, which is mediated by complement activation, begins within hours of antibody-induced immunological injury, usually peaks in intensity by 24 hours, and subsides by 48 hours. A special case of immediate hypersensitivity, induced by antigen, IgE, and mast cells, and *not* mediated by complement, arises within minutes of antigen–IgE binding, subsiding several hours later. Delayed hypersensitivity first becomes apparent 1–2 days after T-cell-induced immunological injury, peaking in intensity at 48–72 hours, and subsiding thereafter.

E.   IgE antibodies on the surfaces of mast cells bind antigens from multicellular parasites and initiate mast-cell degranulation. As a result, histamine and heparin are released, thereby causing vasodilation and smooth-muscle contraction (Essential Concept 1–8B5). Although the full functional significance of the IgE system is still a mystery, it is believed that this process promotes the expulsion of parasites from organs that are surrounded with smooth muscle, such as the gastrointestinal tract and uterus. Blood IgE levels rise significantly in individuals with gastrointestinal parasites such as worms and helminths. These individuals have high concentrations of intestinal mast cells coated with IgE. Blood IgE levels also are high in allergic individuals.

1–10 Effector T cells cooperate with B cells to produce a humoral immune response

A.   Antibody molecules are synthesized only by the progeny of B cells. However, certain effector T cells serve to facilitate the differentiation of B cells into plasma cells. Cooperation between B and T cells requires an antigen that carries at least two different antigenic determinants, which suggests that the antigen functions as a bridge. In many immunizations with a hapten conjugated to a carrier, it has been demonstrated that T cells specific for carrier determinants cooperate with B cells specific for hapten determinants. The subclass of effector T cells that cooperate with B cells in antibody formation is called T helper (T_H) cells. T_H cells are essential for IgG, IgA, and IgE immune responses; most IgM responses are T_H-cell-independent.

B.   T and B cells require other accessory cells for effective antigen-specific collaboration. Specific T_H cells recognize and respond to antigen only when it is presented by macrophages. Antigen-activated T_H cells also require accessory cells, perhaps macrophages or dendritic reticular cells, to trigger specific B cells. Accessory cells are not antigen-specific,

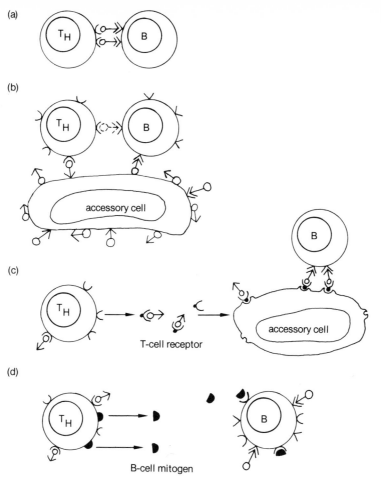

Figure 1–42 Models of T cell–B cell interactions. (a) T$_H$ cells and (b) possibly accessory cells may concentrate antigen for presentation to B cells. (c) T cells may release antigen-specific factors that bind to accessory cells or (d) other factors that act directly as mitogens specific for B cells that bind antigen (see text).

in that they will perform their accessory functions even if derived from a host that cannot respond to the specific antigen. In contrast, antigen-specific T$_H$ and B cells both must be present to produce an antibody response.

C.   Two kinds of models for T$_H$–B cell interactions have been proposed. The first kind of model postulates that antigen-specific T$_H$ cells attach via an antigen bridge to antigen-specific B cells. This bridging could be a two-cell interaction (Figure 1–42a), or a three-cell interaction wherein an antigen-bearing accessory cell holds antigen-specific T$_H$ and B cells together (Figure 1–42b). The second kind of model postulates that antigen-activated T$_H$ cells release factors that interact with accessory cells and/or antigen-specific B cells to trigger the B-cell response. The T-helper factors could be antigen-specific T-cell receptors that bind antigen to accessory cells in a multivalent array (Figure 1–42c), or they could act as B-cell mitogens that specifically trigger those B cells that bind antigen (Figure 1–42d).

D.   Most T cells are segregated from B cells within lymphoid organs, yet immune responses that require a T-B collaboration take place in these organs. Two alternative explanations for this apparent discrepancy have been proposed. One explanation is based on the observation that T and B cells entering a lymphoid organ traverse a field of antigen-charged macrophages together before migrating to their specific domains. Antigen-specific T and B cells may be retained on these accessory cells, as in Figure 1–42b. Alternatively, antigen-activated T_H cells may enter B-cell domains and there trigger B cells directly (Figure 1–42a or b) or via soluble factors (Figure 1–42c or d). The latter alternative is consistent with the universal appearance of T cells in the germinal centers of secondary follicles during an immune response (Essential Concept 1–6B).

E.   Whereas most humoral immune responses are T-cell dependent, antigens that have repeating, identical antigenic determinants (e.g., polysaccharides or proteins with identical subunits) can elicit an antibody response in the absence of T cells (Figure 1–43). If accessory cells or T cells act to convert a monovalent determinant to a multivalent cell-surface array, as suggested in the preceding section (Figures 1–42b and c), then it would be understandable that a multivalent polymeric antigen could bypass T-cell participation. However, these antigens primarily stimulate IgM synthesis and fail to generate memory B cells. This fact suggests that repeating antigens may be unable to stimulate T_H cells. If so, then their behavior would be consistent with the relative T_H-cell independence of the IgM response and dependence of the IgG response. According to the models of antigen-dependent B-cell maturation (Figure 1–28), T_H cells might act to trigger differentiation of B_γ cells from a B_μ precursor, or differentiation of B_γ cells to PC_γ cells. The possibility that T_H cells could act to switch PC_μ to PC_γ cells seems less likely.

F.   In addition to T_H cells, which stimulate antibody production, there is a class of *suppressor T* (T_S) *cells* that specifically inhibit antibody production. T_S cells are generated by antigenic stimulation, and are antigen-specific in their suppression. It is not yet known whether they act upon antigen-charged accessory cells, T_H cells, or B cells. If they act on lymphocytes, they could recognize either cell-bound antigen or the idiotypic determinants of T- or B-cell receptors.

   1.   Unlike T_H cells, T_S cells are generated in immune responses to antigens with repeating identical antigenic determinants. Removal of T_S cells leads to an augmented IgM response to these antigens, but still does not result in an IgG response.

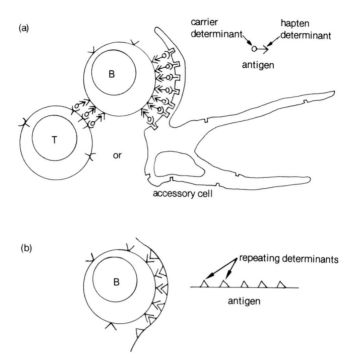

Figure 1–43 Models for T-cell-dependent and T-cell-independent antibody responses (see text). (a) Accessory cells and T cells may be required to present monovalent antigens as a multivalent array to B-cell receptors. (b) Multivalent antigens can activate B cells independently of accessory cells and T cells.

    2. Suppressor T cells are believed to play an important role in regulating the immune response, and may be involved in the mechanism of tolerance.

    3. As in T_H-B interactions, it is not known whether T_S cells interact with other lymphoid cells through cell-surface components or through soluble factors.

1-11 Two categories of genes control the B-cell immune response to antigen

A. The two categories of genes that control the B-cell immune response are *structural genes* for the antibody polypeptide chains and *immune response* (Ir) *genes.*

    1. Structural genes for several antibody idiotypes have been mapped genetically in the mouse and shown to be linked to antibody constant-region genes. The properties of immunoglobulin structural genes are discussed in Chapter 3.

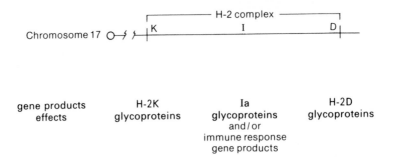

Figure 1–44   A genetic map of the major histocompatibility complex on Chromosome 17 of the mouse. Chromosome 17 carries genes for a variety of different cell-surface molecules, which are discussed further in Chapter 4.

2.   Immune response genes have been investigated in various inbred strains of mice. One well-studied locus, the Ir-1 locus, is situated in the middle of the major histocompatibility complex (MHC) and is unlinked to any of the loci that code for antibody polypeptides (Figure 1–44). The Ir-1 locus regulates the amount of IgG (and perhaps IgA and IgE) antibody that is synthesized in response to certain specific antigens that are T-cell dependent. Ir-1 alleles are inherited as dominant or codominant characters. Mice with different Ir-1 alleles can be grouped into two classes: *high responder* mice synthesize 10 to 20 times as much specific IgG antibody as do *low responder* mice. Mice that are high responders to some antigens may be low responders to others. Therefore Ir genes do not code for general immune responsivity, but show some degree of antigenic specificity. Mice that are low responders to a particular antigen may give a high response if the antigen is linked to an immunogenic carrier. Consequently a low response cannot be due solely to limitations of the animal's repertoire of antigen-specific B cells.

B.   Three general models have been proposed to explain the action of Ir genes.

1.   The Ir locus actually may code for T-cell antigen-specific receptors, which then would constitute a second antigen recognition system distinct from that of the immunoglobulins expressed in B cells (Figure 1–45a). Ir deficiencies would result in a decreased repertoire of antigen-specific T_H cells, which would be expressed as a failure of the corresponding antigen-specific B cells to produce either IgG antibodies or memory cells.

2.   The Ir locus may code for cell-surface receptors that are required for the interactions of T_H cells with accessory cells, T_H cells with B cells, and B cells with accessory cells (Figure

1–45b). In this model the postulated receptors could be required on any or all cell types necessary for an IgG response, but not on those necessary for most IgM responses. Because Ir defects are antigen-specific, antigens to which response is low would have to interfere somehow with these cellular interactions.

3. The Ir locus may control some aspect of suppressor T-cell function (Figure 1–45c). According to this model, low responsivity would represent too much suppression by T_S cells rather than too little help from T_H cells.

C. Some genes within the I region of the MHC are known to code for cell-surface molecules. In general, gene products of the MHC are polymorphic; that is, for each locus or sublocus a large number of distinct alleles are present in the population. Therefore the I-region gene products from one individual will be antigenic to other individuals in the species. Such I-region antigens are called Ia antigens. The characterization of Ia determinants and genes is still incomplete, but it is clear that the I region codes for a multiplicity of cell-surface molecules present on subclasses of T cells, B cells, accessory cells, and even sperm and epidermal cells. It appears that at least some Ia determinants are differentially expressed on different subclasses of a particular cell type. For example, B_γ cells express a set of Ia antigens generally not expressed by B_μ cells, and T_S cells express a set that is not found on T_H cells. If all these Ia molecules are products of

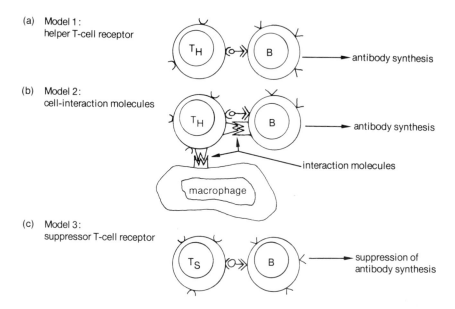

(a) Model 1:
helper T-cell receptor

(b) Model 2:
cell-interaction molecules

(c) Model 3:
suppressor T-cell receptor

Figure 1–45 A diagram of three models for the function of Ir genes (see text).

Ir genes involved in immune response regulation, Model 1 (Figure 1–45) must be either extended to cells other than T cells, or modified, or abandoned.

1–12 Two distinct T-cell lineages cooperate in a cellular immune response

A.   In addition to the helper (T_H) and suppressor (T_S) T-cell functions, which operate in a humoral immune response, there are two other T-cell effector functions, which are involved in the generation of cellular immunity. These functions are development of local chronic inflammatory responses by T_D cells and direct lysis of foreign antigenic cells by T_C cells.

An additional class of T cells, called T_A cells, serves an amplifier function in the maturation of antigen-specific killer T_C cells. T_A cells apparently recognize a macrophage-processed or native cell-surface antigen, and then somehow stimulate T_C-cell precursors that recognize other antigens on the same target cell to proliferate and differentiate to T_C effector cells.

B.   Serological studies in mice seem to show that the various classes of T cells divide into two major cell categories, which have been designated the T_H category and the $T_{C,S}$ category, distinguishable by their Ly antigens. Table 1–2 lists the various T-cell classes with their functions and serological markers. The classes within the two categories are distinguishable so far only on the basis of their functions. All classes probably include memory cells in addition to effector T cells.

> **1.**   The T_H category, which consists of Ly-1 cells, gives rise to the helper T_H cells, which cooperate with B cells in the humoral response, and to the T_A cells, which play an analogous helper role in killer T_C-cell maturation. The T_H category includes T_D

Table 1–2
Classes of effector T cells

Category	Class of cells	Function	Ly phenotype in mice
T_H	T_H	Stimulation of B-cell differentiation	Ly-1
	T_A	Stimulation of T_C precursor cell differentiation	Ly-1
	T_D	Transfer of delayed hypersensitivity	Ly-1
$T_{C,S.}$	T_C	Lysis of specific antigenic target cells	Ly-2,3
	T_S	Suppression of immune responses	Ly-2,3

cells, which are responsible for the establishment of local chronic inflammatory responses such as delayed hypersensitivity.

2. The $T_{c,s}$ category includes suppressor T_s cells as well as precursors of T_c cells. The cells in this category appear to be predominantly of the Ly-2,3 phenotype, although recent experiments have detected both T_c and T_s cells of Ly-1,2,3 phenotype as well.

C. The T cells that mediate delayed hypersensitivity release a variety of polypeptides called *lymphokines* (Table 1–3). Most work on lymphokines so far has been done with species in which markers to distinguish T_H and $T_{c,s}$ categories have not been identified. Therefore, production of the various lymphokines cannot yet be assigned to a particular T-cell line.

Lymphokines are believed to attract macrophages and other cells to the site of T_H-cell interaction with antigen, activate these macrophages to a phagocytic stage of differentiation, and prevent their departure from the site. In addition, other lymphokines are thought to stimulate division of itinerant lymphocytes; these lymphokines could include the proposed B-cell mitogens released by antigen-activated T_H cells. The lymphokines also may include agents that nonspecifically damage all cells except lymphocytes, and agents such as *interferon* that prevent intracellular viral multiplication. It is not yet known which of these agents are active *in vivo*, but it has been demonstrated that lymphokines

Table 1–3
Characteristics of some T-cell lymphokines

Lymphokine	Properties
Macrophage chemotactic factor (CF)	Attracts macrophages *in vitro*
Macrophage migration inhibition factor (MIF)	Inhibits macrophage movement *in vitro*
Macrophage aggregation factor (MAF)	Agglutinates macrophages *in vitro*
Lymphocyte blastogenic factor (BF)	Induces lymphocyte DNA synthesis *in vitrc*
Lymphotoxin (LT)	Acts *in vitro* as a slow general cytotoxin which spares lymphocytes.
Interferon	Prevents viral replication in target cells
Transfer factor	Transfers delayed hypersensitivity to specific antigens from one person to another; dialyzable factor

induced in tissue culture will initiate delayed hypersensitivity if injected into the skin, and that antibodies to lymphokines will prevent the expression of delayed hypersensitivity when injected together with antigen.

D.   The observation that T_C and T_S cells belong to the same category suggests that T_S cells also might be specifically cytotoxic and might carry out suppression of B-cell immune responses by killing appropriate cells. However, a possible distinction between T_S and T_C cells in mice recently has been reported. T_S cells bear a specific Ia antigen not found on T_C cells from the same animal. It will be important to verify that this distinction is general, rather than a special case of the particular system used in the assays.

E.   In mice, nearly 50% of peripheral T cells are neither T_H nor $T_{C,S}$ cells. These lymphocytes are Thy-1 and Ly-1,2,3, and their functions are incompletely understood. They may be precursors of the T_H and $T_{C,S}$ categories, or they may represent a separate lineage with distinct properties. Lineage relationships between T cells of the three known Ly subsets, Ly-1,2,3, Ly-1, and Ly-2,3 have not been clearly worked out, although it is known that cells of the latter two subsets are stable and do not give rise to cells of other subsets.

1–13   Some T cells recognize a gene product of the major histocompatibility complex as well as a specific antigenic determinant

A.   When lymphocytes from two genetically different individuals of a species are mixed in cell culture medium, the T cells of each individual recognize and respond to antigens of the major histocompatibility complex (MHC) presented by cells of the other. In the course of this process, called the *mixed lymphocyte response* (MLR), small T_A cells react first by enlarging, dividing, releasing lymphokines, and stimulating maturation of T_C effector cells. In mice, T_A cells generally respond to Ia antigens on macrophages and B cells to a greater degree than to antigens coded by the D or K regions (D/K antigens; see Figure 1–44). Conversely, T_C cells generally recognize and respond to D/K antigens to a greater degree than to Ia antigens. This distinction may be analogous to the differing recognition specificities of T_H and B cells in the humoral response to a hapten-carrier antigen. In both responses T_A and T_H cells recognize one set of determinants (Ia antigens or carrier) and stimulate mature T_C or B_γ cells, which recognize a second set of associated determinants (D/K antigens or haptens), to differentiate to effector cytotoxic T_C cells and IgG-secreting PC_γ cells, respectively.

B.   In the mixed lymphocyte reaction, the MHC determinants of one individual represent foreign antigens to the T cells of the other.

However, some kind of recognition of *self*-MHC determinants also appears to be important in normal humoral and cellular immune responses.

1.   In a humoral response to a hapten-carrier antigen, T_H cells recognize and respond to processed carrier antigen on macrophages. Recent experiments with mice have shown that this response usually requires that the T_H cells and the macrophages be genetically identical in the I region of the MHC. In an individual mouse this identity is assured. If T_H cells from one mouse of an inbred strain are tested *in vitro* with antigen-fed macrophages of another genetically identical animal, they will function normally. However, antigen-specific T_H cells usually will not respond to the antigen-bearing macrophages from a host that differs genetically in the I region. Genetic identity in the D and K regions is not required for T_H-macrophage cooperation.

2.   In the cellular response to host cells that carry foreign cell-surface antigens (e.g., virus-infected cells that carry cell-surface viral determinants), antigen-specific effector T_C cells recognize, react with, and destroy the antigen-bearing cells. Experiments analogous to those described in the preceding paragraph have shown that this cytolysis reaction will occur only if the effector T_C cells recognize viral antigens on cells that share D or K MHC antigens with the cells that stimulated these T_C cells; for virus infections within an individual, effector T_C cells and target cells must be genetically identical in the D and K regions of the MHC. Identity in the I region is not required for effector T_C-target cell interaction.

3.   These observations suggest that both T_H-macrophage and T_C-target cell interactions involve specific MHC gene products, as well as antigens and antigen-specific receptors. This phenomenon has been termed *associated* or *dual recognition.* An alternative nomenclature may be used to describe associated recognition. When the immune system is stimulated to respond to exogenous antigen, T_H cells can do so only in the appropriate *context* of I-region gene-product interaction, and T_C cells can do so only in the appropriate *context* of D/K-region gene-product interaction. Neither the mechanism nor the biological function of associated recognition is yet understood, but both raise questions of major importance in understanding the immune system.

4.   Although most T_C and T_H cells recognize foreign antigens in the context of self-MHC gene products, a subset of these cells can recognize foreign antigens in the context of particular nonself MHC gene products. Under appropriate conditions, these cells can give rise to the predominant clones capable of reacting to a particular foreign antigen. This finding seems to rule out like–like molecular interactions in T_H-macrophage and T_C-target cell interactions, and therefore implies that this recognition involves specific receptor–ligand interactions.

D.   Immunologists currently are exploring three models for the mechanism of associated recognition by T cells. Each model places different restrictions on the nature of the antigen-specific T-cell receptors and the form of the antigens they recognize (Figure 1–46).

1.   The first model postulates that each T cell carries two types of surface receptors. One type specifically recognizes a self-MHC gene product. The receptors of this type presumably could be the same on most T cells of a given class, such as T_C cells. The other type is the antigen-specific cell-surface receptor discussed previously. From this model it is predicted that the antigens recognized by T-cell receptors will have no necessary association with MHC gene products in the target cell membrane, and that two distinct types of T-cell receptors will be identified.

2.   The second model postulates that T cells have only a single type of receptor and that most T cells recognize a self-MHC product that has been altered by reaction with a specific antigen. Such covalent alterations could include direct covalent linkage of the two molecular species, or enzymatic modification of one by the other. This model predicts that the cell surfaces of macrophages and target cells will carry antigenically modified MHC gene products and specific antigens, and that only these molecules will be recognized by cognate T cells.

3.   The third model postulates that T cells have a single type of receptor, which recognizes both a self-MHC gene product and a specific antigen when the two are complexed together

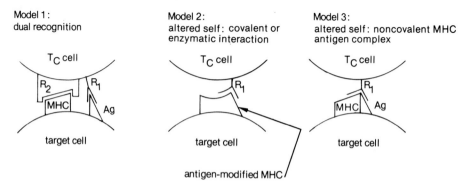

Figure 1–46   Three models for the mechanism of associated recognition of MHC and non-MHC antigenic determinants at the cell membrane (see text).

on the cell surface. According to this model, antigen and MHC product either could form a stable noncovalent complex on the target-cell surface, or could stabilize their association by interaction with the T-cell receptor when the cells were in contact. This model predicts that the cell surfaces of macrophages and target cells will carry unmodified MHC gene products and antigens, either separate or associated with each other. Only associated heterodimeric molecules will give high avidity binding to the cognate T-cell receptor.

E.   Knowledge of the nature of T-cell receptors would help to provide the basis for a choice among the foregoing models. Preliminary evidence indicates that some antigen-specific T-cell surface receptors share idiotypic determinants with humoral antibodies that are specific for the same antigens. If this observation turns out to be general, then a component of T-cell receptors may be coded by immunoglobulin V-region genes, and T-cell receptors may be immunoglobulin-like molecules. Different molecules bearing similar idiotypes conceivably could arise by convergent evolution of two independent gene families, but this possibility seems unlikely.

F.   The differentiation of T_C and T_H cells bearing receptors specific for self- or nonself-MHC gene products occurs in the thymus. Thus bone marrow thymocyte precursors from strain $(A \times B)F_1$ maturing in an A strain thymus will give rise to T_C and T_H cells, which can recognize foreign antigens in the context of strain A (but not strain B) MHC gene products. This finding has two important consequences. First, since all foreign antigens are unlikely to be present in the thymic maturational microenvironment, selection is likely to be via anti-MHC (self or nonself) receptors only. This has been taken as evidence for Model D.1 on p. 66. Second, immunological reconstitution of thymus-deficient animals or patients by thymic transplantation (Essential Concept 2–4) may only be effective if donor and host share MHC alleles.

G.   The biological function of MHC gene products in associated recognition still is a matter for speculation.

1.   One plausible function for I-region gene products could be to enable T_H lymphocytes to identify the cells with which they interact. Ia antigens are found almost exclusively on macrophages, B cells, and T cells. T_H cells must interact with macrophages in the process of surveillance for foreign antigens, and then must interact with B cells and T_C precursor cells to stimulate their differentiation into plasma cells and T_C effector cells, respectively. I-region determinants could constitute an identification system that would restrict the interactions of T_H cells to functionally significant contact with macrophages, B cells, and T_C precursor cells.

However, other considerations suggest that the I-region determinants are more than simple identification tags for different cell types in the immune system. Ia antigens show a high degree of polymorphism within a species, and differences in Ir genes of the I region cause differences in immune response that are antigen-specific (Essential Concept 1–11). These findings have led to the suggestion that I-region genes may code for the T-cell antigen-specific receptors themselves, as well as for the cell-surface molecules that restrict T-cell interactions to macrophages and B cells.

2. The function of D- and K-region determinants in the interaction of T_C cells with target cells is even less clear at present. D/K determinants are found on most cells of the body; consequently it is unlikely that they serve as markers to restrict T_C surveillance to certain classes of cells. Because D/K determinants show a very high degree of polymorphism, they could constitute identification for distinguishing self cells from foreign cells. However, it would seem logical that T_C cells be programmed to attack any cell that displays a foreign antigen, regardless of whether it also displays self-identification, so that self-identification would be unnecessary.

It is possible that associated recognition protects T cells from inappropriate interactions with soluble antigens. For example, T_C cells must identify and eliminate cells that carry viral antigens, yet not be inappropriately triggered by free viral antigens. Similar arguments could be made for the interaction of T_H cells with antigen-charged macrophages or with specific B cells.

Clues as to the function of the I region and the D/K region eventually may come from understanding the unusual properties of MHC determinants as immunogens, discussed in the following paragraph, from further insight into the mechanism of tolerance (Essential Concept 1–14), and from an understanding of the evolution of the MHC from subvertebrate ancestors, considered in Chapter 4.

H.   An unexpectedly high proportion of T cells recognizes and responds to the MHC products of different individuals of the same species. Clonal selection predicts that about one in 10^4 virgin cells should respond to any antigenic determinant, and that less than 1% of these virgin cells could respond to the multideterminant MHC differences (*haplotypes*) that distinguish two allogenic individuals of a species. Yet in mice and rats, 1–12% of the T cells (either T_H or T_C) respond to any MHC haplotype difference (Figure 1–47). Because there are over 30 distinct MHC haplotypes in each species investigated, and about 10% of the lymphocyte population responds specifically to

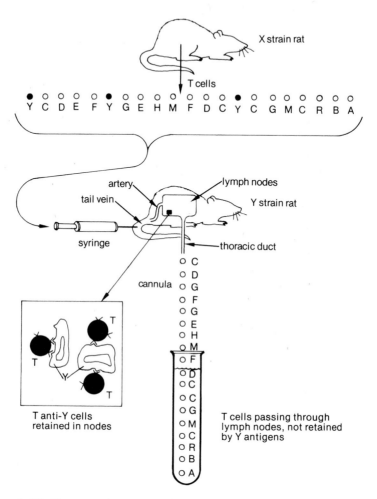

Figure 1–47 Diagrammatic representation of an experiment illustrating that 5–10% of the lymphocyte population responds to each major histocompatibility haplotype. Thoracic duct lymphocytes from rat X contain T lymphocytes specifically reactive to strain Y MHC antigens (●), and lymphocytes reactive to other antigens (○). Injection of these cells into the tail vein of a rat whose thoracic duct is cannulated allows recirculating lymphocytes to traverse rat Y's lymphoid tissues over a 24-hour interval and then enter the cannula. Those reactive to Y's MHC antigens are retained by Y's lymphoid tissues, whereas the others enter the thoracic duct. In this hypothetical example, nearly 15% of the cells were retained. [Based on experiments by W. L. Ford and colleagues.]

each, it seems at first sight either that the sum of lymphocyte specificities is more than 100%, or that the one lymphocyte–one receptor specificity hypothesis must be violated. However, there are several possible explanations for this apparent paradox:

1. A haplotype includes a large number of antigenic determinants. Although each of the 30 or more distinct haplotypes must include unique determinants, it also can include determinants that are common to one, two, three, four, or more of the other haplotypes (Figure 1–48). Thus a given subset of T cells may respond to several MHC haplotypes. Nevertheless, it is still puzzling that the set of MHC determinants appears to fill the universe of T-cell receptor specificities. One possible explanation would be that the microorganisms that infect a species may bear or induce determinants that cross-react with the MHC determinants of that species, so that the responding cells are not virgin T cells, but rather antigen-specific memory T cells that already represent amplified clones.

2. Each T cell may carry more than one type of receptor for antigens, as postulated in Essential Concept 1–12D. If so, a significant proportion of cells could bear one type of receptor for a particular MHC haplotype, and another type of receptor for a specific non-MHC antigen. Stimulation by the MHC antigen would be sufficient to activate these clones, which should contain T cells reactive to any specific non-MHC antigen at the same frequency as in the total T-cell population.

3. Each T cell may have a single class of antigen receptors, all of which have the capacity for associated recognition of MHC and specific non-MHC antigens, as proposed in Essential Concept

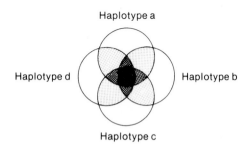

Haplotype a

Haplotype d

Haplotype b

Haplotype c

Figure 1–48 A Venn diagram illustrating cross reactions among four different hypothetical haplotypes. The set of determinants for each haplotype is represented by a circle. Clear spaces within a circle represent *private* determinants for a particular haplotype. Light stippling and dark stippling represent *public* determinants shared by two or three haplotypes, respectively, and blackened regions represent determinants common to all four haplotypes.

1–13D. If so, a related MHC haplotype could be recognized mistakenly as altered self MHC by a high proportion of T-cell clones that previously were activated and expanded by exposure to altered self antigens. Again, these clones should contain cells specific for any given non-MHC antigen at the same frequency as in the total T-cell population.

1-14 Normally the immune system does not respond to self-antigens

A.   The immune system can respond in two ways when exposed to an antigen. A positive response leads to differentiation of T and B effector cells, to antibody synthesis, and to immunologic memory. A negative response leads to active suppression or inactivation of specific lymphocytes, and to *tolerance.* Tolerance can be defined as the failure of an organism to mount an immune response against a specific antigen. Normally an organism is tolerant of its own antigens. Immunologic defenses are based on the ability of an organism to distinguish between self and foreign molecules; the effector mechanisms of the immune system, if activated, could destroy self-molecules and cells as effectively as their foreign counterparts. When tolerance to self-antigens is lost, autoimmune disease may ensue.

Both the immune response and tolerance are specific for individual antigens; both are acquired through appropriate antigenic exposure; and both are mediated by lymphocytes. Immunologic memory and tolerance both are active responses of the vertebrate immune system.

B.   A vertebrate has the genetic information necessary to synthesize antibodies against self-antigens, but it prevents the expression of this information in effector cells. The mechanism of the tolerance reaction is unclear, but as a consequence of this response, lymphocytes that carry cell-surface receptors specific for self-determinants either are eliminated or rendered incapable of activation (*paralyzed*) by exposure to these determinants. At any early stage in their differentiation from precursor lymphocytes, B and T cells appear to be particularly sensitive to antigen. Contact at this stage with even low concentrations of self-antigens paralyzes or eliminates immature B and T cells that are self-specific. Since lymphocytes continue to differentiate in the bone marrow and thymus throughout the lifetime of an individual, this process, termed *clonal abortion,* must be an active and continuous check against production of antiself immunity (Figure 1–49a). Maintenance of tolerance requires continued presence of the tolerance-inducing antigen.

C.   During early fetal development the immune system normally is exposed almost exclusively to self-antigens, which react with and paralyze or eliminate all self-specific clones of immature lymphocytes. Later in life it is less clear how the organism distinguishes self from

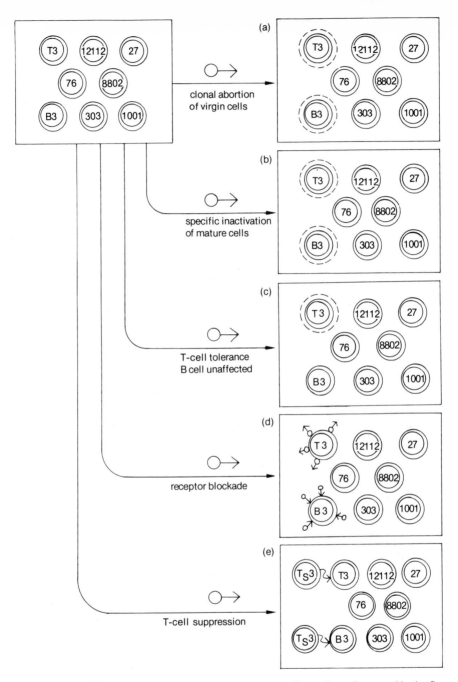

Figure 1–49 Five models for induction of tolerance. The antigen diagramed in the figure has two antigenic determinants, one recognized by B-cell clone 3 and the other by T-cell clone 3. Inactivation of a clone is indicated by a dashed circle. (a) Clonal abortion of virgin lymphocytes, usually accomplished with very low antigen concentrations. (b) Paralysis or inactivation of mature lymphocytes, usually requiring high concentrations of antigen. (c) Tolerance at the level of T cells, but not at the level of B cells. This type of tolerance also prevents B-cell activation for responses that are T-cell dependent. (d) Blockade of receptors by antigen, which leads to paralysis. (e) Activation of specific T_s cells, which prevent specific T_H- or B-cell activation.

foreign determinants. Some insight into this question has come from experiments on induction of tolerance in mature animals. Certain antigens administered under certain conditions can induce tolerance by eliminating or paralyzing mature lymphocytes (Figure 1–49b).

1.   Mature lymphocytes are far more difficult to inactivate with a tolerance-inducing antigen than are immature lymphocytes. T and B cells of adult animals respond differently to the induction of tolerance. Very low (subimmunogenic) doses of an appropriate antigen can inactivate only T cells (*low zone tolerance*), whereas high doses produce a more rapid and prolonged tolerance in T cells than in B cells. Since B and T cells must cooperate to produce most humoral immune responses, tolerance in either cell type can block the synthesis of specific antibodies (Figure 1–49c). Unfortunately, it is not yet clear how experimental induction of tolerance in mature lymphocytes relates to the natural induction of tolerance in immature lymphocytes. Recent evidence indicates that low zone tolerance can be induced in B_μ, but not $B_{\mu+\delta}$ or other B cells expressing IgD as a receptor immunoglobulin.

2.   The form of an antigen may determine whether it elicits a positive or a negative immune response. Aggregated protein antigens, for example, are always immunogenic at all concentrations, whereas soluble monomeric forms of the same determinants may be immunogenic or tolerance-inducing (*tolerogenic*), depending on the dose administered. In general, a high dose of a monomeric antigen favors a negative response. Some self-antigens always will be present at higher levels than most foreign antigens. Conceivably, the immune system also has mechanisms for presenting self-antigens in more tolerogenic forms.

3.   One type of experimentally induced tolerance is somewhat better understood and may have important clinical applications. Very high doses of polysaccharide antigens cause paralysis of most of the antigen-specific B cells by binding to all their surface receptors (Figure 1–49d). This binding is reversible, but if the antigen is present at high enough levels it nevertheless can prevent B-cell activation by a mechanism that is still unknown (*receptor blockade*). A small amount of humoral antibody is produced, but then is absorbed by the excess of antigen.

Unnatural D-isomers of polypeptide antigens also induce tolerance by blockade of B-cell receptors. The blockade is irreversible, because mammals lack proteases that can degrade polypeptides of D-amino acids. This situation can be exploited clinically to induce tolerance to an allergen or a drug to which a patient normally mounts an immune response. Penicillin, for example, can be linked chemically to a D-polypeptide. When the resulting compound is injected in high doses into a sensitive individual, the penicillin-specific B-cell receptors become blockaded, and the allergic reaction to penicillin is eliminated.

4. Induction of tolerance in later life may be a cooperative phenomenon, rather than a direct antigen-mediated elimination or paralysis of reactive clones. Selective activation of T_s cells suppresses immune responses to specific antigens; this process is operationally equivalent to tolerance (Figure 1–49e). The two types of tolerance may be distinguished by mixing lymphocytes from a tolerant host with lymphocytes from a normal host. Tolerance mediated by T_s cells will prevent normal lymphocytes from reacting to the tolerance-inducing antigen, whereas clonal deletion or clonal abortion leaves a tolerant-cell population that will not transfer tolerance to normal lymphocytes. Both types of tolerance have been demonstrated by this test.

Selected Bibliography

Where to begin

Burnet, F. M., "A modification of Jerne's theory of antibody production using the concept of clonal selection," *Austral. J. Sci.* **20,** 67 (1957).

Edelman, G. M., "The structure and function of antibodies," *Sci. Am.* **223,** 34 (1970).

Jerne, N. K., "The immune system," *Sci. Am.* **229,** 52 (1973).

Raff, M. C., "Cell-surface immunology," *Sci. Am.* **234,** 30 (1976).

General

"Origins of Lymphocyte Diversity," *Cold Spring Harbor Symp. Quant. Biol.* **41** (1976). Most aspects of immunology are represented in these proceedings of a recent important symposium. For an impression of the development of immunology over the past decade, see Volume 32 of the same series.

Katz, D. H., *Lymphocyte Differentiation, Recognition, and Regulation,* Academic Press, New York, 1977. A comprehensive and up-to-date description of the cells and cellular interactions involved in the immune response.

Landsteiner, K., *The Specificity of Serological Reactions,* Harvard University Press, Cambridge, Mass., 1945. The basis of immunological specificity, as described by the investigator most responsible for its definition.

Origins and development of the hematolymphoid system

Ford, C. E., Micklem, H. S., Evans, E. P., Gray, J. G., and Ogden, D. A., "The inflow of bone-marrow cells to the thymus. Studies with part body-irradiated mice injected with chromosome-marked bone marrow and subjected to antigenic stimulation," *Ann. N. Y. Acad. Sci.* **129**, 283 (1966).

Till, J. E., and McCulloch, E. A., "A direct measurement of the radiation sensitivity of normal mouse bone marrow cells," *Radiat. Res.* **14**, 213 (1961).

Wolf, N. S., and Trentin, J. J., "Hemopoietic colony studies V: Effect of hemopoietic organ stroma on differentiation of pluripotent stem cells," *J. Exp. Med.* **127**, 205 (1968).

Wu, A. M., Till, J. E., Siminovitch, L., and McCulloch, E. A., "A cytological study of the capacity for differentiation of normal hemopoietic colony-forming cells," *J. Cell. Physiol.* **69**, 177 (1967).

Wu, A. M., Till, J. E., Siminovitch, K., and McCulloch, E. A., "Cytological evidence for a relationship between normal hematopoietic colony-forming cells and cells of the lymphoid system," *J. Exp. Med.* **127**, 455 (1968).

These papers describe research that helped put hematolymphoid differentiation on an experimental and quantitative cellular basis. The experiments by Till's and Ford's groups deal with the total differentiative potential of hematopoietic stem cells. The paper by Wolf and Trentin describes the microenvironmental induction of a particular differentiation pathway.

Lymphocytes as specific elements of the immune system

Billingham, R. E., Brent, L., and Medawar, P. B., "Quantitative studies on tissue transplantation immunity II: The origin, strength, and duration of actively and adoptively acquired immunity," *Proc. R. Soc. Lond.* [Biol.] **143**, 58 (1954).

Gowans, J. L., McGregor, D. D., Cowen, D. M., and Ford, C. E., "Initiation of immune responses by small lymphocytes," *Nature* **196**, 651 (1962).

These two germinal papers introduced the concept of afferent, central, and efferent limbs of the immune response; the concept of specific and nonspecific cellular elements in the immune response; and the concept that primary, secondary, and tolerance responses are properties of immuno-specific lymphocytes.

The thymus and T lymphocytes

Cantor, H., and Boyse, E. A., "Functional subclasses of T lymphocytes bearing different Ly antigens I: The generation of functionally distinct T cell subclasses is a differentiative process independent of antigen," *J. Exp. Med.* **141,** 1375 (1975).

Miller, J. F. A. P., "Immunological function of the thymus," *Lancet* **ii,** 748 (1961).

Weissman, I. L., "Thymus cell migration," *J. Exp. Med.* **126,** 291 (1967).

These papers define the role of the thymus in immunological maturation, the cellular basis for the development of peripheral T cells, and the division of peripheral T lymphocytes into functional subpopulations.

Development and function of B lymphocytes

Manning, D. C., "Heavy chain isotype suppression: A review of the immunosuppressive effects of heterologous anti-Ig heavy chain antisera," *J. Reticuloendothel. Soc.* **18,** 63 (1975).

Möller, G. (Ed.), "Subpopulations of B lymphocytes," *Transplant. Rev.* **24** (1975).

Szenberg, A., and Warner, N. L., "Dissociation of immunological responsiveness in fowls with a hormonally arrested development of lymphoid tissues," *Nature* **194,** 146 (1962).

These sources describe the development of B-cell lines, the controversy as to their sites of development, their functional subpopulations, and some preliminary research into their maturational sequences.

Physiology of the lymphocyte and compartmentalization in lymphoid organs

Ford, W. L., "Lymphocyte migration and immune responses," *Prog. Allergy* **19** 1 (1975).

Gowans, J. L., and Knight, E. J., "The route of recirculation of lymphocytes in the rat," *Proc. R. Soc. Lond.* [Biol.] **159,** 257 (1964).

Weissman, I. L., Gutman, G. A., and Friedberg, S. H., "Tissue localization of lymphoid cells," *Ser. Haematol.* **8,** 482 (1974).

These papers define the types of antigen-independent cellular interactions between lymphoid and nonlymphoid cells that result in the establishment and maintenance of lymphocyte migration pathways in peripheral lymphoid organs.

Lymphocyte interactions in immune responses

Cantor, H., and Asofsky, R., "Synergy among lymphoid cells mediating the graft-versus-host response III: Evidence for interaction between two types of thymus-derived cells," *J. Exp. Med.* **135**, 764 (1972).

Katz, D. H., and Benacerraf, B., "The function and interrelationships of T-cell receptors, Ir genes, and other histocompatibility gene products," *Transplant. Rev.* **22**, 175 (1974).

Mitchell, G. F., and Miller, J. F. A. P., "Cell-to-cell interaction in the immune response II: The source of hemolysin-forming cells in irradiated mice given bone marrow and thymus or thoracic duct lymphocytes," *J. Exp. Med.* **128**, 821 (1968).

Sprent, J., and von Boehmer, H., "Helper function of T cells depleted of alloantigen-reactive lymphocytes by filtration through irradiated F_1 hybrid recipients. Failure to collaborate with allogeneic B cells in a secondary response to sheep erythrocytes *in vivo*," *J. Exp. Med.* **144**, 617 (1976).

These papers describe T–B and T–T cell interactions in the immune response, as well as some restrictions placed upon their interactions by gene products of the MHC.

T-cell recognition of antigen and its relationship to the immune response genes

Benacerraf, B., and McDevitt, H. O., "The histocompatibility-linked immune response genes," *Science* **175**, 273 (1972).

Binz, H., and Wigzell, H., "Shared idiotypic determinants on T and B lymphocytes reactive against the same antigenic determinants," *J. Exp. Med.* **142**, 197 (1975).

Doherty, P. C., Blanden, R. V., and Zinkernagel, R. M., "Specificity of virus-immune effector T cells for H-2K or H-2D compatible interactions, implications for H-antigen diversity," *Transplant. Rev.* **29**, 89 (1976).

Howard, J. C., and Wilson, D. B., "Specific positive selection of lymphocytes reactive to strong histocompatibility antigens," *J. Exp. Med.* **140**, 660 (1974).

McDevitt, H. O., "The evolution of the genes in the major histocompatibility complex," *Fed. Proc.* **35**, 2168 (1976).

These papers present the discovery of MHC-linked immune response genes, and the current understanding of entities recognized by T-cell receptors.

Antibodies and effector mechanisms

Griffin, F. M., Griffin, J. A., and Silverstein, S. C., "Studies on the mechanism of phagocytosis," *J. Exp. Med.* **144**, 788 (1976).

Mayer, M., "The complement system," *Sci. Am.* **229**, 54 (1973).

Medicus, R. G., Schreiber, R. D., Götze, O., and Müller-Eberhard, H. J., "A molecular concept of the properdin pathway," *Proc. Natl. Acad. Sci. USA* **73**, 612 (1976).

Spiegelberg, H. L., "Biological activities of immunoglobulins of different classes and subclasses," *Adv. Immunol.* **259**, 19 (1974).

These articles describe recent knowledge of several of the effector mechanisms triggered by combination of antibodies with target antigens.

Self–nonself discrimination and immunological tolerance

Billingham, R. E., Brent, L., and Medawar, P. B., "Actively acquired tolerance of foreign cells," *Nature* **172**, 603 (1953).

Owen, R. D., "Immunogenetic consequences of vascular anastomoses between bovine twins," *Science* **102**, 400 (1945).

Triplett, E. L., "On the mechanism of immunologic self recognition," *J. Immunol.* **89**, 505 (1962).

Chiller, J. M., Habicht, G. S., and Weigle, W. O., "Cellular sites of immunologic unresponsiveness," *Proc. Natl. Acad. Sci. USA* **65**, 551 (1970).

Gershon, R. K., and Kondo, K., "Infectious immunological tolerance," *Immunology* **21**, 903 (1971).

Katz, K. H., Davie, J. M., Paul, W. E., and Benacerraf, B., "Carrier function in anti-hapten responses IV: Experimental conditions for the induction of hapten-specific tolerance or for the stimulation of antihapten anamnestic responses by "nonimmunogenic" hapten–polypeptide conjugates," *J. Exp. Med.* **134**, 201 (1971).

The first three papers define natural and experimentally induced tolerance in the framework of self–nonself discrimination. The last three papers present more complex views of the underlying mechanisms at the cellular level.

Problems

1–1 Indicate whether each of the following statements is true or false. Explain the error in each statement you consider to be false.
(a)   An antibody molecule has one type of antigen-binding site.
(b)   A large antigen generally can combine with many different antibody molecules.
(c)   Antigens combine with a specific antibody and stimulate the production of antibody.

(d)   A hapten can stimulate antibody production but cannot combine with antibody molecules.

(e)   In a secondary immune response, IgM is the major class of antibody synthesized.

(f)   Antibodies generally do not react with self-molecules because genes that code for self-antibodies are not inherited.

(g)   Antigenic stimulation of macrophages in the thymus will trigger their differentiation into T cells.

(h)   T cells are derived from hematopoietic stem cells.

(i)   When triggered by a cognate antigen, B_γ lymphocytes may differentiate to give plasma cells that secrete IgM antibody.

(j)   B cells that enter the spleen home to the lymphoid white pulp of the periarteriolar sheath.

(k)   Immunologic memory can last twenty years or more.

(l)   The T-cell receptor molecule has not yet been identified conclusively.

(m)   Blast transformation is an antigen-driven differentiation process that occurs in B and T cells.

(n)   Plasma cells are the major effector cells of the B-cell response; several classes of small lymphocytes are the effector cells of the T-cell response.

(o)   The fixation of complement is triggered by the interaction of antibody with antigen.

(p)   Some antigens can evoke an antibody response in B cells that do not require T-cell cooperation.

(q)   Mice that show a low immune response (low responders) to artificial polypeptides lack the genes for the corresponding antibody molecules.

(r)   Tolerance is an active process that exhibits a high degree of specificity.

(s)   The typical antibody response to a single antigen is heterogeneous.

(t)   The polypeptide called secretory component, which mediates the transport of IgA from blood to epithelial surfaces, is a T-cell lymphokine.

(u)   Activation of the third component of complement, C3, occurs only when an antigen interacts with specific antibody of a class that can fix complement.

(v)   Delayed hypersensitivity lesions contain cellular infiltrates composed of lymphocytes and macrophages.

(w)   In the presence of antigen a purified population of T and B cells may cooperate *in vitro* to produce a B-cell immune response.

(x)   Genes that code for antibody combining-site specificities, and thereby control the immune response to specific antigens, are linked to MHC genes.

(y)   Killer cells may derive from either T-cell or macrophage lineages.

(z)   In mice, T cells that mediate delayed hypersensitivity (T_D cells) may undergo antigen-driven maturation to killer T (T_C) cells.

1-2   Supply the missing word or words in each of the following statements.

(a)   When haptens are attached to a larger _____ molecule, they become immunogenic.

(b)   The major class of antibody synthesized in a _____ immune response is IgG.

(c)   _____ is the process whereby a lymphocyte undergoes an antigen-driven differentiation.

(d)   _____ are the terminal effector cells of B-cell differentiation.

(e)   The process whereby antigens and receptors coalesce into a single aggregate at one pole of the lymphocyte is termed _____.

(f)   T cells mediate _____ immunity.

(g)   The B-cell response usually requires the cooperation of _____, _____, and _____.

(h)   T-cell-independent antigens evoke the synthesis of antibody of the _____ class.

(i)   Genes that regulate the antibody response to many antigens and are linked to the major histocompatibility genes of the mouse are called _____ genes.

(j)   Immunological _____ is the process that normally prevents lymphocytes from reacting with self-antigens.

(k)   The clonal selection theory contends that lymphocytes commit themselves to the synthesis of one type of antibody molecule prior to exposure to _____, but that _____ triggers the final stage of differentiation, called blast transformation.

(l)   Accessory cells involved in antigen processing include _____ and _____.

(m)   _____ are the blood counterparts of tissue mast cells.

(n)   _____ immunity is protective against extracellular bacterial infections.

(o)   The effector functions of an immunoglobulin are defined by the class of its _____ chains.

(p)   The _____ subcomponent of complement binds to the Fc portion of IgG in IgG–antigen complexes.

(q)   C8 and C9 effect the _____ function of the complement pathway.

(r)   The _____ of anti-hapten antibodies increases late in an immune response, after peak titers are reached.

(s)   Administration of Dnp-d (glu, lys) to mice will lead to Dnp tolerance caused by B lymphocyte _____.

(t)   The presence of specific immunoglobulin responses to antigen in the animal kingdom is thought to be limited to _____.

(u)   Mast cells possess surface receptors for _____ antibodies.

(v)   In the two-signal model of T-cell-dependent B-cell triggering, antigen binds to B-cell surface _____, and T cells or accessory cells give a second signal to B-cell _____ receptors.

(w) _____ immunoglobulins are transported across the placenta.

1-3   The apparent range of different specificities in the immune system is enormous. The average concentration of serum antibody is about 15 mg/ml. Assume a molecular weight of 160,000 daltons for the antibody molecule, and assume that the average human has 5 liters of serum.

(a)   How many antibody molecules are present in each milliliter of serum? In the average human?

(b)   Assume that there are 1,000,000 different types of antibody molecules and that each is represented equally in the population. How many molecules of each type are present in 1 ml of serum?

1-4   When white blood cells from Person X are mixed with white blood cells of Person Y, the X lymphocytes will proliferate and some of them will become T_C cells, able to lyse lymphocytes from Person Y. The generation of these specific killer T cells will be most enhanced if the histocompatibility genes of X and Y differ (1) at the I locus, (2) at the D and K loci, (3) at both I and D/K loci, or (4) at neither locus.

(a)   Which of the above four choices is the best answer?

(b)   Describe which kinds of cells from Person X specifically recognize Person Y's MHC antigens and trigger the production of specific T_C cells.

(c)   Describe lineage relationships, cellular interactions, MHC products recognized, and effector cell functions in all of Person X's reactions to Person Y's cells.

1-5   *E. coli* cells grown in minimal medium, or in medium containing less than 10^{-5} *M* methyl-β-D-thiogalactoside (TMG), produce no β-galactosidase. Transferred to medium containing 10^{-4} *M* TMG, the bacteria quickly start to produce the enzyme. After a brief interval that corresponds to only a fraction of a division cycle at this concentration of TMG, a subculture returned to medium containing 8×10^{-6} *M* TMG continues for a prolonged period to synthesize the enzyme. A variety of compounds related to TMG induce the same enzyme. What points of similarity and of difference do you discern between this system and the vertebrate immune system?

1-6   (a)   For many years the function of the thymus was unknown. Although the gland was found to consist of a mass of rapidly dividing lymphocytes within an epithelial meshwork, no antibody synthesis could be detected in the thymus, nor did it display any histological changes upon antigenic challenge. Surgical removal of the thymus (thymectomy) had no effect on the immune capabilities of adult animals. However, in 1960 an

Australian scientist, J. F. A. P. Miller, thymectomized some mice within 16 hours of birth. Within three months, most of these mice began to lose weight, suffer from chronic diarrhea, and become "runted" or "wasted" in appearance, and eventually all died. A strictly germ-free environment, however, prevented this wasting. What inferences can you draw about the nature of the wasting disease? What other experiments could you do to investigate your inferences further?

(b)   Table 1–4 gives data showing the survival of foreign skin grafts on normal and thymectomized mice. Sham-thymectomized mice are controls that were subjected to the same surgical procedures as thymectomized mice except that their thymuses were not removed. *Allogeneic grafts* are those exchanged between individuals that are not genetically identical; *syngeneic grafts* are those exchanged between genetically identical individuals.

Compare the median survival time of allogeneic skin grafts on normal mice and on neonatally thymectomized mice. What seems to be the effect of neonatal thymectomy? What other immunologic functions would you expect to be impaired in neonatally thymectomized mice?

(c)   Compare groups A, B, and E in Table 1–4. What do you infer from these data about the timing of the role of the thymus in the development of cellular immunity? Now consider Figure 1–50, which shows cumulative percent mortality as a function of age at thymectomy for several strains of mice. Suggest explanations both for the shape

Table 1–4
Survival of allogeneic skin grafts in mice thymectomized in the neonatal period (Problem 1–6)

Group	Age at operation	Strain of mice	Skin graft donor strain	Number of grafts	Number of grafts accepted	Median Survival time of graft (days)
A Thymectomized	1–16 hours	C3H	Ak	7	5	45–101[a]
		Ak	C3H	6	4	41–90[a]
		(Ak × T6)F$_1$	C3H	8	8	50–118[a]
B Thymectomized	5 days	C3H	Ak	5	0	11 ± 0.7
C Thymectomized and thymus-grafted 3 weeks later	5 hours	C3H	Ak	5	0	11–15
D Sham-thymectomized	1–16 hours	C3H	Ak	6	0	11 ± 0.6
		Ak	C3H	3	0	10 ± 0.8
E Intact		C3H	Ak	61	0	11 ± 0.6
		Ak	C3H	45	0	10 ± 0.9
		(Ak × T6)F$_1$	C3H	10	0	11 ± 0.1

[a]These figures apply only to mice that accepted the foreign transplant.
[From J. F. A. P. Miller, *Lancet* **2**, 749 (1961).]

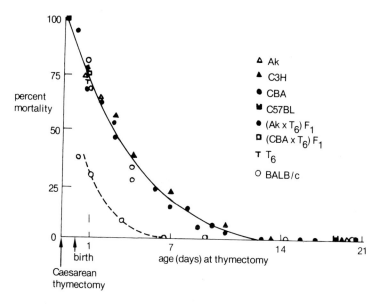

Figure 1–50 Mortality from wasting disease in thymectomized mice of several different strains (Problem 1–6). [From J. F. A. P. Miller, A. H. E. Marshall, and R. G. White, *Adv. Immunol.* **2**, 111 (1962).]

of the curve and for the difference between BALB/c mice and the other strains. Suppose Miller had used BALB/c mice originally; what might he have thought?

1–7   In related experiments, Miller tested the effect of neonatal thymectomy on humoral antibody formation. Rather than measure directly the amount of specific antibody produced in response to antigenic challenge, he chose to measure the number of spleen lymphocytes that could be induced to secrete antibody specific for sheep red blood cells (SRBC) injected into the mice. To quantitate these spleen cells, he used the so-called Jerne plaque assay, described in the Appendix to Chapter 2 (Essential Concept A2–3B3).

   After immunizing the mice with SRBC, Miller tested spleen cells from sham-thymectomized mice, from neonatally thymectomized mice, and from neonatally thymectomized mice that subsequently were reconstituted with syngeneic thymic or thoracic duct lymphocytes, to determine the ability of these cells to substitute for the ablated thymus cells.

(a)   Figure 1–51 shows the results of this experiment. What do you conclude about antibody production in mice subjected to these procedures? What do Curves 1, 2, and 3 in Figure 1–51 indicate? Given that thymic lymphocytes do not synthesize antibody, how may one explain the experimental data?

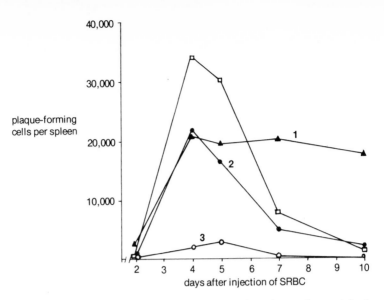

Figure 1–51 Plaque-forming cells (PFC) produced in the spleens of neonatally thymectomized CBA mice at various times after injection of sheep red blood cells (SRBC) and
syngeneic thymus or thoracic duct cells (Problem 1–7). □-□, sham-operated controls given
SRBC only; o-o, neonatally thymectomized mice given SRBC only; ●-● neonatally
thymectomized mice given 10 million CBA thymus cells and SRBC; ▲-▲, neonatally
thymectomized mice given 10 million thoracic duct cells and SRBC. [From J. F. A. P. Miller
and G. F. Mitchell, *J. Exp. Med.* **128,** 801 (1968). © 1968 by The Rockefeller University
Press.]

Table 1–5

Distribution of labeled cells following infusion of ³H-nucleosides into the thymus
(Problem 1–8)

| Organ and tissue | Percentage thymus-derived cells[a] | | | |
| | Adult | | Newborn | |
	Adenosine label	Thymidine label	Adenosine label	Thymidine label
Thymus	100	100	100	100
Splenic white pulp	2.9	0.024	9	18
Splenic red pulp	0	—	0	—
Mesenteric node, whole	0.51	—	19	12
Mesenteric node, diffuse cortex	2.7	0.12	—	—
Cervical node, whole	0.44	—	—	—
Cervical node, diffuse cortex	1.6	—	—	—
Bone marrow	0.017	—	0	—
Intestinal mucosa	0	—	0	—

[a]Measured by autoradiograph of tissue slices (see Essential Concept A2–3C2) 24 hours
after administration of labeled nucleoside; normalized to 100% for whole thymus.
(—) indicates not measured.
[From I. L. Weissman, *J. Exp. Med.* **126,** 291 (1967). © 1967 by The Rockefeller
University Press.]

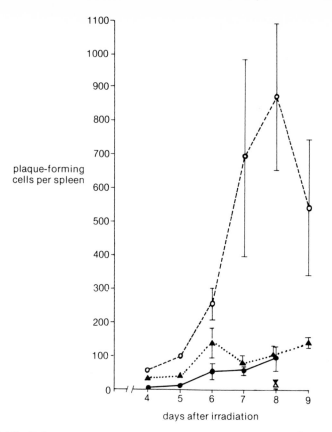

Figure 1–52 PFC produced in the spleens of heavily irradiated CBA mice injected, after irradiation, with SRBC alone (△), SRBC and 1 million syngeneic thoracic duct cells (●—●), SRBC and 10 million syngeneic bone marrow cells (▲•••▲), or SRBC and a mixed inoculum of 1 million syngeneic thoracic duct cells and 10 million syngeneic bone-marrow cells (o- - -o) (Problem 1–7). Vertical bars indicate the magnitudes of the standard errors. [From J. F. A. P. Miller and G. F. Mitchell, *J. Exp. Med.* **128,** 801 (1968). © 1968 by The Rockefeller University Press.]

(b) Figure 1–52 illustrates the response to SRBC of heavily x-irradiated mice, some of which were reconstituted with various lymphoid cells. Heavy x-irradiation kills a high proportion of lymphoid cells of all classes. What is the basic difference between the experimental protocol here and the protocol in Part (a) of this problem? What do you infer from the cell types required for an antibody response? Does this modify your conclusions from Part (a)?

1–8 A cellular immunologist wished to trace the fate of thymocytes in adult and newborn mice. He labeled thymus cells in living animals by infusing ^{3}H-adenosine or ^{3}H-thymidine into the thymus with a microneedle, and then 24 hours later measured the percent of thymus cell migrants among the cells of various tissues (Table 1–5).

(a) What can you conclude about the homing specificity of thymus cell migrants from the data in Table 1–5?

(b)   How might you explain the differences between the results of adenosine and thymidine labeling in adults?

(c)   Compare the results obtained with adults and newborns, and propose an hypothesis to explain any differences you observe.

1–9   Research with hapten–carrier conjugates has revealed a curious phenomenon termed the "carrier effect." An animal immunized with Hapten A attached to Carrier B and then challenged with the same A–B conjugate will produce copious anti-hapten (and anti-carrier) antibody. However, if the same animal is challenged instead with Hapten A attached to a different carrier, C, it will produce little anti-hapten antibody in the secondary response. Figure 1–53 shows an experiment using 2,4-dinitrophenol (Dnp) as a hapten and ovalbumin (OVA) and bovine gamma globulin (BBG) as carriers. (CFA designates complete Freund's adjuvant.

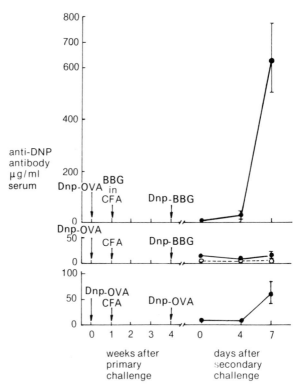

Figure 1–53   A study of the carrier effect in inbred guinea pigs (Problem 1–9). Primary immunization with Dnp-OVA was performed at week 0. One week later supplemental immunization with either 50 μg of **BBG** emulsified in CFA or with a saline-CFA emulsion was carried out. Four weeks after primary immunization, the animals were challenged with either Dnp-**BBG** or Dnp-OVA. Serum anti-Dnp antibody concentrations just prior to challenge and on days 4 and 7 are illustrated. In the middle panel, the results indicated by o- - -o were observed in animals that were passively immunized with anti-BBG serum 24 hours before administration of Dnp-**BBG**. [From D. Katz, W. Paul, E. Goidl, and B. Benacerraf, *J. Exp. Med.* **132**, 261 (1970). © by the Rockefeller University Press.]

Adjuvants usually are oily substances which, when mixed and injected with antigen, serve both as a tissue depot that slowly releases the antigen and also as a lymphoid system activator, which nonspecifically enhances the immune response.)

(a)   What is the significance of the experiment in the lower panel of Figure 1–53?

(b)   What is the difference between the experimental protocols in the upper and middle panels of Figure 1–53? What sorts of cell populations appear to be necessary for a secondary anti-hapten response? If one omitted the first immunization with Dnp-OVA, what sort of anti-Dnp response do you think would result?

(c)   In the experiment shown in the upper panel of Figure 1–53, the animals are actively immunized against BGG. In the experiment shown in the middle panel, the animals are passively immunized with antiserum against the heterologous carrier. What does the difference in the two results imply? What result would you expect if the animals had been passively immunized by transfer of lymphocytes from a donor that had been immunized with BGG?

1–10   Another approach toward analysis of the carrier effect uses a procedure termed *adoptive transfer* to place hapten-specific and carrier-specific lymphocytes derived from different mice together in a third mouse. The procedure employs inbred mice all of whose genes and surface antigens are identical, so that cellular transplants will not be subject to graft rejection. The recipient mice are heavily irradiated so that a high proportion of their own lymphocytes are destroyed. The irradiated mice then can be reconstituted immunologically by transfer of spleen lymphocytes from normal mice. In the experiment, lymphocytes from one mouse immunized with Dnp–OVA and lymphocytes from a second mouse immunized with BGG are transferred into the same irradiated host. Such reconstituted mice give a large secondary anti-hapten response to a Dnp–BGG conjugate. Pretreatment of the Dnp–OVA-primed lymphocytes with anti-Thy-1 antiserum and complement has no effect on the response of the reconstituted mice. However, pretreatment of the BGG-primed lymphocytes with anti-Ly-1 antiserum and complement before transfer into the irradiated host destroys the host's ability to respond to the Dnp–BGG conjugate. What do these experiments reveal about the nature of the carrier-specific cells and the hapten-specific cells in this immune response?

1–11   Histologists use the term "blast" to denote large, rapidly dividing cells whose descendants usually are further differentiated. Such cells often are seen in lymph nodes that are responding to an antigenic challenge. Specific antigens provoke the appearance of blast cells in cultures derived from specifically immunized individuals, but not in cultures from unimmunized individuals. The degree of blast transformation can be quantified by adding ^{3}H-thymidine to these cultures. Only the actively

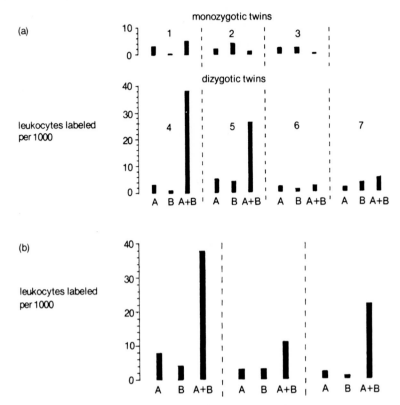

Figure 1–54   ³H-thymidine labeling of lymphocyte cultures (Problem 1–11). (a) Cultures from pairs of twins. (b) Cultures from three pairs of unrelated individuals. In each experiment, A and B are the unmixed controls; A + B is the corresponding mixture. [From B. Bain, M. R. Vas, and L. Lowenstein, *Blood* **23,** 108 (1964). Used by permission from Grune & Stratton, Inc.]

replicating blast cells take up ³H-thymidine. These radiolabeled cells can be counted by radioautography or by other methods. In one study, researchers cultured mixtures of lymphocytes from pairs of individuals. In each pair the lymphocyte donors were either monozygotic twins, dizygotic twins, or unrelated individuals. After five days, ³H-thymidine was added to each culture for a short period. The number of labeled cells in each culture was found to be as shown in Figure 1–54.

(a)   Compare the results obtained with monozygotic twins to those obtained with unrelated individuals. What does this pattern of reactivity suggest about the nature of this immune reaction?

(b)   The major histocompatibility complex in man (HLA) is polymorphic; that is, there are many allelic variants of the genes in this complex among the population. Given this property of the HLA complex, how can you explain the variability in the dizygotic twin results?

(c)   Suppose that a person had suffered acute kidney damage and needed a transplant to survive. In addition, suppose that this person had several siblings, all willing to donate a kidney. How could you decide which sibling to use as a donor?

(d)   Assume that the mixed lymphocyte reaction is determined by identity or nonidentity at a single locus, and that the products of this locus are expressed in a codominant fashion on the surfaces of cells in a heterozygote. What sort of reaction would you expect if you mixed lymphocytes from a child with lymphocytes from one of its parents? Why?

1–12   The large lymphocytes generated in a mixed lymphocyte response begin mitosis after four days in culture. If the lymphocytes in a mixed culture come from donors of different sexes, the response of each donor's lymphocytes can be assayed independently by determining the karyotypes of the mitotic cells. This technique was used to examine mixed lymphocyte reactions between parental and F_1 lymphocytes. Using inbred rats of four strains—L, DA, BN, and F—various male–female parental–F_1 combinations were tested with the results shown in Table 1–6. Remember that inbred animals are essentially homozygous at all loci.

(a)   Describe the pattern of reactivity. What do you infer from the results with regard to the rats' histocompatibility genes?

(b)   Suppose the reactions between parental and F_1 lymphocytes were examined using outbred humans as donors. How and why would the results differ from those obtained with inbred rats?

(c)   Suppose that the parental human cells were inactivated by x-irradiation or treatment with mitomycin C, a fungal antibiotic, to prevent DNA synthesis and mitosis. What result would you expect in a mixed lymphocyte reaction between inactivated parental cells and untreated

Table 1–6

Mixed lymphocyte reactions between cells from inbred parental (homozygous) rats and their F_1 (heterozygous) offspring (Problem 1–12)

Culture mixture	Sex	Number of mitoses on day:				Totals
		5	6	7	11	
L/L (♀) + DA/L (♂)	♀	1	19	38	0	58
	♂	0	1	7	0	8
L/BN (♀) + L/L (♂)	♀	0	0	0	0	0
	♂	1	9	49	2	61
F/BN (♀) + F/F (♂)	♀	0	0	0	0	0
	♂	3	24	23	4	54
L/BN (♀) + DA/L (♂)	♀	4	19	23	0	46
	♂	8	15	14	0	37

[From D. B. Wilson, W. Silvers, and P. Nowell, *J. Exp. Med.* **126**, 655 (1967). © 1967 by the Rockefeller University Press.]

cells from an F_1 individual? What results would you expect if the F_1 lymphocytes were inactivated and the parental lymphocytes were untreated?

(d)   Can you think of a situation in which measuring the response of each donor's lymphocytes independently would be important?

1–13   One technically simple way to assess the number of mature T cells in a population of lymphocytes is to test for their ability to mount a graft-versus-host response (GVHR). Mature T cells injected into an allogeneic, immunologically incompetent host (e.g., an immature newborn or a suitably irradiated adult) will react against the host. The GVHR is directed against all tissues, and within seven days can cause marked loss of body weight due to liver and gastrointestinal tract damage. In this same period of time there is a great enlargement of the spleen, termed splenomegaly, due initially to proliferation of the injected T cells that migrate to the spleen. Later, damage to host spleen cells results in inflammation, repair, and regeneration. The increase in spleen weight commonly is used to indicate the magnitude of the GVHR, which in turn provides an estimate of the proportion of mature reactive T cells among the injected lymphocytes.

Table 1–7

Stimulation of GVHR of allogeneic bone-marrow cells by thymosin *in vitro* (Problem 1–13)

Injected cells experimental groups	Number of host animals	Spleen weight (mg)/ body weight (g)	p Values[a]	Spleen index[b]
(C57BL × CBA)F₁ bone-marrow cells (syngeneic)	60	2.08 ± 0.10	—	—
CBA bone-marrow cells (allogeneic), preincubated with:				
saline	62	2.65 ± 0.10	—	1.27
100 μg thymosin	28	3.74 ± 0.36	<0.01	1.80
10 μg thymosin	21	3.99 ± 0.30	<0.01	1.92
1 μg thymosin	9	3.78 ± 0.37	<0.01	1.82
100 μg spleen extract	8	3.23 ± 0.40	0.05	1.55
10 μg spleen extract	12	2.97 ± 0.17	>0.2	1.43
1 μg spleen extract	8	2.45 ± 0.23	>0.5	1.18

[a]p value is a statistical measure of the probability that the observed difference between experimental and control values could be due to statistical fluctuations alone rather than to a real difference in the mean values. A p value of 0.05 means that the results could have happened by chance 5% of the time; this difference is considered significant. A p value of 0.01 or less is considered highly significant.

[b]Spleen index = $\dfrac{\text{allogeneic (spleen weight/body weight)}}{\text{syngeneic (spleen weight/body weight)}}$

[From A. L. Goldstein, A. Guha, M. L. Howe, and A. White, *J. Immunol.* **106**, 777 (1971).]

One research group, investigating how T-cell precursors mature in the thymus, isolated from calf thymus a humoral factor named thymosin. The group incubated CBA mouse bone-marrow cells with this factor, and then injected the cells into adult, irradiated (C57Bl × CBA) F$_1$ hosts. The magnitudes of the ensuing GVHR's are given in Table 1–7.

(a)   Why is the ratio of spleen weight to body weight used in measuring the GVHR, rather than simply the absolute spleen weight?

(b)   What does Line 1 in Table 1–7 indicate?

(c)   What seems to be the effect of thymosin? Give two hypotheses for thymosin action.

1–14   One of the most fruitful approaches in exploring the nature of killer cells activated by the immune response has been to generate cytotoxic lymphocytes *in vitro* in mixed lymphocyte cultures and then to measure the effectiveness of their cytotoxicity by the ^{51}Cr-release assay. For this assay the target cells are incubated in Na^{51}CrO$_4$, which is taken up and apparently binds nonspecifically to cytoplasmic proteins. After washing, the labeled target cells are added to a lymphocyte population. When a target cell is lysed, the labeled cytoplasmic proteins leak out into the culture fluid, so that the amount of radioactivity in the supernatant fraction after the cells have been centrifuged out is directly proportional to the degree of cell lysis.

In the experiment summarized in Figure 1–55, 60 × 10^6 CBA spleen cells were cultured with 15 × 10^6 mitomycin-C treated BALB/c cells, and ^{3}H-thymidine incorporation was monitored every 12 hours. Aliquots of cells from the mixed lymphocyte cultures were added to ^{51}Cr-labeled target cells that carry the same H-2 antigens as BALB/c cells, at a lymphocyte:target-cell ratio of 100:1.

(a)   What does the ^{3}H-thymidine incorporation measure? What does the ^{51}Cr-release measure?

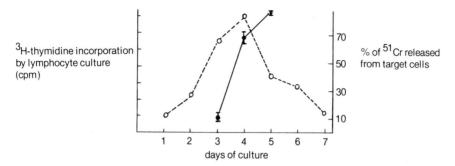

Figure 1–55 Comparison of the proliferative response and the generation of cytotoxic lymphocytes *in vitro* (Problem 1–14). ○------○, ^{3}H-thymidine uptake; ●——●, ^{51}Cr release. [From H. Wagner, *J. Immunol.* **109**, 633 (1972).]

(b)   What do the results in Figure 1–55 suggest about the order of events in differentiation of cytotoxic cells?

(c)   Notice that 100 lymphocytes were added for each target cell. Why do you think such a high ratio is needed to get a large degree of cytotoxicity?

1–15   Many investigators have tried to determine how cytotoxic lymphocytes kill target cells. In one experiment, lymphocytes from inbred Wistar rats were incubated on a monolayer of lethally irradiated mouse fibroblasts. After six days, the lymphocytes were removed and added to a new monolayer consisting of ^{51}Cr-labeled fibroblasts and unlabeled fibroblasts intermixed. The types of fibroblasts used and the results of these experiments are given in Table 1–8.

(a)   What are the specific targets of the sensitized rat lymphocytes?

(b)   Why were experiments in Line (b) of Table 1–8 carried out?

(c)   What apparently happens in the experiment summarized in Line (c) of Table 1–8? What does this result suggest about the mechanism of cytotoxicity?

Table 1–8
Cytotoxic tests (Problem 1–15)

| Sensitizing fibroblasts | Mixed fibroblast target monolayer | | % ^{51}Cr release |
	^{51}Cr-labeled	unlabeled	
(a) mouse	mouse	mouse	31 ± 0.3
(b) mouse	Lewis rat	Lewis rat	10 ± 0.6 p < 0.01[a]
(c) mouse	Lewis rat	mouse	21 ± 0.3

[a]See footnote [a] in Table 1–7.
[From I. R. Cohen and M. Feldman, *Cell. Immunol.* **1**, 527 (1971).]

1–16   Simply injecting large amounts of antigen into an animal does not always insure a strong immune response. Normal adult rabbits were injected subcutaneously with one gram of BSA six times a week for six weeks. At various times, individual rabbits were sacrificed, their spleens removed, and the number of indirect plaque-forming cells (cells that secreted either IgM or IgG specific for BSA) was measured. Figure 1–56 shows the results.

(a)   Compare the primary and secondary responses to 20 mg of BSA with the response to 1 g of BSA given 6 days per week for 6 weeks. What seems to have happened?

(b)   Some of the rabbits unresponsive to BSA were immunized with 5 mg of human gamma globulin (HGG) on Day 30, and they responded normally to the HGG. Why is this an important control and what does it prove?

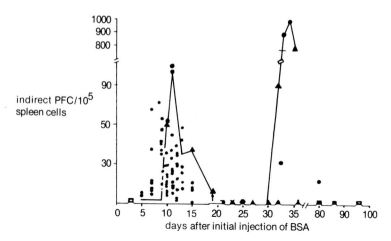

Figure 1–56 Quantitation of indirect plaque-forming cells (PFC) following injection of bovine serum albumin (BSA) (Problem 1–16). Rabbits were given daily subcutaneous injections of 1 g BSA for 6 weeks. Each solid circle represents the number of PFC directed against BSA from spleen cells of an individual rabbit so treated. The solid line represents the response of a rabbit given a single intravenous injection of 20 mg of soluble BSA on Day 0 and again on Day 30. [From J. M. Chiller, C. G. Romball, and W. O. Weigle, *Cell. Immunol.* **8**, 29 (1973).]

(c)   Some newborn rabbits were injected subcutaneously with 150 mg and 250 mg of soluble BSA on the first and third days of their life, respectively. Absolutely no plaque-forming cells were detected for over a month after the last injection. What do you conclude about neonatal animals? (Immunization with 0.5 mg BSA normally elicits a vigorous immune response in neonatal rabbits.)

1–17   An interesting experiment was done to investigate the question of whether tolerance, or immunological unresponsiveness, is an active or a passive state. Normal adult mice were thymectomized, irradiated, and then reconstituted with syngeneic bone-marrow cells so that they lacked T cells. Thirty days later, all the mice were given 3×10^7 normal thymocytes intravenously. Group 1 also received 8×10^7 spleen cells from mice immunized with sheep red blood cells (SRBC), while Group 3 received spleen cells from mice tolerant to SRBCs. Group 2 mice received only the thymocytes. All the mice then were challenged with SRBC, and at an appropriate time thereafter their anti-SRBC antibody titers were measured by hemagglutination (Essential Concept A2–3A). Figure 1–57a indicates total antibody titers; Figure 1–57b shows the titers of mercaptoethanol-resistant antibody (IgM activity is destroyed by reducing agents such as mercaptoethanol; hence the level of resistant antibody corresponds roughly to that of antibody of the IgG class.)
(a)   Compare the responses of Groups 1 and 2 in Figure 1–57. Does the difference seem reasonable?

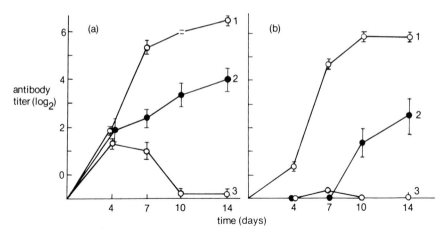

Figure 1–57 The anti-SRBC response of thymus-deprived mice given normal thymo-cytes and spleen cells from three different donors (Problem 1–17). Groups 1, 2, and 3 were described in the text. (a) Total antibody.(b) Mercaptoethanol-resistant antibody. [From R. Gershon and K. Kondo, *Immunology* **21**, 903 (1971).]

(b)   Now compare Groups 2 and 3 in Figure 1–57. What response would you expect if normal thymocytes alone were injected? If the tolerant spleen cells were injected alone? What do you conclude about the interaction between the two cell populations? Can you propose a mechanism to explain this effect? Suggest an experiment to test your proposed mechanism.

1–18   Pregnancy presents the immune system with a special challenge. The immune system normally recognizes and reacts against foreign antigens, yet during pregnancy the mother's immune system must *not* react against the foreign paternal antigens expressed on fetal cells. The following experiments illustrate one immunologic control mechanism that may help to protect the fetus.

From five pregnant women who had already borne several children, lymphocytes were taken during the third trimester of pregnancy and then again two months *postpartum* (after delivery). Each batch of cells was incubated with a sample of the father's lymphocytes, which had been inactivated by mitomycin C. After 24–48 hours, the release of macrophage migration inhibition factor (MIF) was measured. MIF release after only 24–48 hours in culture is an indication that the maternal lymphocytes had previously been sensitized to the paternal antigens. Either 15% autologous plasma (from the same mother) or 15% homolo-gous plasma (from another pregnant but unrelated woman) was included in each mixed lymphocyte culture. (Plasma is the supernatant fluid that remains when blood is centrifuged to remove all cells.) The results are shown in Figure 1–58.

(a)   Consider the cultures incubated with homologous plasma (solid circles). How do you interpret these results? Were the maternal cells sensitized to paternal antigens? If so, how might they have become sensitized?

(b)   Which paternal cell-surface antigens most probably are being recognized by the maternal lymphocytes?

(c)   Consider the cultures to which autologous plasma was added (open circles). Was MIF released by the maternal cells in these cultures? Suggest an explanation for the results.

(d)   When the autologous plasma was fractionated on a Sephadex G-200 column, the active fraction was found to elute with IgG. How may further proof be obtained that the active factor is an immunoglobulin?

(e)   The results in Figure 1–58 demonstrate that maternal lymphocytes can recognize and respond *in vitro* to paternal antigens, and yet the fetal "allograft," which expresses these antigens, is not rejected. Using all the information presented, propose as complete a model as you can for the control mechanism involved. What is the active factor that suppresses the normal response? Where did it come from? Is it immunologically specific? Does it exert its effect on afferent (antigen processing and presentation), central (T and B lymphocyte recognition and response), or efferent (effector cell or product interaction with antigen) arms of the immune response? Is the mother "tolerant" to paternal antigens?

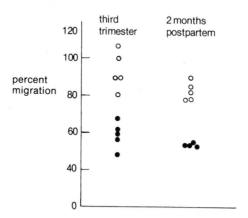

Figure 1–58 Migration of macrophages in supernatant fluid from mixed lymphocyte cultures (Problem 1–18). Percentages were determined by comparison to migration in control supernatant fluid derived from cultures of maternal lymphocytes alone. Open circles (○) indicate values obtained with mother:father cultures in autologous plasma. Solid circles (●) indicate values obtained with the same cultures in homologous plasma. [From H. Pence, W. Petty, and R. Rocklin, *J. Immunol.* **114,** 525 (1975).]

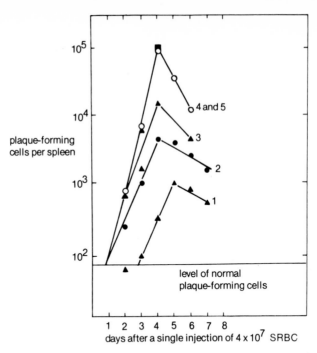

Figure 1–59 Primary responses of mice to a single intravenous injection of 4×10^7 SRBC (Problem 1–19). In each of four experiments, 0.1 ml of anti- SRBC antibody was given intravenously: 1 hour before SRBC (Curve 1); 4 hours after SRBC (Curve 2); 1 day after SRBC (Curve 3); or 2 days after SRBC (Curve 4). As a control, no antibody was given (Curve 5). [From C. Henry and N. Jerne, *J. Exp. Med.* **128**, 133 (1968). © 1968 by the Rockefeller University Press.]

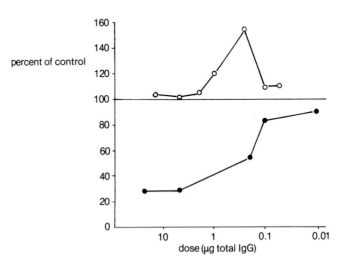

Figure 1–60 Immune response to a fixed dose of antigen in the presence of varying concentrations of IgG_1 and IgG_2 antibodies (Problem 1–19). The control (no antibody) level of plaque-forming cells is represented as 100% on the ordinate, and the levels in IgG_1-treated (solid circles) and IgG_2-treated (open circles) cultures are expressed as percent of the control value. [From J. Gordon and R. A. Murgita, *Cell. Immunol.* **15**, 392 (1975).]

1-19   The two preceding problems underscore the interdependence of the humoral and cellular components of the immune system. A facet of this interaction is the ability of antibody itself to influence the humoral response. One research group passively immunized AKR mice with anti-SRBC IgG just prior to, or shortly after, a single injection of SRBC. Figure 1–59 gives the numbers of plaque-forming spleen cells at various times after immunization with SRBC, determined by the Jerne plaque assay (Essential Concept A2–3B).

(a)   What do you conclude from the data shown?

(b)   What simple explanation can you suggest for this effect?

(c)   A second research group extended these experiments to an *in vitro* system in which they cultured spleen cells with SRBC and anti-SRBC IgG. In addition, these researchers fractionated the anti-SRBC IgG into IgG_1 and IgG_2 subclasses, and added anti-SRBC antibody of each subclass separately to spleen cell cultures. The observed production of plaque-forming cells is plotted against antibody concentration in Figure 1–60. How do you interpret these results?

(d)   The researchers then added anti-SRBC antibodies to some cultures containing chicken red blood cells (CRBC) instead of SRBC. Figure 1–61 shows the anti-CRBC responses they obtained. What is the significance of this experiment?

(e)   Are the results in Part (c) consistent with your answer to Part (b)? If not, how would you modify your answer to Part (b)?

(f)   Gordon and Murgita also tested $F(ab')_2$ fragments of the IgG antibodies from each subclass, but these fragments had no significant effect, either positive or negative. Remember that $F(ab')_2$ fragments

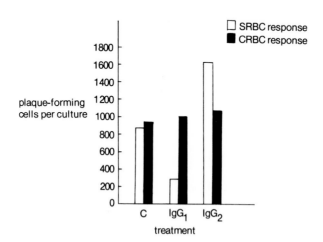

Figure 1–61   The plaque-forming cell response to sheep red blood cells (SRBC) or chicken red blood cells (CRBC) in the presence of IgG_1 or IgG_2 anti-SRBC antibodies (approximately 0.5 μg) (Problem 1–19). C indicates a control in which no antibodies were added. [From J. Gordon and R. A. Murgita, *Cell. Immunol.* **15,** 392 (1975).]

lack much of the heavy-chain constant regions, but they still contain both antigen binding sites, and they specifically bind antigen almost as well as complete immunoglobulin molecules. How does this observation bear on your explanation of the results in Figure 1–61?

1–20   The control mechanisms demonstrated in the preceding problems all share the characteristic of immunological specificity. The phenomenon of antigenic competition provides an interesting counterpoint. How do animals respond when challenged with two different antigens, one after another? In one such experiment, mice were immunized with either sheep red blood cells (SRBC) or horse red blood cells (HRBC) and then, several days later, were challenged with the other antigen. Table 1–9 shows the resulting splenic response (production of plaque-forming cells) five days after the last injection.

(a)   What is the apparent effect of these temporal sequences of immunizations?

(b)   When the mice in Group I were immunized with bovine serum albumin, HeLa cells (a human cell line), or *Brucella abortus* (a gram-negative bacterium) instead of SRBC on Day 0, the results were essentially the same. What does this observation indicate about the immunologic specificity of the effect?

(c)   Several hypotheses have been advanced to explain this effect. One possibility is that lymphocytes specific for the two antigens compete *in vivo* for space, for some limiting nutrient, or for some helper-cell population (T cells or accessory cells such as macrophages). Prior exposure to one antigen gives the corresponding lymphocytes a competitive advantage and hence reduces the response to the second antigen. Alternatively, this phenomenon could reflect a positive control mechanism. Specifically stimulated lymphocytes could inhibit the initiation of new responses, via nonspecific soluble factors or other means. Discuss the critical variables which must be considered in the design of experiments which discriminate between these two alternatives.

Table 1–9

Antigen competition between sheep red blood cells (SRBC) and horse red blood cells (HRBC) (Problem 1–20)

	ASSAY		ASSAY (Day 8)	
Group	Immunizing antigen and time of administration		Test antigen	PFC/10^6 spleen cells
I	Antigen 1 (Day 0)	Antigen 2 (Day 3)		
	—	HRBC	HRBC	205 ± 45
	SRBC	HRBC	HRBC	13 ± 5
II	—	SRBC	SRBC	626 ± 58
	HRBC	SRBC	SRBC	78 ± 15

[From G. Möller and O. Sjoberg, *Cell. Immunol.* **1**, 110 (1970).]

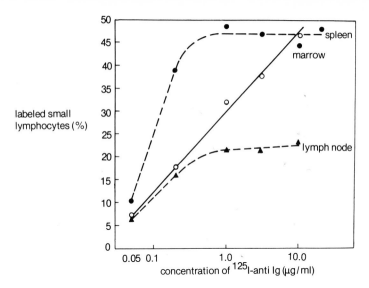

Figure 1–62 The incidence of labeled small lymphocytes in suspensions of cells from lymphoid tissues of CBA mice following exposure to rabbit ^{125}I-anti-mouse globulin at various concentrations (Problem 1–21). [From D. G. Osmond and G. J. V. Nossal, *Cell. Immunol.* **13**, 117 (1974).]

1–21 The preceding problems present several unusual situations in which an organism fails to respond to a set of antigenic determinants. How does the immune system normally become tolerant to its own self-antigens while retaining the ability to respond to nonself-antigens? An Australian scientist and his colleagues investigated this process. They began by looking at the surface immunoglobulin (sIg) on bone-marrow (BM) and peripheral lymphocytes of mice. To mouse lymphocyte suspensions they added increasing concentrations of ^{125}I-antiglobulin (^{125}I-labeled rabbit antibodies specific for mouse immunoglobulin), and recorded the percentages of radiolabeled cells (sIg$^+$) in each population, as shown in Figure 1–62. In this assay, there is an inverse linear relationship between the amount (or density) of sIg on a cell and the minimum concentration of ^{125}I-antiglobulin that labels the cell: the greater the amount of sIg on a cell, the lower the concentration of ^{125}I-antiglobulin required to label it. Consider the data on lymph node and spleen cells in Figure 1–62.

(a) Is there a variation in the amount of sIg per cell among sIg$^+$ spleen and lymph-node cells?

(b) Can you deduce the approximate percentage of B cells in each population?

(c) Compare these populations with bone-marrow cells. Do these data provide a reliable estimate of the number of BM sIg$^+$ cells?

(d) Is the variation in the amount of sIg per sIg$^+$ cell comparable for bone-marrow cells and the other two cell populations? (*Note:* At antiserum concentrations greater than 10 μg/ml, nonspecific binding

becomes significant and consequently limits the assay.)
(e)   What do these data suggest to you about the maturation of lymphocytes in the bone marrow?

1–22 (a)   The Australian researchers next studied the maturation of bone-marrow cells by *in vivo* labeling with ^{3}H-thymidine. They found that one hour after intraperitoneal injection of ^{3}H-thymidine, large bone-marrow lymphocytes (diameter > 8 μ) had been labeled but not small lymphocytes (diameter < 8 μ). When these same cells were treated with ^{131}I-antiglobulin, only the small lymphocytes were labeled. Rarely was a doubly labeled cell detected. What can you infer about the biochemical events that occurred in the large and small lymphocytes?
(b)   Some mice were given ^{3}H-thymidine at eight-hour intervals over a four-day period. Analyses of their bone marrow cells gave the following results: first, the proportion (and absolute number) of small lymphocytes labeled with a 1 μg/ml concentration of ^{131}I-antiglobulin remained approximately constant; second, the percentage of small lymphocytes labeled with ^{3}H-thymidine increased monotonically, 83% of the cells having been labeled after 84 hours; third, the proportion of doubly labeled cells also increased monotonically, but only after a considerable time lag, as shown in Table 1–10.

What does the increase in the number of small lymphocytes labeled by ^{3}H-thymidine suggest?
(c)   What does the time lag before the appearance of doubly labeled cells suggest?
(d)   New cells apparently are being produced, yet the proportion and absolute number of bone-marrow sIg$^+$ cells remain roughly constant. How may this constant pool size be maintained?

Table 1–10
Percentages of bone-marrow small lymphocytes labeled after administration of ^{3}H-thymidine *in vivo* and exposure to ^{131}I-antiglobulin *in vitro* (Problem 1–22)

| Duration of ^{3}H-thymidine labeling (hr) | Double label experiments[a], using ^{131}I antiglobulin concentrations of: | | | | | |
| | 1.0 μg/ml | | | 0.2 μg/ml | | |
	^{3}H	^{131}I	^{131}I + ^{3}H	^{3}H	^{131}I	^{131}I + ^{3}H
12	17.5	31.8	0			
26	41.7	24.0	0.5	44.2	17.2	0
33	51.7	35.1	1.2	51.8	20.8	0
50	64.8	27.9	6.6	63.5	16.6	1.8
57	71.8	20.3	11.5	68.5	17.5	3.7
74	77.6	15.9	17.8	70.4	11.3	5.0
83	82.6	10.3	16.4			

[a]Numbers indicate percentages of cells singly labeled with ^{3}H, singly labeled with ^{131}I, and doubly labeled with ^{131}I and ^{3}H as indicated by column headings.
[From D. G. Osmond and G. J. V. Nossal, *Cell. Immunol.* **13**, 132 (1974).]

(e)   After 84 hours of continuous labeling, only 5% of the small lymphocytes in the periphery (blood, lymph nodes, and spleen) were labeled. What additional facts do you need to compare the number of labeled cells that migrate to the periphery with the number of new cells generated in this period?

1–23   The same investigators carried out several experiments to test the immunologic capabilities of bone-marrow cells. They injected marrow or spleen cells into irradiated syngeneic hosts after culture *in vitro* for up to three days before adoptive transfer. They then challenged the recipient animals with 5 μg of Dnp conjugated to polymerized *Salmonella* flagellin (Dnp–POL). Nine days later they determined the numbers of anti-Dnp plaque-forming cells in the host spleens. Table 1–11 summarizes several experiments with this system. Notice that in Experiment III varying concentrations of Dnp conjugated to horse γ globulin (Dnp–HGG) were added during the *in vitro* incubation period.
(a)   What effect does *in vitro* incubation have on the spleen cell response? How may this result be explained?
(b)   How do the marrow cells respond to culture? How may you explain this result? What do the kinetics of this effect suggest?
(c)   Now consider Experiment III in Table 1–11. What may be the relevance of the data?
(d)   What do you think may have happened to the 800 potential plaque-forming cells whose development was inhibited by 0.4 μg Dnp–HGG in Experiment III? Do your answers to Problems 1–21 or 1–22 provide a possible explanation?

Table 1–11
Adoptive transfer experiments with bone-marrow and spleen cells (Problem 1–23)

Cell source	Number of cells	Hours incubated *in vitro*	Antigen concentration added *in vitro*	Anti-Dnp plaque-forming cells on Day 9
I spleen	10^7	0	—	1600
		3	—	1400
		24	—	900
		72	—	400
II bone marrow	2×10^7	0	—	400
		3	—	400
		24	—	400
		48	—	700
		72	—	1200
III bone marrow	2×10^7	72	—	1200
		72	0.004 μg/ml Dnp–HGG	900
		72	0.04 μg/ml Dnp–HGG	650
		72	0.4 μg/ml Dnp–HGG	400
		72	4.0 μg/ml Dnp–HGG	250

[Data adapted from G. J. V. Nossal and B. Pike, *J. Exp. Med.* **141,** 904 (1975). © 1975 by the Rockefeller University Press.]

(e)   How could you determine whether the nonresponsiveness is due to a suppressor cell population? Assuming that there is no suppressor cell population, what experimental results would you expect?

1-24   There are two general mechanisms by which tolerance may be established in the developing organism. Potentially reactive cells could be killed or irreversibly paralyzed, or they could be reversibly suppressed. The latter mechanism would require the constant presence of a suppressive factor, either humoral or cellular. A group of Israeli researchers interested in this problem incubated thymocytes from a Lewis rat with the thymic reticulum (thymic epithelial tissue) from the same rat *in vitro*. They then measured the ability of these lymphocytes to mount a graft-versus-host response (GVHR) in syngeneic animals, after varying intervals in culture. They injected the treated lymphocytes into a rat's right footpad and untreated control lymphocytes into the left footpad. After several days, they compared the number of cells in the lymph node that drains the right foot with the number of cells in the corresponding left lymph node to determine the magnitude of the GVHR. They also measured the cytotoxic potential of the lymphocytes in the right lymph node against syngeneic or allogeneic fibroblasts, with the results shown in Table 1-12.

(a)   Should thymocytes generate a GVHR in syngeneic recipients, or, specifically, lyse syngeneic target cells? What do these data show?

(b)   Outline the sequence of events that must occur to develop a GVHR. Which of these events occur *in vitro*, and which occur *in vivo* in this experiment? Does this suggest something about one mechanism of tolerance?

(c)   What is the minimum incubation time *in vitro* necessary to develop a strong response? How does this interval compare with the average

Table 1-12
Kinetics of autosensitization of Lewis thymus lymphocyte cells against Lewis fibroblasts (Problem 1-24)

| | POPLITEAL LYMPH NODE ASSAY | | |
| Sensitization time *in vitro* (hr) | Average cells per right lymph node[a] | Lysis of target fibroblasts[b] | |
		Lewis	BALB/c
0	3×10^6	11.9 ± 1.2	10.9 ± 0.4
2	3×10^6	9.1 ± 0.7	10.4 ± 0.6
6	8×10^6	17.0 ± 1.5	8.8 ± 1.7
24	12×10^6	21.6 ± 0.6	10.5 ± 2.0

[a]The control left lymph nodes contained an average of 2×10^6 cells per node.
[b]$5 \times 10_6$ lymphocytes from the right lymph nodes of each group were incubated with BALB/c or syngeneic Lewis mouse target cells for 65 hours. The lysis of Lewis fibroblasts was significantly greater than that of the BALB/c controls at 6 and 24 hours ($p < 0.01$).
[From I. R. Cohen and H. Wekerie, *J. Exp. Med.* **137,** 224 (1973). © 1973 by the Rockefeller University Press.]

generation time of lymphocytes, which is 10–16 hours? Could you attribute the appearance of anti-self reactive cells to the differentiation of precursor cells *in vitro*? If not, how else could you explain this phenomenon?

(d)   Combine your answers in Parts (a–c) to formulate a model for the development of natural tolerance.

1–25   Immunization of Lewis rats with Brown Norway (BN)-rat fibroblasts elicits a T-cell response as well as production of antibodies specific for those antigens that distinguish Lewis rat cells from BN rat cells. Following such an immunization experiment, the specific anti-BN antibodies were isolated by adsorbing the Lewis antiserum with BN cells and then eluting the specifically bound antibodies. These Lewis anti-BN antibodies then were injected into $(L \times BN)F_1$ rats. The F_1 rats should have reacted against any antigenic determinants that are present on the Lewis anti-BN antibodies and that normally are not present on $(L \times BN)F_1$ immunoglobulins. These immunized F_1 rats and nonimmunized F_1 control rats then were injected with either L or BN parental lymphocytes, and the resulting GVHR was measured. The assay was the same as that used in the preceding problem, except that the weight of the lymph node was measured and plotted against the number of cells injected, as shown in Figure 1–63.

Can you explain the differences in GVHR generated by Lewis lymphocytes in immunized versus nonimmunized hosts? Can you explain the differences in the GVHR of Lewis and BN lymphocytes in immunized hosts? What do these results suggest about the similarity of T-cell-surface receptors?

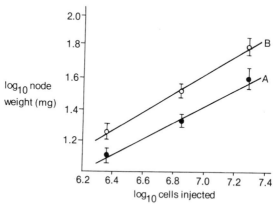

Figure 1–63   The local popliteal node GVHR produced by Lewis and BN spleen cells in L × BN) F_1 hosts (Problem 1–25). The response (the weight of the nodes in milligrams) is plotted against the number of cells injected. Curve A shows the response produced by Lewis cells in immunized F_1 hosts. Curve B shows the response of Lewis cells in nonimmunized hosts; these responses were all equivalent (p > 0.4). Curve A differs significantly from curve B (p < 0.02). The points plotted are means ± standard error of mean. [From T. McKearn, *Science* **183**, 94 (1974). Copyright 1974 by the American Association for the Advancement of Science.]

Answers

1–1   (a)   True
(b)   True
(c)   True
(d)   False.   A hapten cannot stimulate antibody production by itself, but it can combine with specific antibody.
(e)   False.   IgG is the major class of antibody synthesized in a secondary response.
(f)   False.   Genes that code for antiself-antibodies are inherited. Tolerance probably results from the elimination or paralysis of lymphocyte clones that produce antiself-antibodies.
(g)   False.   Macrophages do not belong to the lymphocyte lineage and never differentiate into T cells.
(h)   True
(i)   False. B_γ cells are committed to give rise to IgG-secreting plasma cells only.
(j)   False.   B cells that enter the spleen home to follicles on the outside of the sheath.
(k)   True
(l)   True
(m)   True
(n)   True
(o)   True
(p)   True
(q)   False.   In low responder mice, a normal spectrum of antibodies to artificial polypeptides are synthesized, but in low amounts.
(r)   True
(s)   True
(t)   False.   SC or T piece is synthesized by epithelial cells, not by T cells.
(u)   False.   C3 also can be activated by the alternate (properdin) pathway.
(v)   True
(w)   False.   Macrophages also are required for a B-cell immune response.
(x)   False.   The genes that code for antibody combining-site specificities (variable-region genes) are linked to allotypic markers, which represent antibody constant-region genes. Ir genes are linked to the major histocompatibility complex.
(y)   True
(z)   False. T_D cells (Ly-1) and T_C cells (Ly-2,3) represent separate lineages that do not interconvert.

1-2   (a)   carrier
       (b)   secondary
       (c)   Blast transformation
       (d)   Plasma cells
       (e)   capping
       (f)   cellular
       (g)   T cells, B cells, and macrophages
       (h)   IgM
       (i)   immune response (Ir)
       (j)   tolerance
       (k)   antigen; antigen
       (l)   macrophages and dendritic
              reticular cells

       (m)   Basophiles
       (n)   Humoral
       (o)   heavy
       (p)   Clq
       (q)   lytic
       (r)   affinity
       (s)   receptor blockade
       (t)   vertebrates
       (u)   IgE
       (v)   immunoglobulins;
              mitogen
       (w)   IgG

1-3   (a)   The number of antibody molecules in 1 ml of serum is

$$\frac{15 \times 10^{-3} \text{ gm/ml}}{16 \times 10^4 \text{ gm/mole}} \times \frac{6 \times 10^{23} \text{ molecules}}{\text{mole}}$$

$$\cong 6 \times 10^{16} \text{ antibody molecules/ml}$$

In an average human, the total number of antibody molecules is

$$\frac{6 \times 10^{16} \text{ molecules}}{\text{ml}} \times 5 \times 10^3 \text{ ml} = 3 \times 10^{20} \text{ antibody molecules}$$

(b)   There are $6 \times 10^{16}/10^6 = 6 \times 10^{10}$ molecules of each type of antibody in 1 ml of serum.

1-4   (a)   3

(b) T_A and T_C precursor cells specifically recognize MHC antigens. Accessory cells also may be involved, but not in the specific recognition and response to antigens. B cells are not involved.

(c) T_A cells from Person X recognize Ia antigens from Person Y and proliferate. These T_A cells stimulate the T_C cell precursors of Person X that recognize D/K antigens of Person Y, thereby causing formation of specific T_C cells from these precursors. T_D cells of Person X respond to Ia antigens of Person Y and become poised to effect delayed hypersensitivity. T_H cells of Person X recognize Ia antigens of Person Y and help the B cells of X respond to the D/K antigens of Y by proliferating, differentiating to plasma cells, and secreting antibody.

1-5   This induction of β-galactosidase synthesis seems similar to an immune response in the following ways: induction results in the elaboration of a specific protein in response to a specific stimulant; it is an expression of genetic information that is already in the system and that can be "turned on" by the specific stimulant; under the culture conditions described, induction results in a long-term modification of the cellular system—a kind of "memory." Induction of β-galactosidase differs from a typical immune response in that the protein formed is not tailored specifically to the stimulant; the same protein is formed in response to a variety of compounds related to lactose. Furthermore, the data given do not indicate that there is a memory that leads to a more rapid response upon second exposure to the stimulant. The main difference between the two systems may be the homogeneity in the response of the *E. coli* culture, compared with the great heterogeneity of an antibody response in the vertebrate immune system.

1–6   (a)   The protective effect of a sterile environment clearly indicates that the symptoms of the thymectomized mice are caused by external microbial agents rather than internal causes (spontaneous cancers, hormonal deficiencies, histological damage, and so on). This increased susceptibility to infections suggests that the immune system may have been impaired. To test this suggestion further, you could survey the immunologic status of these mice by testing for transplant rejection, delayed hypersensitivity, and antibody production, and by examining the histology of the lymphoid organs.

(b)   The extended survival of allogeneic skin grafted onto neonatally thymectomized (NTx) mice demonstrates a marked depression of cellular immunity in these mice. Therefore delayed hypersensitivity responses also should be diminished. Even if thymectomy affects only cellular immunity, antibody formation nevertheless should be reduced in accordance with the requirements for T-cell and B-cell cooperation.

(c)   By five days after birth the thymus has fulfilled a major part of its role in the development of the cellular immune system. Thus adult thymectomy has little effect. The shape of the curve can best be explained by assuming that the immune system needs a population of cells that differentiate in the thymus. Over a period of days, these cells leave that organ and migrate elsewhere to proliferate and develop further. The effect of thymectomy decreases with age as an increasing number of differentiated cells leave the thymus and become established in peripheral organs. There is no satisfactory explanation why this developmental process seems to occur several days earlier in BALB/c mice than in most other strains. If Miller had used BALB/c mice in his original experiments, he might have concluded that the thymus was less important, since the effects he saw would have been much reduced. This observation points up the possibility that even closely related organisms may vary, and illustrates the possible role of luck in the choice of an experimental system.

1–7   (a)   Spleen cells from neonatally thymectomized mice are unable to produce antibodies specific for SRBC. Intravenous injection of thymus cells, or thoracic duct lymphocytes, can restore this ability. Because thymic lymphocytes do not synthesize antibody (at least while in the thymus), there are two possible explanations: (1) the thymic lymphocytes make anti-SRBC antibody, but only after they have migrated from the thymus to peripheral organs; (2) thymus-derived cells must cooperate, in some undefined manner, with antibody-producing lymphocytes before those cells actually can make antibody. In either case, a high proportion of thoracic duct lymphocytes seem to be thymus-derived.

(b) In (a), the lymphocytes in the bone marrow, nodes, and spleen were unaffected; only the thymus-specific component of the immune system was ablated. X-irradiation ablates the entire system. The data show an impressive synergistic interaction between bone-marrow and thymus cells, but thymus cells alone are ineffective. This result excludes the first explanation offered in the answer to Part (a). Because antibody formation by bone marrow-derived lymphocytes is well known, it can be inferred that these cells produce antibody only following some sort of cooperative interaction with thymus-derived lymphocytes.

1–8   (a) Thymus cell migrants home to lymph nodes and spleen, but not to intestine. In spleen, they home to white pulp, and in lymph nodes, to diffuse cortex. White pulp and diffuse cortex are the thymus-dependent areas (domains) of spleen and lymph nodes, respectively.

(b) Thymus cells labeled *in situ* with ^{3}H-adenosine migrate rapidly to the periphery, whereas cells labeled with ^{3}H-thymidine migrate much more slowly. Because ^{3}H-adenosine is incorporated into both DNA and RNA, it probably labels all thymus cells. ^{3}H-thymidine labels only cells that are in the process of dividing and are synthesizing DNA. These cells apparently must undergo some thymic maturation prior to migration.

(c) A higher proportion of peripheral lymphocytes are thymus cell migrants in newborns as compared to adults. Moreover, most of these migrants appear to be cells that were in the process of DNA synthesis and division during the labeling period, since they are labeled approximately equally by adenosine or thymidine. The higher proportion of migrants in newborns could be explained by either a higher rate of thymus cell production and migration, or by entry of migrants into a smaller pool of preexisting cells. It is not yet known which of these explanations is correct.

1–9   (a) This is a control experiment that illustrates the normal secondary response when animals immunized with Dnp–OVA are challenged with Dnp–OVA.

(b) The middle panel of Figure 1–53 shows the absence of a secondary response when animals immunized with Dnp–OVA are challenged with Dnp–BGG. The upper panel shows the result of preimmunizing with the heterologous carrier. Preimmunization generates a population of

BGG-immune ("BGG-primed") lymphocytes. Consequently both hapten-primed cells (generated by the first immunization with Dnp–OVA) and carrier-primed cells seem necessary for a secondary anti-hapten response. Without the first Dnp–OVA immunization, there would be no Dnp-primed cells; therefore only a primary anti-Dnp response would be expected.

(c)   An animal can be immunized passively by transfer of humoral antibodies, either purified or as an unfractionated antiserum, or by transferring lymphocytes. Because passive immunization with antibody against heterologous carrier did not increase the secondary anti-hapten response (middle panel of Figure 1–53), the carrier effect appears to be a manifestation of cellular immunity. This notion could be tested by adoptively immunizing with BGG-primed lymphocytes, which would be expected to enhance the secondary anti-hapten response. The results of these experiments support the conclusion that T_H cells specific for carrier determinants somehow cooperate with B-cells specific for hapten determinants to produce the secondary anti-hapten response.

1–10   Treatment with anti-Ly-1 antiserum plus complement lyses thymus-derived lymphocytes, which express the Ly-1 antigen on their surface. Since the Dnp-primed cells are unaffected by this treatment, they must be B cells. This result is expected, because these cells actually produce the anti-hapten antibody. The destruction of BGG-primed cells by the antiserum provides additional evidence that these BGG-primed specific cells are T cells.

1–11   (a)   Cells from genetically identical monozygotic twins hardly respond to one another, whereas cells from unrelated donors undergo active lymphocyte proliferation when mixed. This observation implies that lymphocytes react only to genetically disparate cells, in a manner reminiscent of transplant rejection *in vivo*.

(b)   At any particular genetic locus, dizygotic twins will be identical or quite different. Thus some pairs will be identical at their HLA loci and hence will not react with each other, whereas other pairs will differ and hence will react.

(c)   A sibling who is identical to the prospective recipient at the HLA locus should be chosen. Identity can be assayed by culturing the recipient's lymphocytes with the cells from each sibling. The mixture that gives the lowest reactivity will identify the sibling whose HLA locus is most similar to that of the recipient. The kidney should be transplanted from the most similar donor to minimize the possibility of rejection.

(d)   Since histocompatibility genes are codominant, F_1 lymphocytes will express both maternal and paternal histocompatibility antigens. Therefore, unless the parents had closely similar histocompatibility genotypes, the F_1 lymphocytes will differ from either parent's cells, and a vigorous mixed lymphocyte reaction should ensue.

1–12 (a)   Parental lymphocytes account for 173 of the 181 mitotic figures observed. Clearly, F_1 lymphocytes are not stimulated to undergo blast transformation by parental cells, whereas parental cells respond strongly to F_1 cells. This result shows that lymphocytes are stimulated only by foreign histocompatibility antigens. Quantitative differences in the antigens expressed do not trigger a response.

(b)   Unlike inbred rats, humans are likely to be heterozygous, particularly at the highly polymorphic histocompatibility loci. Thus F_1 lymphocytes will probably carry some, but not all, of each parent's histocompatibility antigens. Hence, F_1 cells should respond actively against parental cells.

(c)   Inactivation of human parental lymphocytes would allow direct demonstration of the result predicted in Part (b), that F_1 cells generally will react to parental cells. If the F_1 cells were inactivated, the response of the parental cells could be determined. In general this technique allows independent determination of the two responses in a mixed lymphocyte reaction under conditions where karyotype analysis cannot distinguish the two cell populations.

(d)   For organ transplants, it is necessary to know whether the donor's kidney cells will trigger an immunologic response in the recipient. Whether recipient cells can trigger the donor's lymphocytes is irrelevant, because no donor lymphocytes are transferred. If the donor lymphocytes are inactivated, as in Part (c), then a mixed lymphocyte reaction between these cells and lymphocytes of the recipient will furnish the required information.

1–13 (a)   Use of the spleen/body weight ratio is intended to correct for variations in the normal body weights and spleen weights of individual mice. It also magnifies the observed response, because the GVHR causes an increase in spleen weight and a decrease in body weight.

(b)   Line 1 in Table 1–7 provides a control value for recipient mice in which no GVHR should have occurred, because these mice received syngeneic cells.

(c)   Thymosin somehow increases the magnitude of the GVHR. One possible explanation is that it induces maturation of at least some bone-marrow cells into functional T cells. If so, thymus-cell differentiation antigens (e.g., Ly-1,2,3; TL) and other T-cell characteristics also should be expressed. An alternative possibility is that thymosin acts on the few immunocompetent cells in bone marrow to increase their activity or their number. The difference in the effects of thymosin and spleen extract are quantitative, but not qualitative, suggesting that thymosin activity may not be confined to the thymus.

1-14   (a)   The ^{3}H-thymidine incorporation indicates amount of DNA synthesis and hence proliferation in the CBA lymphocyte population, and the ^{51}Cr release is proportional to the number of CBA lymphocytes specifically cytotoxic for cells that bear the BALB/c histocompatibility antigens.

(b)   DNA synthesis precedes the appearance of specifically cytotoxic lymphocytes. Perhaps expression of the specialized cytotoxic functions requires a round of cell division, although it was not shown directly in this experiment that DNA synthesis occurred in precursors of cytotoxic cells.

(c)   Assuming that the clonal selection theory holds for the cellular immune system, only a small proportion of the T cells will be able specifically to react selectively against any particular antigen or set of antigenic determinants. Consequently large numbers of T cells are needed to produce a detectable reaction *in vitro*.

1-15   (a)   The specific targets of the sensitized rat lymphocytes are the mouse fibroblasts.

(b)   Line (b) in Table 1-8 indicates the background of nonspecific cytotoxicity.

(c)   In Experiment (c) of Table 1-8, both specific and nonspecific target cells are added to the sensitized rat lymphocytes. Notice, however, that only the rat fibroblasts, the nonspecific target cells, were labeled with ^{51}Cr; thus the percent of ^{51}Cr released is a measure solely of nonspecific cytotoxicity. The data show a marked and highly significant increase in nonspecific cytotoxicity when specific targets also are added. This could be explained by assuming that the cytotoxic reaction has two stages: cytotoxic lymphocytes must first be stimulated specifically by their appropriate target, but then they release a nonspecific effector molecule that can kill any cell in the vicinity. The addition of specific target cells would greatly increase the amount of effector molecules released and, therefore, also would increase the nonspecific cytotoxicity. In support of this notion, two proteins called lymphotoxins have been isolated and partially characterized. These proteins are released by human lymphocytes and are nonspecifically cytotoxic to most mammalian cells.

1-16   (a)   The massive doses of BSA inhibit the development of a normal immune response. The rabbits have become unresponsive (tolerant) to the antigen. This result is a typical example of high-zone tolerance.

(b)   The control result proves that the BSA has not suppressed the whole immune system. Rather, the unresponsiveness, or tolerance, is specific for the tolerance-inducing antigen. The animals still can react normally to other antigens.

(c)   Neonatal animals are more sensitive to the induction of tolerance than are adults. Their immune system has not yet matured and apparently is paralyzed easily by moderate amounts of antigens.

1–17 (a) That specifically SRBC immune spleen cells would augment the response to SRBC seems reasonable.

(b) The results of Group 2 illustrate the response of mice injected with thymocytes alone. A very poor response would be expected if only the tolerant spleen cells had been injected. From the results observed with Group 3, it appears that the tolerant spleen lymphocytes also actively suppress the response of the normal thymocytes. The active suppression affects IgG production more severely than IgM production. This result might have been expected, because T cells are not absolutely required for a primary IgM response. One might hypothesize that the suppressor T cells kill or inhibit cells that secrete IgG specific for SRBC. The proposed specificity of this effect could be tested by simultaneously administering SRBC and a second, unrelated antigen. In fact, there does seem to be a generalized, nonspecific depression of the immune system in such experiments. These observations emphasize the important regulatory role that T cells may play in the immune response, but they also emphasize the need for specificity controls in these types of experiments.

1–18 (a) Supernatant fluid from cultures containing homologous serum significantly inhibited macrophage migration. This result indicates the presence of MIF and thus demonstrates that the maternal lymphocytes were sensitized to paternal antigens. This sensitization probably occurred during one or more previous pregnancies.

(b) Because the major histocompatibility antigens usually are immunologically dominant, the mother probably is responding primarily to paternal HLA antigens.

(c) Supernatant fluid from these cultures had essentially no effect on macrophage migration. Hence autologous plasma somehow inhibited the sensitized maternal lymphocytes from reacting to the paternal cells. This finding may be interpreted to demonstrate the existence of a mechanism to protect the fetus from reactive maternal lymphocytes. Moreover, the observation that only autologous sera inhibit indicates that this mechanism may be immunologically specific.

(d) If the inhibitory factor is an immunoglobulin, then removal of immunoglobulins with appropriate anti-Ig antisera should abolish the inhibition of MIF release by autologous sera. Alternatively, purified immunoglobulin from autologous sera should inhibit release of MIF.

(e) The active factor probably is IgG, and the effect is immunologically specific. Thus autologous IgG molecules appear to prevent MIF release and, by inference, the total immunological response. Both these humoral factors and the sensitized maternal lymphocytes arise in response to paternal antigens on fetal cells, which presumably somehow have entered the maternal circulation. Thus both could be specific for paternal antigens. If so, specific IgG could bind to paternal antigens and block recognition by maternal lymphocytes. To prove this hypothesis, one could absorb autologous serum with paternal cells. The specific IgG should bind to the cells, and the serum, which still would contain all other IgG molecules, should have no protective effect. With regard to the question of tolerance, the mother's system may not recognize small doses of paternal antigens, but her lymphocytes can respond to those antigens and probably could reject a skin transplant. Consequently the mother is, to a limited extent, unresponsive, but she is not truly tolerant.

1-19 (a)   Injection of anti-SRBC antibody one hour before or four hours after SRBC diminishes the number of plaque-forming cells, reflecting a decreased number of specifically stimulated B cells. Therefore specific IgG reduces the primary humoral (IgM) response to the same antigen.
(b)   The simplest explanation is that the specific IgG interferes with the afferent arm of the response to SRBC. The IgG could bind to the SRBC and prevent recognition by other specific B cells or helper T cells. Alternatively, the IgG may act by promoting the phagocytosis and digestion of the SRBC before they could elicit an immune response.
(c)   Specific IgG_1 antibodies inhibit the response, but specific IgG_2 antibodies actually stimulate the response significantly.
(d)   The anti-SRBC antibodies had negligible effects on the anti-CRBC response, thereby demonstrating that the inhibitory effect of added antibody is specific.
(e)   The inhibition by IgG agrees with the previous results, but the stimulation by specific IgG_2 antibodies indicates that a more complex explanation is required. If the only differences between specific IgG_1 and IgG_2 antibodies are subtle variations in the heavy-chain structure, then the simple "recognition–interference" hypothesis seems invalid.
(f)   The finding that specific $F(ab')_2$ fragments of either subclass are neither stimulatory nor inhibitory underscores the importance of the heavy chains in this control mechanism and strengthens the argument against the simple recognition interference explanation in Part (b).

1-20 (a)   The response to the second (competing) antigen is sharply reduced, regardless of which antigen is administered first and which second.
(b)   This effect does not depend on relatedness of the antigens. The mechanisms underlying this so-called antigen competition must be nonspecific.
(c)   The central problem is to distinguish between an active suppression and a failure to compete successfully for some limiting factor. Unfortunately, there is considerable experimental evidence on both sides of the question. Clearly, suppressor cells do exist, and some groups have

reported the adoptive transfer of antigenic competition by T cells. Other groups report that addition of normal T cells relieves antigenic competition, which suggests that T cells are the limiting factor. Still other experiments strongly suggest that limitation of binding sites for T-cell receptors on accessory cells is the cause. Important variables seem to be the exact timing and dose of antigen, the physical state of the antigens, whether the competing antigenic determinants are on the same or different molecules, whether the experiment is done *in vivo* or *in vitro* (the microarchitecture of the lymph nodes may influence this phenomenon critically), and finally whether accessory cells such as macrophages are present.

1–21 (a) There is some variation in the sIg per cell, but both populations show a plateau at about 1 μg/ml antiserum.

(b) The percentages of lymphocytes labeled at the plateau is a good measure of the total number of sIg^+ cells or B cells. Hence about 45% of the splenic lymphocytes and 20% of the lymph node lymphocytes are B cells.

(c) These data do not allow an estimate of the number of B cells, because no plateau is evident. The assay would have to be carried out to higher antiserum concentrations to determine whether the marrow curve would reach a plateau. However, at antiserum concentrations greater than 10 μg/ml, nonspecific labeling becomes significant and invalidates the assay.

(d) The lack of a plateau up to 10 μg/ml antiserum demonstrates a greater variation in the amount of sIg per cell among sIg^+ marrow cells. An even greater variation is implied, in that there may be cells with still smaller amounts of sIg that are not labeled by even 10 μg/ml antiserum.

(e) If there is a continuous variation in the surface density of sIg, from cells with no sIg to cells with large amounts of sIg, then perhaps the density of sIg is a measure of the cells' maturity. The acquisition of sIg may be a critical step in lymphocyte maturation.

1–22 (a) The large lymphocytes synthesized DNA, which implies that they are rapidly dividing cells, whereas the small lymphocytes are not.

(b) Bone-marrow small lymphocytes are derived from dividing precursors; if there is no migration of cells into bone marrow these small lymphocytes must be descendants of the rapidly dividing large marrow lymphocytes. Furthermore, the pool of small lymphocytes must be turning over rapidly: within four days, the majority of the unlabeled small lymphocytes were replaced by labeled small lymphocytes recently generated from the large blast cells.

(c) This lag indicates that newly formed small lymphocytes have little, if any, sIg. Apparently, it takes 30–40 hours before the sIg density is sufficient for the cell to be labeled by 1 μg/ml antiglobulin. This observation further supports the idea that lymphocytes mature and acquire increasing amounts of sIg over 3–4 days in the bone marrow.

(d)   Mature cells could migrate from the marrow and enter the blood-stream or peripheral lymphoid organs. Alternatively, some lymphoid cells could differentiate into other cell types, or could simply die.

(e)   You would need to know the size of the peripheral lymphoid pool (which includes the nodes, spleen, peripheral blood, interstitial fluids, lymph vessels, thymus, and gut-associated lymphoid tissue) and the percent of those cells that are labeled. [Notice that recently migrating cells may preferentially home to one organ (e.g., the spleen) so that measurement of only one organ may give erroneous results.] Then you would have to calculate the number of small lymphocytes generated in all of the bone marrow and estimate the number of labeled cells that should have migrated in $3\frac{1}{2}$ days. If this number greatly exceeded the number of labeled cells in the periphery, then you should look for evidence of cell death.

1–23   (a)   *In vitro* incubation significantly decreases the spleen cell response. Cell death *in vitro* may explain this result.

(b)   *In vitro* incubation significantly increases the bone-marrow cell response, particularly during the last 24–72 hours. This period is the same time at which ^{3}H-thymidine-labeled BM cells acquire detectable amounts of sIg (recall Problem 1–22). These kinetics suggest that new B cells matured during the culture interval.

(c)   The molar concentrations of the added Dnp-HGG range down to $10^{-10} M$. Many serum proteins are present at these or much greater concentrations, even early in ontogeny. This result, which shows that developing B cells are inhibited by minute amounts of their specific antigens *in vitro*, may reflect the process by which tolerance to self-antigens is induced *in vivo*.

(d)   The potential anti-Dnp B cells may have been irreversibly inactivated or forced out of the bone marrow into the periphery. Alternatively, binding to antigen early in development may cause cell death.

(e)   A mixture of one culture incubated with antigen and one incubated without should give results equivalent to the average of those obtained with the two cultures separately.

1–24   (a)   Thymocytes should not react in any way against syngeneic cells, yet the data show a strong graft-versus-host response (GVHR) and specific cytotoxicity.

(b)   In a GVHR, the lymphocytes first must be triggered by binding to their specific antigens. Then the cells undergo blast transformation and several rounds of division. (During this stage, other white blood cells are attracted to the site, probably by chemotactic lymphokines.) Finally, effector cells (e.g., cytotoxic lymphocytes) appear. In this experiment only the triggering occurs *in vitro*; the proliferation and generation of effector cells occur *in vivo*. This result implies that tolerance normally is maintained by interfering with the triggering of self-specific lymphocytes.

(c)   Two to six hours is the minimum incubation time required, much shorter than the average generation time for lymphocytes. Therefore it is unlikely that this effect can be explained by the *in vitro* differentiation of precursor cells. It seems more likely that naturally occurring antiself-reactive clones are reversibly suppressed *in vivo*, and that this suppression is lost *in vitro*.

(d)   Any model should incorporate reversible suppression of self-reactive cells mediated by some factor that interferes with recognition or triggering, and not with proliferation or effector function. This factor could be antibodies directed against self-components, soluble antigen–antibody complexes, self-antigens shed into the serum and present in amounts which induce low-zone tolerance, or something more exotic (see Problem 1–25). Other mechanisms probably are used concomitantly, thereby giving the organism several control mechanisms to prevent autoimmune reactions.

1–25   BN lymphocytes generate GVHR of similar magnitude in immunized and nonimmunized F_1's. The reaction generated in nonimmunized hosts by Lewis lymphocytes also is similar. However, in immunized hosts, the Lewis lymphocyte GVHR is significantly inhibited. Consider exactly what antibodies are elicited in the F_1 host by immunization with the Lewis anti-BN antibodies. The only antigenic determinants on these antibodies normally not found on the F_1 immunoglobulins should be their idiotypic determinants, that is, those of the actual antigen-binding site. Thus the F_1 rats are making antibodies against those particular antigen-binding sites on Lewis immunoglobulins that are specific for BN antigens. Those Lewis rat T cells that are specific for BN histocompatibility antigens probably have receptors (either antibodies or other molecules) whose active sites closely resemble the antigen-binding sites on the anti-BN antibodies, and hence cross-react with the antibodies raised in the F_1's. Thus, when Lewis lymphocytes are injected into an immunized F_1, the F_1 antibodies could combine with those Lewis anti-BN receptors and presumably block the triggering process. This would not happen in nonimmunized F_1's, and the BN lymphocytes, carrying noncross-reactive receptors for Lewis antigens, would not be affected in immunized or nonimmunized hosts.

These results suggest that the same antibodies in F_1 hosts recognize both Lewis anti-BN idiotypes and Lewis anti-BN T-cell-surface receptors. Thus receptors on B cells and T cells that are specific for the same antigens must be very similar in structure, if not identical.

2 IMMUNOPATHOLOGY

Diseases of the immune system can be grouped into two general classes. *Deficiency* diseases result when a component of the system fails to function. These diseases all manifest themselves clinically by low resistance to infection and loss of other immunologic surveillance functions. *Hypersensitivity* diseases result when the system reacts under inappropriate conditions. These diseases lead to a variety of pathologic symptoms. Some diseases of both classes are congenital, whereas others are acquired. This chapter considers the causes and consequences of immune deficiency and hypersensitivity. The first half deals primarily with the cellular or molecular bases of deficiency diseases. The second half describes the inappropriate responses of T cells and B cells in hypersensitivity diseases, and concludes by returning to a recurrent theme in modern immunology: the role of gene products coded by the major histocompatibility complex in normal and pathological immune responses. An appendix describing the nature of antigen–antibody reactions and their use for immunoassay and immunodiagnosis is included at the end of the chapter.

Essential Concepts

2-1 Lowered resistance to infection may result from defects in general host defenses that do not involve the lymphoid system

Immunity to infection depends upon a combination of nonspecific innate functions and specific T- and B-cell adaptive immune responses. The nonspecific functions prevent invasion by the vast majority of microorganisms. Some of the most important of these functions are: maintenance of epithelial surface integrity; action of antibacterial substances such as lysozyme (an enzyme in secretions that attacks bacterial cell walls) and C-reactive protein (an inducible serum factor that binds to bacterial cell-wall phosphorylcholine residues and activates complement-mediated opsonization and lysis); maintenance of local pH conditions, for example acidity in the stomach and vagina; and mechanical expulsion of microorganisms by various mechanisms such as ciliary movement on respiratory tract epithelium and the sneeze reflex. Failure of any of these innate defenses may lead to infection in the absence of any immunologic deficiency disease.

If microorgansims successfully invade epithelial barriers, most of them are removed by the phagocytic system, which also stimulates the specific functions of T- and B-cell immunity. Because most immunologic reactions also end with phagocytosis and degradation of the antigenic microorganisms, it is appropriate to begin the discussion of lymphoid system deficiencies with malfunctions of phagocytic cells.

2–2   Diseases that interfere with phagocytic functions usually result in lethal bacterial infections

A.   The elimination of invading microorganisms by phagocytic cells is a multistep process. It includes chemotactic attraction of phagocytes to the site of infection, phagocytosis of invading microorganisms, intracellular union of phagosomes and lysosomes, and lysosomal destructive action involving enzymatic iodination of microorganism cell walls leading to their breakdown by various acidic hydrolases. In normal hosts most types of microorganisms are eliminated by this process. Consequently these microorganisms are nonpathogenic (not disease generating). A few types of microorganisms regularly survive these events, and hence are pathogenic. Patients with malfunctioning phagocytic cells have recurrent infections, usually caused by normally nonpathogenic organisms, which become pathogenic in these hosts. Such phagocytic malfunction diseases are relatively rare, and usually are inherited. Practical diagnosis of these disorders involves isolation and testing of blood phagocytes for (a) motile responses to chemotactic factors, (b) ability to phagocytize a range of microorganisms, (c) ability to kill phagocytosed microorganisms, and (d) ability to generate hydrogen peroxide, H_2O_2, which is required in the iodination of microorganisms, and can be measured *in vitro* using the redox-sensitive dye, nitroblue tetrazolium.

B.   Two forms of phagocytic-cell disease have been described in humans.

1.   One of these diseases involves a defect of lysosomal structure in phagocytes and other cells. These cells have abnormally large lysosomes that lyse bacteria ineffectively, and fuse sluggishly with phagosomes, although phagocytosis is normal. Humans with this disease, called *Chediak-Higashi syndrome,* are also partial albinos, presumably due to a related defect of structures similar to lysosomes in the pigmented cells of the retina and skin. The

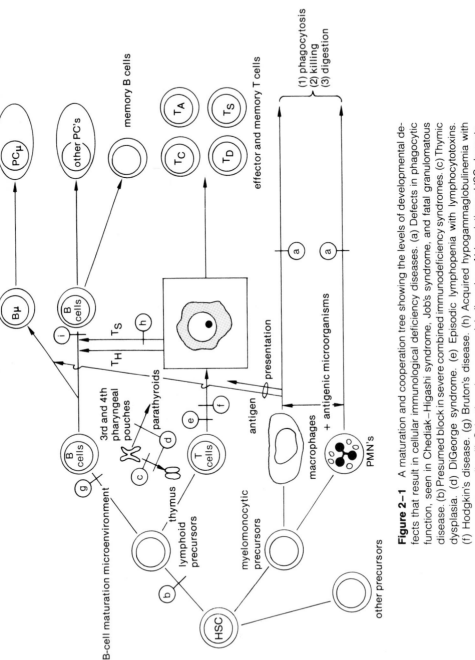

Figure 2–1　A maturation and cooperation tree showing the levels of developmental defects that result in cellular immunological deficiency diseases. (a) Defects in phagocytic function, seen in Chediak–Higashi syndrome, Job's syndrome, and fatal granulomatous disease. (b) Presumed block in severe combined immunodeficiency syndromes. (c) Thymic dysplasia. (d) DiGeorge syndrome. (e) Episodic lymphopenia with lymphocytotoxins. (f) Hodgkin's disease. (g) Bruton's disease. (h) Acquired hypogammaglobulinemia with suppressor cells. (i) Selective dysgammaglobulinemias. Abbreviations: HSC, hematopoietic stem cell; T, T cell; B, B cell; PMN, polymorphonuclear leukocyte; PC, plasma cell.

disease usually is fatal in childhood. Related disorders have been found in mink (Aleutian mink disease), cattle, and mice.

2. A second form of phagocytic malfunction is due to defects in the lysosomal enzymes that produce H_2O_2, or those that act on H_2O_2 to produce oxygen free radicals required in the iodination of microorganisms. Cells from patients with this disease phagocytize, but do not kill most bacteria, which continue to grow inside the phagocytes and induce a prolonged local inflammatory reaction. The combination of activated phagocytes and surrounding cells growing in a nodule is identifiable histologically as a *granuloma*. Such granulomatous diseases usually are fatal in childhood, and can exhibit either of two modes of inheritance: an X-linked recessive form is known as *chronic granulomatous disease*, and an autosomal recessive form is known as *Job's syndrome* (Figure 2–1a).

2-3   Some patients lack both T- and B-cell systems

Congenital lack of lymphocytes, known as *severe combined immunodeficiency*, may result from any one of several defects. Three distinct genetic bases for these diseases are known: an X-linked recessive, an autosomal recessive defect of the enzyme *adenosine deaminase*, and an autosomal recessive of unknown primary effect. How or why each of these defects eliminates only the lymphoid compartment of the hematolymphoid system is unknown.

Patients with these defects are extraordinarily susceptible to microorganisms that grow either inside host cells—mainly viruses and a few types of bacteria—or outside host cells—mainly bacteria. These patients lack a lymphoid thymus, and their blood (Table 2–1), spleen, lymph nodes, Peyers patches, tonsils, and appendix also lack lymphocytes. They have no serum immunoglobulins. In some patients, bone-marrow cell transplants may completely repopulate both T- and B-cells systems. Because both T and B cells but no other blood cell types are missing in these patients, the defect apparently is at the level of cells that are committed to lymphoid maturation, but are not yet committed to either T- or B-cell lineages (Figure 2–1b). The syndrome may not represent the same defect in all cases.

2-4   Some patients lack only the T-cell system

A. Individuals who lack T cells are especially susceptible to viral and bacterial intracellular infections. Vaccination of these individuals with live, attenuated (nonpathogenic) viruses usually is fatal. In general, T cells are absent from their blood and lymphoid tissues, and they

Table 2-1

Properties that can be assayed in diagnostic tests for human blood lymphocyte classes

Properties	T cells	B cells	Monocytes
Percentage representation among nucleated blood mononuclear cells (excludes granulocytes)	60–70%	10–15%	10–20%
Presence of cell-surface:			
κ or λ chains	−	+(10–15%)[a]	−
μ chains + δ chains	−	+(5–8%)	−
γ chains	−	+(0.02–1.0%)	−
α chains	−	+(0.2–1.0%)	−
Fc receptors	−(<5%)	+(10–15%)	+
C3 receptors[b]	−(<5%)	+(6–12%)	+
native sheep RBC receptors	+(>80%)	−(<1%)	−
human T-cell-surface antigens	+(>90%)	−(<1%)	−
Mitogenic response to:			
concanavalin A (Con A)	+	−	
phytohemagglutinin (PHA)	+	−	
pokeweed mitogen (PWM)	+	+	

[a]Percentages in parenthesis indicate the % of all mononuclear blood cells that possess the marker.

[b]Including cells that possess receptors for the two split products of C3 (C3b and C3d). Different assays can distinguish among B cells with C3b receptors, B cells with C3d receptors, and monocytes with C3b receptors.

lack testable T-cell functions, such as graft rejection and activation of blood lymphocytes in response to the T-cell mitogenic lectins concanavalin A and phytohemagglutinin (Table 2–1 and Essential Concept 1–6C).

B.   Several congenital defects can lead to specific lack of T cells.

1.   One such defect, characterized by disorganized tissue in the thymus, is known as *thymic dysplasia* (Figure 2–1c).

2.   A second defect is characterized by lack of the thymic (and parathyroid) inductive microenvironment, presumably a result of improper formation of the third and fourth pharyngeal endodermal pouches during embryogenesis (Figure 2–1d). This congenital abnormality, known as the *DiGeorge syndrome,* is not heritable. Children with this abnormality can be recognized clinically because they also lack parathyroid hormones and therefore cannot maintain appropriate calcium levels in the blood. Consequently, soon after birth they go into muscle spasm (hypocalcemic tetany).

3. A defect in the formation of the thymic inductive microenvironment also is found in mice; however, this abnormality is heritable. The epithelial cells of the affected animals have several defects, including the absence of hair follicles. Consequently these mice are hairless, and the autosomal recessive gene responsible for their multiple defects is called *nude* (nu).

C. Some *acquired* diseases also result in a total or partial lack of peripheral T cells.

1. Some patients show episodic decreases in T cells, accompanied by the expected range of immunodeficiencies. During these episodes the patients produce a serum autoantibody that lyses T cells in the presence of complement. This disease is known as *episodic lymphopenia with lymphocytotoxins* (Figure 2-1e).

2. An acquired T-cell deficiency also occurs in patients with *Hodgkin's disease,* a cancer of lymph-node cells. Although the malignant cells may be limited to a single lymph node, these patients exhibit a whole-body deficiency of T-cell functions: for example, delayed allograft rejection, weak contact sensitivity, and decreased resistance to intracellular infections such as tuberculosis and Herpes viruses. These patients have normal numbers of peripheral T cells as measured by anti-T-cell antisera, but these cells respond weakly to T-cell mitogens, and do not exhibit the normal ability to bind sheep red blood cells nonspecifically. The surface receptors of T cells from these patients appear to be blocked by serum factors that are elevated markedly in Hodgkin's disease (Figure 2-1f).

2-5   Some patients lack only the B-cell system

A. A total congenital lack of B cells, their progeny and their products, can result from another X-linked recessive gene. Patients with this syndrome, called *infantile sex-linked agammaglobulinemia* or *Bruton's disease* (Figure 2-1g), are especially susceptible to pyogenic (pus-causing) bacterial infections of the skin and respiratory tracts, beginning at about six months of age, when placentally transferred maternal immunoglobulin has disappeared. The lives of these patients can be saved by inoculation with gamma globulin pooled from several different donors, which usually prevents infections.

B. Several *acquired* B-cell defects also are known. These diseases, all poorly understood, include both complete and partial defects of B cells and their immunoglobulin products.

1. One class of patients with *acquired agammaglobulinemia* has normal levels of B cells, but no plasma cells (Figure 2-1h). *In* *vitro* analysis has demonstrated that these patients possess a class of T_S cells that prevents stimulation of antibody formation. Thus this disease may be classified more properly as a T-cell abnormality.

2. Selective deficiencies of IgA, or IgA and IgG, often are associated with gastrointestinal tract disorders, such as diarrhea and poor intestinal absorption of fats and fat-soluble vitamins, by mechanisms that are not understood. Patients with these deficiencies have normal numbers of B_α cells, and these cells can be stimulated to become IgA-secreting plasma cells *in vitro* (Figure 2–1i). Several other such *selective dysgammaglobulinemias* (dysfunctions of particular immunoglobulin classes in the blood) have been reported, including deficiencies in IgM alone, IgM and IgA, or IgM and IgG. Deficiencies in IgM and IgG usually are accompanied by susceptibility to pyogenic infections.

2-6   Some immune deficiencies are secondary to other diseases, or are unexplained

A.   Immunological deficiency may be secondary to diseases which result in the accumulation of immunosuppressive products. Thus defective function of the kidney or liver leads to an accumulation of toxic substances which may depress immune responses. Patients ill with virus infections often release immunosuppressive products into the blood, as do many patients with advanced cancers.

A well-known multisystem disease that involves a deficiency in immunity is called *Cushing's disease.* It is caused by the excess secretion of cortisone and cortisol, two hormones of the adrenal cortex. These hormones have several effects at these increased concentrations: potent anti-inflammatory actions, direct lysis of most T and B cells, and decreased levels of blood monocytes. Patients with Cushing's disease become extremely susceptible to infection, particularly to those agents usually controlled by the T-cell system. The increased secretion of the two hormones sometimes may be episodic, related to periods of emotional or physical stress.

B.   Because the immune system employs cellular biochemical mechanisms common to several other cell systems, it frequently may be affected by defects in these mechanisms. Such a defect may first become apparent clinically as failure of immunity, leading to early infection, and careful analysis may be required to show that the defect in fact is more general.

1.   *Adenosine deaminase deficiency* is one example of a general defect that is manifested most clearly as an immune-system abnormality. Patients who are deficient in this enzyme, usually present in tissues and red cells, lack both T and B cells.

2.   Patients with *ataxia-telangiectasia* are defective in their ability to repair x-ray-induced damage to DNA. In early life their immune system appears normal. As they grow older, they develop pathological alterations in their small veins with the formation of *telangiectases* (*tel*: end; *angio*: vessel; *ectases*: stretching out), which are highly dilated, tortuous venous networks. These alterations first become apparent as effects on the cerebellum, resulting in disorders of balance and movement (ataxia). Later, telangiectases become visible in the skin and the whites of the eyes. Beginning in about the fifth year of life, these patients develop a progressive immune deficiency that is characterized by defective cellular immunity and, often, by a total lack of IgA (and sometimes IgE). The thymus is alymphoid in these patients by the time the immunological defects appear. No clear relationship between the x-ray sensitivity of the cells from these patients and their subsequent pathology has yet been established.

3.   Another unexplained, multisystem, progressive disease that results in the loss of T cells is called *Wiskott–Aldrich syndrome,* or *immunodeficiency with thrombocytopenia and eczema.* "Thrombocytopenia" means lack of platelets, and eczema is a skin disorder characterized by an inappropriate response of the IgE system to antigens. Patients with this disease are born normal, but at an early age they have problems of bleeding due to lack of platelets, which are important in the blood clotting process. They develop eczematous skin rashes and later show a progressive loss of T-cell functions. The underlying pathological process that causes this distinctive combination of immunodeficiency, thrombocytopenia, and eczema is unknown.

2-7   Most immunological deficiencies result from medical therapy for other diseases

Many therapeutic treatments involve suppression of the immune system, either intentionally or inadvertently. These treatments may have dangerous side effects related to the resulting immunodeficiency. Diseases *caused* by medical therapy are called *iatrogenic* diseases.

1.   The potent anti-inflammatory effect of the adrenocortical hormones, cortisone and cortisol, and of their inducer, ACTH (*a*drenoc*orticot*ropic *h*ormone), has led to widespread use of these agents in the control of diseases that have a major inflammatory component. Prolonged use of these hormones has the same effects as Cushing's disease, and may make infections fatal.

2.   Chemotherapy and x-ray therapy of most cancers (see Chapter 5) involve the use of agents that inactivate dividing cells. Because cell division is necessary to generate most effector cells of the immune system, the prolonged use of anticancer agents depletes cells important for host immunity.

3.   Transplantation operations to replace defective organs often introduce foreign antigenic tissue into the recipient. Adrenocortical hormones and anticancer drugs, as well as antisera against lymphocytes of the T-cell series, all are used to suppress the host rejection reaction. All these agents cause nonspecific immunosuppression that leads to immunodeficiency.

2-8   Hereditary deficiency of complement system components may be either fatal or trivial

1.   Hereditary deficiencies of several complement components involved in acute inflammation (Essential Concept 1–5) are known. These deficiencies often, but not invariably, are associated with a decreased resistance to bacterial infections, or an increased incidence of hypersensitivity diseases. Deficiencies of other complement components usually are not associated with decreased host immunity (Table 2–2).

2.   Deficiency of a control element in complement activation, C-1 esterase inhibitor, leads to a condition known as *hereditary angioneurotic edema.* It is believed that normally the complement system may be activated and deactivated repeatedly, but that in patients with this condition the reactions go unchecked, thereby causing recurrent episodes of local acute inflammation at sites of activation. The results are vessel dilation and transudation of fluid into the tissue spaces in the upper respiratory tract, gastrointestinal tract, and skin. If activation occurs in the throat at or near the larynx, it may cause death by suffocation.

2-9   Abnormal autoimmune responses can cause disease

A.   Immune responses to self-components (autoimmune responses) usually do not occur. When they do, some autoimmune responses are pathogenic, whereas others are not. It seems probable that only some components of an immune response to self can cause disease.

B.   Autoimmune responses that represent a failure of immunological tolerance may occur in three ways, all of which interrupt *induction* of tolerance, and result in the emergence of "forbidden clones" of T and B cells that bear receptors for self-antigens.

1.   Since the maturation of lymphocytes occurs continuously (Essential Concept 1–4), a constant supply of autoantigen must

Table 2–2

Complement deficiency and associated diseases in man

Deficient component	Associated diseases
C1r	Hypersensitivity diseases, infections
C1s	Hypersensitivity diseases
C2	Hypersensitivity diseases, infections
C3	Infections
C4	Hypersensitivity diseases
C5	Infections

be present to induce tolerance in newly arising virgin lymphocytes. If an autoantigen is not present for an extended period, then breakdown of tolerance will ensue. For example, removal of the pituitary from larval tree frogs results in rejection of the same pituitary when it is reimplanted into the same frog as an adult.

2. An immune response to nonself-antigens may activate lymphocytes that bear antiself-receptors and had formerly been maintained in a state of nonreactivity. Low dose tolerance may involve tolerance at the T-cell but not the B-cell level (Essential Concept 1–14). Therefore, if some breakdown of T-cell tolerance occurs, *humoral* autoimmunity may result from presentation of autoantigens to clones of B antiself-cells via the newly activated T_H cells. Three models of how such an event may occur are shown in Figure 2–2. Panel (a) shows the normal tolerant response to an autologous thyroid protein, thyroglobulin (TG). Panels (b) and (c) show possible consequences of modifying thyroglobulin by combination with Dnp to produce a Dnp–TG conjugate. The Dnp itself may provide an antigenic determinant recognizable by clones of anti-Dnp-TG T_H cells (Panel b), or the Dnp may lead to a conformational change in the TG protein that exposes groups that previously were hidden (Panel c). Such groups would constitute *new antigenic determinants* (NAD) to the immune system, and could be recognized by clones of anti-NAD T_H cells. As shown in Panel (d), injection of TG from another species that has cross-reacting as well as unique antigenic determinants may stimulate T_H clones specific for the unique determinants. As in the situation illustrated by Panels (b) and (c), T_H–B cooperation occurs, and autoantibodies are induced. Once induced, the humoral autoantibodies to TG may eliminate all circulating TG, theoretically permitting the emergence of both T- and B-cell clones that are reactive to self TG.

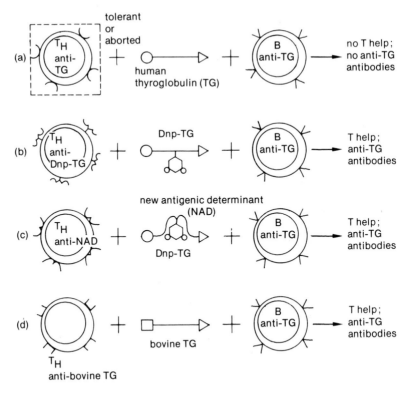

Figure 2–2   Mechanisms by which tolerance to an autologous thyroglobulin (TG) may be broken. (a) Normal tolerance; lack of active T$_H$ anti-TG cells prevents triggering of B anti-TG cells. Hapten modification of TG by Dnp, for example, can result in stimulation of T$_H$ cells which react to either (b) Dnp–TG or (c) to new antigenic determinants revealed on the hapten-modified TG. (d) Injection of TG from another species, bovine TG, for example, may stimulate T$_H$ cells reactive to bovine-TG specific antigenic determinants.

The example in Panel (d) is potentially relevant to patients who receive animal-hormone replacement therapy, for example with bovine insulin or ACTH. A similar situation probably occurs in *rheumatic fever*, in which certain streptococci carry antigenic determinants that cross-react with heart muscle. A similar situation probably also gives rise to the brain and nerve damage that can follow a rabies vaccination if the rabies vaccine is prepared from heterologous brain tissue.

3.   The failure of antigen-specific suppression by T$_S$ cells may allow clones of antiself-lymphocytes to be activated. Loss of specific T$_S$ cells or nonspecific loss of this class of cells could result in the spontaneous appearance of auto-antibodies. This notion is supported by the finding that animals postnatally deprived of their thymus have a higher incidence of auto-anti-bodies, and that animals with a genetic predilection for autoimmune diseases have an accelerated course of these diseases when thymectomized. Whether this result is due to a relatively specific loss of T_S cells or to some other undetermined factors is not known. If it is true that T_S cells express a unique Ia antigen (Essential Concept 1-12), this important question will be open to experimental investigation.

2-10 The T-cell system may react inappropriately to cause disease

Inappropriate T-cell immunity can be defined as a state in which activated T cells initiate or promote disease. This state may come about through immunity to microorganisms, immunity to haptens that couple to endogenous proteins, or immunity to endogenous antigens themselves.

1. An example of immunopathogenic T-cell immunity to microorganisms is the neurological disease induced by the lymphocytic choriomeningitis virus (LCM). This virus infects the choroid membrane of the third and fourth lateral ventricles of the brain and the membranous meninges that cover the brain, inducing infiltration of lymphocytes into these tissues. The neurological damage is not caused by the virus itself, but by the T-cell dependent cellular immune response to the virus-infected cells. Evidence for this conclusion is that the viral infection is not lethal in thymectomized hosts. Thus a specific T-cell immune response may destroy vital cells and cause disease. The observation of T-cell immunity to LCM-infected target cells was the first demonstration of associated recognition (Essential Concept 1-13).

2. T-cell immunity to a microorganism can cause disease if the immune response does not eliminate the microorganism. Tuberculosis provides a good example of this process. The tubercle bacillus primarily infects host macrophages. During its intracellular life it is unaffected by humoral immunity. Most types of tubercle bacilli are killed within activated macrophages. Macrophage activation results from an undefined process that involves interaction with T cells immune to the tubercle bacillus. However, a few resistant strains of tubercle bacilli can proliferate within macrophages in the face of an active and specific T-cell immune response (Figure 2-3a). It has been reported that these pathogenic mycobacteria release substances that prevent fusion of phagosomes with lysosomes. Activated macrophages that carry proliferating tubercle bacilli sometimes are termed epitheloid, because they may assume an abnormal shape resembling that

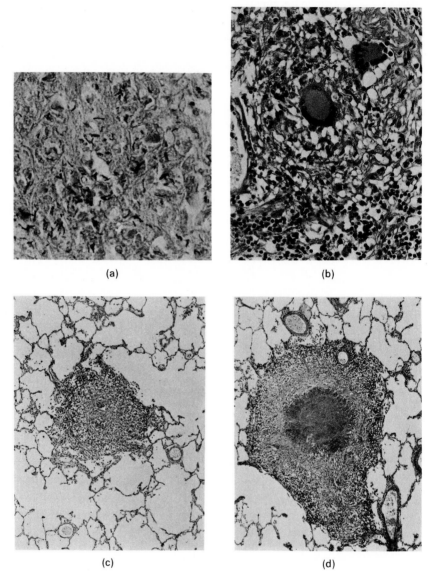

(a)   (b)

(c)   (d)

Figure 2–3   The histological appearance of tuberculosis in the lung. (a) A high-power view of tubercle bacilli inside macrophages, using a dye that stains the rodlike bacilli. (b) A high-power view of cells in an early granuloma. The large multinucleate cells are characteristic of this process. Most of the dark nuclei are lymphocytic; other cells include macrophages and cells involved in repair and regeneration. (c) A low-power view of a central granuloma surrounded by relatively normal lung tissue (large air sacs separated by lacy-thin alveolar walls). The granuloma contains a central zone of giant cells and fibrous tissue, with a shell of lymphocytic infiltrate. (d) A higher-power view of a granuloma containing a core of dead tissue and surrounding fibrous tissue, giant cells, and a shell of lymphocytic infiltrate. [Photographs by R. Rouse and I. Weissman.]

of an epithelial cell. These macrophages also may fuse to form giant syncytial cells (Figure 2–3b).

The result of these conditions is a continuing stimulus for chronic inflammation, with the buildup of a granuloma (Essential Concept 2–2B) of increasing size (Figure 2–3c). As the granuloma enlarges, the signals for repair, which normally accompany chronic inflammation, cause proliferation of fibroblasts at the outer margins of the granuloma, with formation of fibrous tissue. Cells in the central core of the granuloma begin to die (Figure 2–3d), probably due to lack of oxygen, continued proliferation of tubercle bacilli, and release of nonspecific cytotoxins characteristic of chronic inflammation (Essential Concept 1–11). The central core of dead and dying cells may rupture through the fibrous wall of the granuloma, thereby spreading the live tubercle bacilli to neighboring sites. The granulomas form at the expense of valuable lung tissue, and their rupture has two consequences: it spreads tubercle bacilli, initiating new granulomas, and it forms cavities in the old granulomas, which then cannot be reconverted to functional lung tissue. Thus the T-cell immune response to tubercle bacilli can set in motion a destructive chronic inflammatory granulomatous reaction.

The leprosy bacillus, closely related to the tubercle bacillus, causes a destructive reaction much like that of tuberculosis, following preferential infection of macrophages in the skin and around nerves.

3. T-cell immunity to environmental haptens can cause a local, destructive immune response called *contact sensitivity*. Environmental haptens can bind to protein or cell-membrane carriers in the skin and induce a local T-cell immune reaction to the hapten-conjugated proteins or cells. These haptens can be natural products (e.g., the active small molecules in poison ivy and poison oak leaves), or industrial reagents such as picryl chloride (trinitrophenyl chloride or Tnp), which can form Tnp conjugates via a substitution reaction with the ε-amino groups of lysine. Sufficient concentrations of these *contact sensitizing* agents may induce a T-cell immune response that results in a chronic inflammatory focus as well as direct lysis of hapten-conjugated target cells. T_D and T_C cells in animal models of these diseases show associated recognition of MHC gene products (Essential Concept 1–13).

4. T-cell immunity to endogenous antigens can lead to an immunopathologic destruction of vital tissues. The various models of induction of autoimmunity were described in Essential Concept 2–9. The effector phase of T-cell autoimmunity may be directed against organ-specific or multisystem antigens, depending on the antigens involved in the induction process. Experimental organ-specific autoimmunity has been demonstrated many times following the injection of heterologous organ homogenates. Such autoimmune reactions have been studied in detail for adrenals (*adrenalitis,* in which the suffix *itis* indicates inflammation of the affected tissue or organ), thyroid (*thyroiditis*), and nervous tissue (*encephalomyelitis*; encephalo: brain, myelo: spinal cord).

Certain human diseases appear to have organ-specific T-cell immunity as a component. For example, in *Hashimoto's thyroiditis,* all patients exhibit a chronic inflammatory reaction in the thyroid, and T cells from some of these patients are reactive to human thyroid antigens (Figure 2–4). In some cases of adrenal insufficiency (*Addison's disease*), cellular autoimmunity to adrenal cell antigens is present.

5. Both cellular and humoral immunity may be able to cause anemia by an indirect mechanism. Some patients with pernicious anemia are unable to absorb vitamin B_{12}, which is necessary for erythroid and myeloid differentiation in the bone marrow. These individuals usually lack intrinsic factor, a polypeptide produced by parietal cells in the stomach, which binds vitamin B_{12} and allows its absorption across the intestinal epithelium.

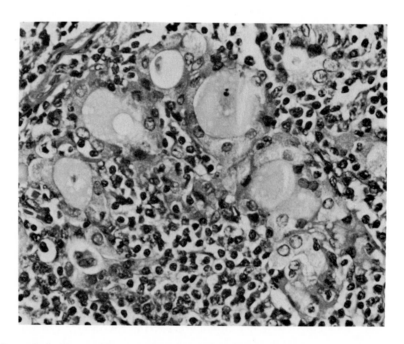

Figure 2–4   Thyroid from a patient with Hashimoto's thyroiditis. The predominant cell types which infiltrate the thyroid are lymphocytes and macrophages. [Photograph by R. Rouse.]

Some of these patients are deficient in parietal cells, presumably as a result of parietal-cell-specific cellular autoimmunity. Others have parietal cells that produce and excrete intrinsic factor, but the factor is neutralized by specific autoantibodies transported to the intestinal lumen.

The foregoing example may be instructive for further investigations into the role of T-cell autoimmunity in human disease. Diseases that have complex, multisystem manifestations that result from loss of an important class of cells may have a T-cell autoimmune origin. A possible example is *juvenile diabetes mellitus,* which is caused by lack of pancreatic islet-of-Langerhans cells. Recent reports indicate that diabetes induced in rats by the drug streptozocin results from the development of cellular immunity to islet cells, probably a consequence of drug-induced damage of these cells.

2-11 Rejection of tissue and organ grafts is mainly a T-cell function

A.   Replacement of defective or severely injured tissues and organs has been a medical objective as long as medicine has been practiced. Grafts from an individual to himself (called *autografts*) almost invariably succeed, and are especially important in treatment of burn patients. Likewise, grafts between two genetically identical individuals (*syngeneic* grafts) almost invariably succeed. However, grafts between two genetically dissimilar individuals of the same species (*allogeneic* grafts), or between individuals of different species (*xenogeneic* grafts), do not succeed. The major reason for their failure is a T-cell-mediated immune response to cell-surface antigens that distinguish donor from host (Figure 2–5). The tissue antigens that induce an immune response in other individuals are called *histocompatibility antigens,* and the genes that specify their structure and synthesis are called *histocompatibility genes.*

   1.   In all species tested, there appear to be two categories of histocompatibility genes. The first category, genes of the major histocompatibility complex (MHC; Essential Concept 1–11), specify antigens that induce rapid rejection of grafts. The second category, termed minor histocompatibility genes, specify antigens that cause a slower graft rejection when acting alone. The MHC is a chromosomal region that comprises a number of closely linked genes which are highly polymorphic within a species, and all of which appear to be involved in immune response and cellular recognition functions. A comparison of the MHC of man and mouse is shown in Figure 2–6. As explained in Essential Concept 1–13, the T-cell immune response to MHC products in the mouse usually involves recognition by T_H, T_D, and T_A cells of I-region-associated antigens, and recognition by T_C and B cells of D/K-

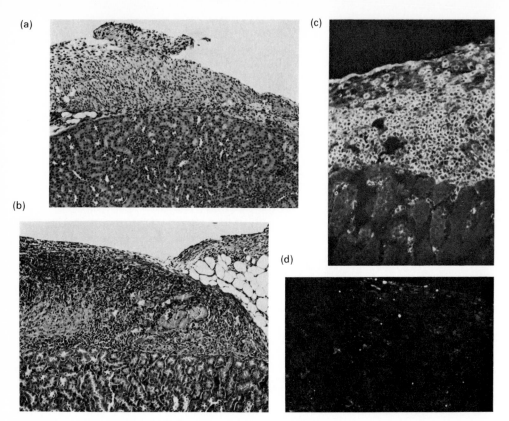

Figure 2–5 A slice of heart tissue from strain C mouse was transplanted under the kidney capsule of another strain C mouse (a), or a strain B mouse (b), 6 days before these sections of tissue were removed for analysis. In (a) the pale tissue on top is heart muscle, and the dark spots are cardiac muscle nuclei. The darker tissue below is normal kidney tissue. In (b) the pale appearance of heart muscle is obscured by the infiltration of many small, dark spots. These are lymphocytes and macrophages. An anti-T-cell stain of another section from (b) is shown in Panel (c), demonstrating that a high proportion of the infiltrating cells are T lymphocytes. An Anti-B-cell stain is used in (d), demonstrating that B cells are rare or nonexistent in the lymphoid infiltrate. By 12 days after grafting, all allogeneic grafts have disappeared and all syngeneic grafts are retained. [Photographs by M. Billingham, R. Warnke, and I. Weissman.]

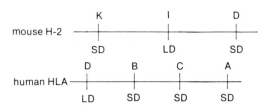

Figure 2–6 The arrangement of subloci in the MHC complexes of mouse and man. In both species antigens specified by the MHC have been identified as serologically defined (SD) antigens (K and D antigens in mouse; B, C, and A antigens in human), or as lymphocyte-defined (LD) antigens (I in mouse; D in human). The SD antigens are found on almost all cells, whereas the LD antigens are present only in some tissues.

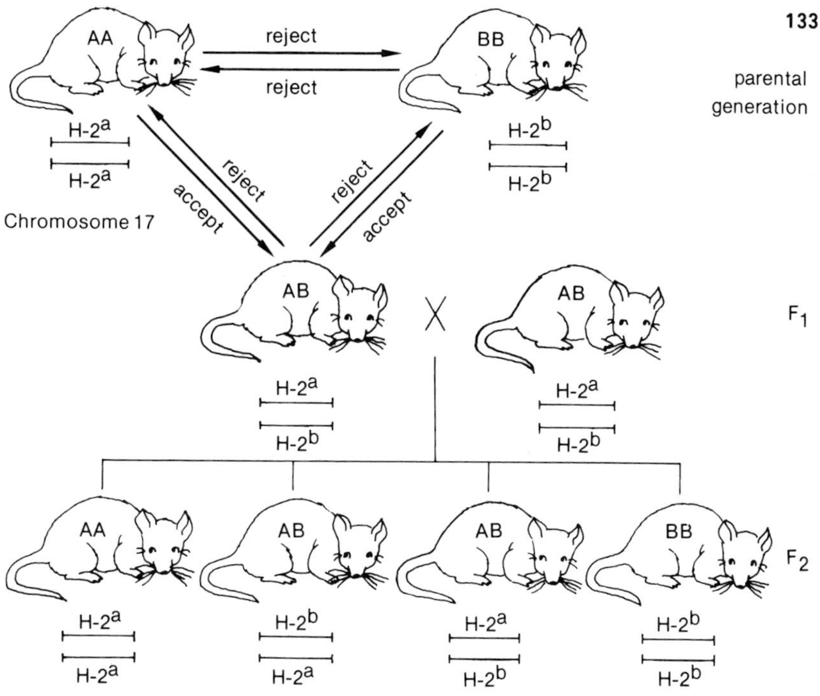

Figure 2-7 The genetics of histocompatibility antigens in inbred mice. Each inbred mouse strain is homozygous for the H-2 complex (e.g., H-2^a or H-2^b). Both sets of products are expressed in the heterozygous F$_1$ hybrids. These mice therefore produce H-2 antigens that stimulate an immune response in either parental strain, whereas neither parental strain expresses H-2 antigens foreign to the F$_1$ hybrid. In the F$_2$ generation there is a classical Mendelian 1:2:1 distribution of homozygous and heterozygous genotypes.

region antigens. T$_C$-cell responses to minor histocompatibility antigens involve associated recognition of the minor antigen and self D/K specificities.

2. The analysis of histocompatibility genetics in mice required the development of inbred strains by repeated brother–sister mating through 20 or more generations. Within such an inbred strain, all mice are virtually identical genetically except for sex. Thus there is MHC (and minor H-gene) identity *within* a strain, and due to the high degree of polymorphism, MHC nonidentity *between* most strains. In mice, the MHC was the second histocompatibility locus named, and is therefore called H-2. Each H-2 haplotype (combination of distinct genes within the MHC) is named by a letter (e.g., H-2^a, H-2^b), and the genetic designation of inbred strains accordingly is H-2$^{a/a}$, H-2$^{b/b}$, and so on.

3. If two strains of mice differ only in the H-2 regions (e.g., H-2$^{a/a}$ and H-2$^{b/b}$), F$_1$ progeny of an intercross (H-2$^{a/b}$) will accept grafts from either parental strain, but either parental strain will reject grafts from an F$_1$ donor (Figure 2–7). Thus MHC

134

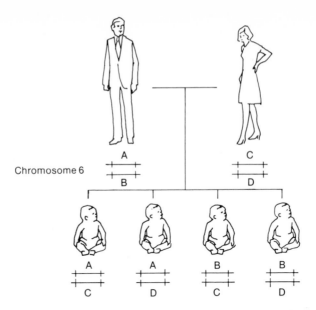

Chromosome 6

Figure 2–8 The genetics of human histocompatibility antigens. Since humans are not inbred, and the HLA system is highly polymorphic, it is likely that any two parents will possess four distinct MHC haplotypes (e.g., A/B, C/D). The F_1 progeny of such a cross will express four distinct haplotype groups: A/C, A/D, B/C, and B/D. Each parent will express one HLA haplotype foreign to each child, and thus parental grafts are rejected by F_1 progeny. Each child will express one HLA haplotype foreign to each parent, and thus F_1 grafts are rejected by parents. On the average, one in four grafts exchanged between F_1 individuals will be histocompatible at the HLA locus.

genes are expressed codominantly. If F_1's are intercrossed to obtain an F_2 generation, three fourths of the offspring will accept grafts from either one of the original parent strains, and half will accept grafts from both (Figure 2–7). In general, the probability of graft acceptance from parent to F_2 in crosses between inbred strains of mice is $(3/4)^n$, in which n = the number of distinct histocompatibility differences between the two strains. In the preceding simplified example, H-2 acts as a single histocompatibility difference. In reality, for two inbred strains chosen at random, $n \geq 30$. Thus there are at least 29 distinct minor H-loci.

4. Humans are an outbred species, and thus almost always will be heterozygous at MHC loci. This fact is critical in the choice of a donor for organ or tissue transplants. Mild immunosuppression (see Essential Concept 2–4D) allows long-term retention of grafts between individuals differing only at minor H-loci, but is insufficient when an MHC difference is involved. Figure 2–8 illustrates the situation in humans. All grafts between parents, from either parent to children, or from children to parents will involve at least one MHC incompatibility. Sibling grafts have a 25% chance of MHC compatibility.

B.   Although most graft-rejection reactions are T-cell mediated, humoral antibodies also can effect rejection in certain cases. The primacy of cellular immunity in graft rejection first was established with skin and tumor grafts. Skin and tumor cells are relatively resistant to antibody-mediated damage, but are susceptible to cell-mediated damage. However, with the advent of organ grafting in man, a new form of antibody-mediated graft rejection occasionally has been found to occur. The reason for this new form of "hyperacute" rejection is illustrated in Figure 2–9. Whereas revascularization of skin and tumor grafts involves host blood vessels, the vascularization of an organ graft is entirely donor in origin. Therefore, in organ grafts anti-MHC antibodies encounter donor MHC antigens on endothelial cells of vessel linings. These cells are susceptible to antibody-mediated damage, presumably via complement activation and antibody-dependent cell-mediated cytotoxicity. Complement components are consumed and localized to vascular endothelial cells of the graft. The resulting combined cytotoxic and acute inflammatory reaction shuts off blood supply to the organ graft, causing graft death.

   1.   Production of high concentrations of anti-donor-MHC antibodies in these cases occurs usually for one of three reasons: insufficient immunosuppression in the grafted host, rejection of a prior transplant that shared some MHC determinants with the new transplant, or immunization with leukocytes that carried cross-reacting MHC antigens. In some instances, cross-reacting leukocytes could have been introduced by previous blood transfusions, although there is no evidence that prior blood transfusion generally hastens subsequent kidney transplant rejection.

   2.   If there has been prior rejection or immunization with inappropriate leukocytes, pre-existing antibodies may act on the new graft as it is being sutured into place, which results in so-called hyperacute rejection. The grafted organ turns gray due to anoxia, and histological examination of the graft vessels demonstrates blood clotting and massive accumulation of polymorphonuclear leukocytes. In addition, immunofluorescence analysis demonstrates immunoglobulin and complement bound to vessels.

   3.   Although antibodies to MHC determinants may cause "hyperacute" rejection of organ allografts, such antibodies may act in different circumstances to interfere with T-cell immunity. This phenomenon, called *immunological enhancement,* is covered in more detail in Chapter 5.

C.   Three methods of immunosuppression have been used to permit allogeneic graft survival in animals. One is used in humans.

   1.   Nonspecific immunosuppression of the host with antimitotic agents, adrenal steroids, and antilymphocyte sera permits long-

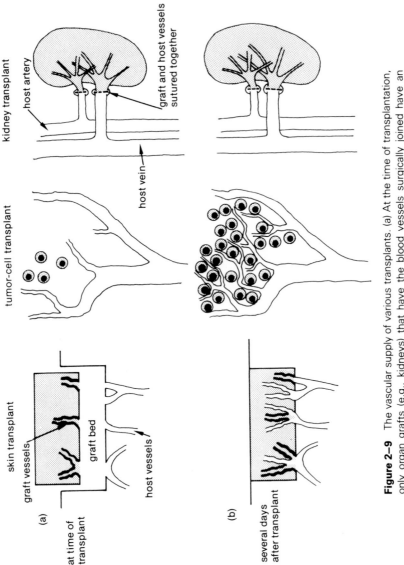

Figure 2–9 The vascular supply of various transplants. (a) At the time of transplantation, only organ grafts (e.g., kidneys) that have the blood vessels surgically joined have an immediate blood supply and therefore do *not* release stimuli for host vessel proliferation and revascularization of donor cells. Both skin grafts and tumor cells induce the release of angiogenic (blood-vessel inducing) factors. (b) Host vessel proliferation may result in the setting up of new channels, or in the natural anastomosis (joining) of host and donor vessels.

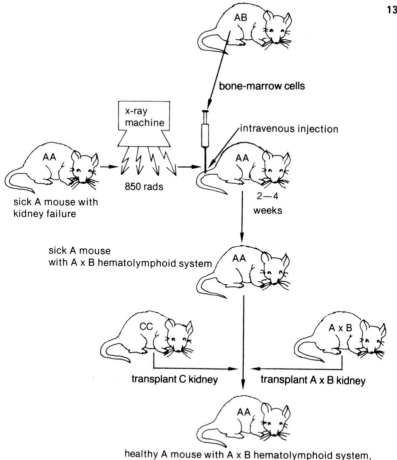

Figure 2–10 A strategy for replacement of the host hematolymphoid system, and subsequent successful allogeneic graft transplantation (see text).

term survival of most MHC-matched allografts, and of about 25% of allografts that differ in MHC determinants. However, all such immunosuppressed patients are immunodeficient (Essential Concept 2–7), and a significant proportion of them suffer life-threatening infections. Even anti-T-cell sera are relatively nonspecific, in that all T cells are susceptible, even to the most highly purified serum. Because most sera are not highly purified, other cell and tissue systems are at risk as well.

2. Replacement of cells in the host hematolymphoid system by donor bone-marrow cells after host marrow has been eliminated by x-radiation permits subsequent successful allogeneic transplantation of donor grafts. As shown in Figure 2–10, an A mouse that has been given an $(A \times B)F_1$ hematopoietic and lymphoid system in this manner accepts an $(A \times B)F_1$ (or even a B) kidney graft but rejects a kidney graft from strain C. If strain B bone-marrow cells had been injected following irradiation, subsequent B kidney grafts also would have been accepted. However, the grafted marrow invariably contains a few T cells, some of which recognize and respond to A-strain MHC antigens. The result is a *multisystem* T-cell *graft-versus-host response* (GVHR), which causes T-cell injury to all organs and usually is fatal. Elimination of donor-marrow T lymphocytes and their precursors is not feasible at this time. Thus the nature of MHC differences in the outbred human population and the dangers of extensive irradiation do not permit this type of marrow transplant in humans.

3. Transplantation tolerance has been created in rodents by transfusion of $(A \times B)F_1$ spleen or bone-marrow cells into fetal or neonatal A hosts. In this procedure, tolerance presumably results from clonal abortion, although other mechanisms, including suppression by T_s cells, have been suggested. This procedure works only in animals that are accessible for transfusion before the full onset of immune competence. Humans probably have passed that stage by the end of the second trimester of gestation, long before organ failure and the need for transplantation have become apparent. Moreover, if a host is sufficiently immature immunologically to accept the donor cellular antigens intended to induce tolerance, then the host also cannot reject donor T cells that are reactive to host MHC antigens. Thus, a lethal graft-versus-host response would follow such a transfusion, unless the tolerance-inducing donor inoculum were genetically (as with inbred rodents) or immunologically unable to respond to host MHC antigens.

D. Despite these problems, modern immunological research eventually may find a safe method of allotransplantation. The goal of this research is selectively to remove or inactivate clones of host T cells that recognize donor MHC antigens, leaving the rest of the T-cell repertoire intact. Two current and promising approaches are development of specific anti-T-cell-idiotype sera, and isolation of MHC antigens in order to make them tolerance-inducing, for example, by changing their form or by coupling them to D-polypeptides for T-cell receptor blockade (Essential Concept 1-13).

2-12 Immune complexes of antigen, antibody, and complement can cause local, destructive, inflammatory lesions

A. Immune complexes (antigen–antibody precipitates) may form in an immune response to a multideterminant antigen if antibody and antigen concentrations are appropriate (Essential Concept A2-1). For antigens

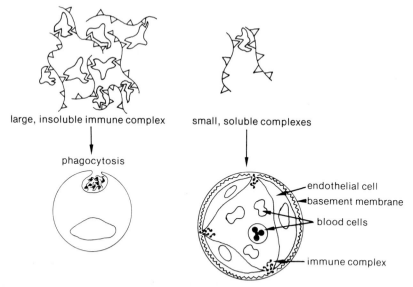

Figure 2–11   Fates of large and small complexes of antigen, antibody, and complement (see text).

confined to lymphoid tissues, complex formation has only minor immunopathological consequences. However, for freely circulating antigens, such as serum proteins, antigen–antibody complexes may be removed both by phagocytic cells and by basement membranes that underlie endothelial cells in blood vessels. There is some discrimination according to the size of these complexes; large complexes are phagocytized, whereas smaller complexes may escape phagocytosis and pass between vessel endothelial cells to deposit on subendothelial basement membranes (Figure 2–11). If these complexes activate complement, they may induce an acute local inflammation at the site of deposition. Usually this effect is transient, as antigen and complexes are cleared and antibody levels rise. However, when the initial antigen load is large the short-term effects may cause serious inflammatory disease. If antigen is reintroduced under these circumstances, chronic or recurrent disease may occur.

   1.   *Serum sickness* is an example of an immune-complex disease in which the initial antigen load is large. The disease is caused by host immune responses to injected antigenic serum proteins. It was most common in the preantibiotic era, when serum from animals (e.g., horses) immunized against particular pathogenic microorganisms was injected into humans to provide passive immunity to the pathogen or to toxins released by the pathogen.

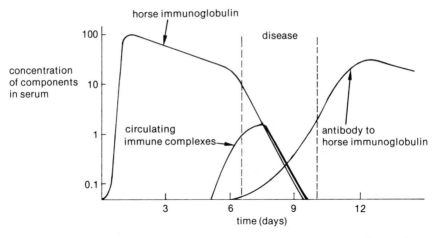

Figure 2–12 The time course of major events in serum sickness (see text).

Figure 2–12 illustrates the course of events in serum sickness following injection of horse immunoglobulin. The levels of horse immunoglobulin at first fall slowly, reflecting the intrinsic degradation rate of these proteins. Beginning at about Day 8, the levels begin to fall more rapidly, as the foreign protein begins to be eliminated by immune complex formation. Concomitant with immune elimination of free horse immunoglobulin is an increase in antigen–antibody complexes, and the appearance of the typical disease pattern: fever, rash, joint lesions, appearance of serum proteins in the urine (proteinuria) and retention in the serum of substances such as urea that normally are cleared by the kidneys. These indications of inflammatory disease subside as immune complexes disappear from the serum and free antibody to horse immunoglobulin appears.

2. Most, if not all, symptoms of serum sickness are due to activation of the complement system by antigen–antibody complexes. Such activation may cause release of vasoactive (*vaso*: vessel) peptides, which induce vasodilation, thereby revealing larger areas of vascular basement membrane. This process is especially notable in the small capillary tufts of the kidney glomeruli where blood filtration takes place (Figure 2–13). Normally, the kidney glomeruli allow passage of small molecules such as urea, but prevent passage of most serum proteins from the vascular lumen into the space that constitutes the beginning of the urinary tubules (Bowman's space). As immune complexes settle on the epithelial side of the glomerular basement membrane, they continue to activate complement, thereby increasing vasodilation and deposition of immune complexes. These complexes

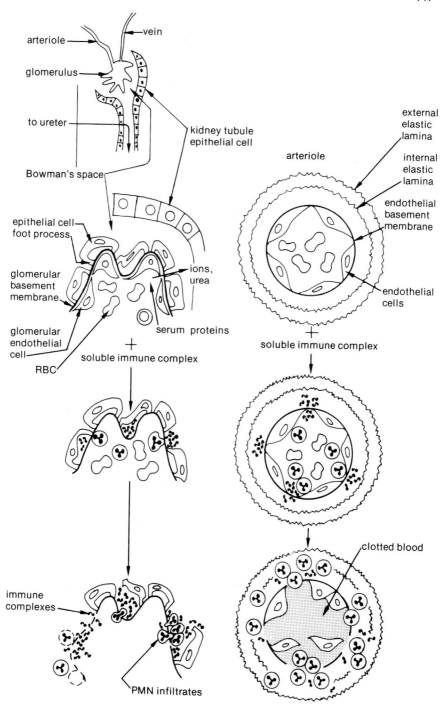

Figure 2–13 Immune complex deposition injury to a kidney glomerulus (left) or to an arteriole (right). See text for details.

induce release of chemotactic factors that attract polymorphonu-clear leukocytes, which tend to disrupt the attachment of epithe-lial-cell foot processes to the glomerular basement membrane. The leukocytes may degranulate, releasing pyrogens (factors that stimulate brain centers to raise body temperature), and hydrolytic lysosomal enzymes that destroy large areas of the basement membrane. At this stage serum proteins leak into Bowman's space, and the kidney's function of clearing small molecules decreases dramatically. However, as phagocytic cells remove bound immune complexes, cells, and tissue debris, the glomerular endothelial and epithelial cells are replaced by cell division. A similar process occurs in arterioles, where the damage is limited to the inner surface of the arteriolar wall (Figure 2–13b).

3. In serum sickness such immune-complex-mediated local acute inflammation can occur within lymph nodes, to cause swollen glands (lymphadenitis), and in joint spaces, to cause arthritis (*arthro*: joint). The acute inflammation of the glomeruli is called *acute glomerulonephritis.* One type is commonly induced by the immune response to a particular protein (M protein) in streptococ-ci. An acute glomerulonephritis that does *not* involve antibody can occur in blood infections by gram-negative organisms, which activate the alternate complement pathway.

B.   Recurrent or continuous immune-complex disease occurs when the inducing antigens are endogenous, are reinjected, or are produced by infecting organisms that cannot be eliminated.

1.   Immune complexes may deposit in skin vessels, to cause local rash and tissue damage (*Arthus phenomenon*), or in systemic blood vessels, to cause *necrotising (necro*: dead or dying) *vasculitis* (*periarteritis nodosa* is an example of a destructive acute inflam-matory lesion of small arteries in nodal foci throughout the body). Immune complexes also may deposit in joints, to cause arthritis. *Rheumatoid arthritis* is a special example in which the antigen may be endogenous IgG, which complexes with circulating IgM antibodies.

2.   Some other diseases consist of immune-complex disease in addition to other pathology. For example, *systemic lupus erythe-matosis* (SLE) is a multisystem autoimmune disorder in which complexes of nucleic acid with specific antibody, or of other tissue components with autoantibody, may affect skin, joints, arteries, muscle, pericardium (tissue surrounding the heart), and glomeruli. The life-threatening immunopathology of SLE usually is either terminal kidney failure or the side effects of immunosup-pressive and anti-inflammatory drugs.

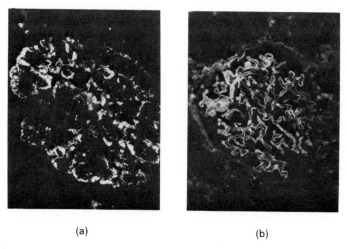

(a)   (b)

Figure 2–14 Immunofluorescence of renal immunoglobulin deposits in glomerulone-phritis. (a) Immune complex nephritis with granular (lumpy-bumpy) deposits of IgG. (b) Good-pasture's syndrome, with linear deposition of IgG on glomerular basement membranes. [Photographs by D. Rice and R. Kempson.]

C.   Immune-complex disease is characterized by granular ("lumpy-bumpy") deposition of immunoglobulin, complement, and antigen on basement membranes underlying the cells that line blood vessels. Because of this characteristic pattern of deposition, immunofluorescence microscopy is often helpful in the diagnosis (Figure 2–14a).

2–13   Antibodies directed against cell-surface or basement-membrane antigens can cause cell death and acute inflammation

Antibodies to cell-surface antigens can cause cell death by direct complement-mediated cytolysis, by antibody-dependent cell-mediated cytotoxicity, and by opsonization. The most common cell types affected are the blood elements—red blood cells (erythrocytes), platelets, polymorphonuclear leukocytes, and lymphocytes. The cell-surface antigens may be haptens (such as penicillin), alloantigens (on transfused or fetal red blood cells), or autoantigens.

> **1.**   If the antigens are on erythrocytes, the usual result is hemolysis (cell lysis that releases free hemoglobin into the serum), and *anemia* (decreased concentration of erythrocytes in the blood). Autoimmune hemolytic anemias often involve hemolysis induced by autoantibodies as well as by antibodies directed against drugs that adsorb to red cells, such as penicillin, quinidine, and α-methyl dopa (Essential Concept 2–9B).

Transfusion of mismatched blood induces formation of antibodies against foreign red blood cell determinants, followed by massive immune hemolysis (*transfusion reaction*). A small transfusion of fetal blood to the mother usually occurs during birth. If an antigen known as Rh is present on fetal blood cells but lacking in the mother, then the mother may produce anti-Rh IgG antibodies. These antibodies can cross the placental barrier and may cause massive antibody destruction of Rh-positive red blood cells in a subsequent fetus (*Erythroblastosis fetalis*). This disease does not occur when there is maternal–fetal incompatibility for the A–B–O blood groups, because all people who lack A or B antigens have significant amounts of "natural" IgM antibodies to the antigens they lack. IgM does not cross the placenta, but will bind to and remove fetal transfusions, thereby preventing the induction of an IgG response.

2. Antibodies to polymorphonuclear leukocytes may be induced by drug treatment: for example, by amidopyrine and sulfa drugs (sulfapyridine, sulfathiazole). The result is *agranulocytosis*, which renders patients highly susceptible to bacterial infections.

3. Autoantibodies to platelets (thrombocytes) may arise after some infections, after some drug therapies, and spontaneously. Such autoantibodies can induce *thrombocytopenic purpura.* The resulting decrease in blood-clotting functions leads to multiple hemorrhages, most visible in the skin and gums as purpura (purple spots). Thrombocytopenic purpura is a general name for platelet-loss diseases, several of which formerly were classed as idiopathic (of unknown origin). Some of these diseases now are known to result from autoimmune responses.

4. Antibodies to vascular basement membranes may cause both complement-mediated lysis and acute inflammation. In a particularly striking form of this condition, called *Goodpasture's syndrome*, autoantibodies are produced against determinants common to glomerular and lung alveolar basement membranes. In the glomerulus, the result is an even, *linear* deposition of immunoglobulin and complement on the endothelial side of the glomerular basement membrane (Figure 2–14b). This deposition may induce infiltration of polymorphonuclear leukocytes and glomerulonephritis. Immunofluorescence microscopy can distinguish this condition from immune-complex glomerulonephritis. Immunopathogenic levels of antibodies to glomerular basement membranes have occurred in kidney transplant patients after kidney rejection, or as a consequence of immunosuppressive treatment with impure antilymphocyte serum (ALS).

2–14 Clinical allergy is caused by an inappropriate IgE response

A.   Some individuals develop exaggerated IgE responses to environmental, drug, or microbial antigens. Reexposure to even minute amounts of these antigens may trigger release of mast-cell products locally or systemically. The specific IgE-mast-cell complexes are so persistent that such a response to an antigen may occur long after the synthesis of IgE directed against that antigen has ceased. Individuals who exhibit such responses are said to be allergic to the inducing antigens. Such reactions often are called *atopic* or *anaphylactic.* The IgE antibodies previously were called *reaginic* antibodies, and antigens that induce these reactions were called *allergens.* The pathological manifestations of IgE-antigen interaction are due to mast cell degranulation resulting in the release of histamine, heparin, slow-reacting substance A (SRS-A), a substance that constricts some smooth muscle cells over a prolonged interval, and a chemotactic factor for eosinophilic leukocytes. Pathological allergic reactions differ from other antibody reactions by their independence of complement, by their induction in response to minute doses of antigen, by their production of vascular and smooth muscle effects that appear in minutes, rather than hours, and by their susceptibility to prevention with antihistamines and to treatment with epinephrine. Epinephrine prevents mast-cell degranulation by raising cellular cAMP levels, and also antagonizes the action on smooth muscle of histamine and SRS-A. Allergic diseases may have systemic or local manifestations, depending on the route of entry of the antigen and the pattern of deposition of IgE and mast cells. Most local manifestations occur on epithelial surfaces, at the site of entry of the allergen. Allergic individuals characteristically give rapid responses in skin testing, have high serum IgE levels, and often have increased blood and tissue concentrations of eosinophilic leukocytes.

   1.   *Systemic anaphylaxis* (anaphylactic shock) results from an IgE-basophil (blood mast cell) response to intravascular antigen. The release of mast-cell mediators produces a biphasic response of vasoconstriction followed by peripheral vessel dilation. The result is a pooling of blood in the periphery and a concomitant drop in blood pressure (shock).

   2.   *Food allergies* involve intestinal IgE-mast cell responses to ingested antigens. These responses may affect the upper gastrointestinal tract, causing vomiting, or the lower gastrointestinal tract, causing cramps and diarrhea. If sufficient antigen is ingested, systemic anaphylaxis and skin reactions may occur.

   3.   Skin reactions of the IgE-mast cell system may be acute or chronic. If acute, they may be a cause of *hives* (urticaria);

if chronic, they may result in atopic dermatitis, a type of eczema. The basis for the latter condition is still unclear.

4.   Allergic reactions of the upper respiratory tract usually are grouped together and called hayfever (*allergic rhinitis*). Some patients affected by this condition develop large nasal polyps, which presumably result from chronic atopic reactions to nasal allergens.

5.   Reactions of the lower respiratory tract usually center in the bronchi and bronchioles, causing constriction and airway obstruction, and are a major cause of *asthma.* The acute effects probably are due to histamine release, and the long-term effects probably are due to SRS-A.

6.   Biting and stinging insects cause more damage by provoking allergic reactions than by direct action of their venom toxins. Individuals who are sensitized to these toxins may suffer fatal anaphylactic shock as the result of a bee sting.

B.   IgE-mediated diseases usually are treated by *desensitization*, the injection at intervals of just suballergic doses of the allergen. There are two likely explanations for the mechanism of desensitization. Treatment could induce an IgG response that competes with IgE for the allergen; or desensitization could induce specific T_S cells that suppress the synthesis of IgE directed against the allergen. Receptor blockade with *monovalent, nonmetabolizable* antigens may prove to be another approach to desensitization. This approach would prevent expression of an existing allergy by inactivating IgE-mast cell complexes, and would prevent further production of IgE antibodies by blockading B_ε cells.

2-15   The predilection for some immunologic diseases is genetically linked to the MHC

A.   The finding that human leukocyte antigens (HLA) are important in tissue transplantation (Essential Concept 2-11) stimulated widespread investigation into the numbers and genetic relationships of these antigens. As previously explained, the MHC which codes for these antigens was found to be highly polymorphic. It was observed that certain MHC determinants occurred with high frequencies in association with certain diseases. Table 2-3 lists diseases that show significant associations with particular MHC determinants. Although this list is based on recent evidence and therefore is certainly incomplete, it indicates that immunopathological injury plays an important role in many diseases.

B.   It is not yet known which of the diseases in Table 2-3 are associated with Ir determinants, which with the human equivalent of D and K

Table 2–3

Examples of associations between particular diseases and the MHC in humans

Disease	Linked MHC determinant (region)	Disease risk of persons who bear determinant (relative to disease risk in the population at large = 1)	Description of disease
Inflammatory diseases:			
Ankylosing spondylitis	W27 (HLA-B)	100–200	Inflammation of the spine, leading to stiffening of vertebral joints
Reiter's syndrome	W27 (HLA-B)	40	Inflammation of the spine, prostate, and parts of the eye (the uvea, which is the iris, the ciliary body, and the choroid)
Acute anterior uveitis	W27 (HLA-B)	30	Inflammation of the iris and ciliary body
Juvenile rheumatoid arthritis (Type II)	W27 (HLA-B)	10–12	A multisystem inflammatory disease of children characterized by joint disease, fever, and rapid onset
Psoriasis	A13 (HLA-B)	4–5	An acute, recurrent, localized inflammatory disease of the skin (usually scalp, elbows, knees), often associated with arthritis.
Celiac disease	A8 (HLA-B)	9–10	A chronic inflammatory disease of the small intestine; probably a food allergy to gluten, a protein in grains
Multiple sclerosis	LD7a (HLA-D)	5	A progressive chronic inflammatory disease of brain and spinal cord that causes hardening (sclerosis) and loss of function in affected foci
Allergy:			
Ragweed hayfever	Many loci; direct linkage shown in family studies	difficult to calculate	An IgE-mediated allergic response to ragweed extracts
Endocrine diseases:			
Addison's disease	A8 (HLA-B)	4	A deficiency in production of adrenal gland cortical hormones
Diabetes mellitus (Juvenile)	A8, W15 (HLA-B) LD8a, LDW15a (HLA-D)	2–5	A deficiency of insulin production; pancreatic islet β cells usually absent or damaged
Graves' disease	LD8a (HLA-D)	10–12	A hyperactivity of the thyroid; patients often produce an IgG antibody that stimulates thyroid function (LATS: long-acting thyroid stimulator)
Malignant diseases:			
Acute lymphocytic leukemia	A2 (HLA-A)	1.2–1.4	A cancer of lymphocytes, usually in children, and usually of the T-lymphocyte series
Hodgkin's disease	A1 (HLA-A)	1.5–1.8	A cancer of lymph node cells; local inflammation is prominent, as well as selective deficiency in cellular immunity and T-cell functions

determinants, and which with closely linked determinants that are neither Ir- or D/K-like. Knowledge of these specific associations undoubtedly will influence investigation into the etiology of the corresponding diseases.

    1.   Diseases associated with I-region determinants could involve too little or too much of an immune response to a particular antigen. If such diseases are found, an understanding of their etiology may depend upon a resolution of the cellular and molecular basis of Ir gene action (Essential Concept 1–11).

    2.   Diseases associated with D/K determinants could involve any of several phenomena. A particular MHC determinant could be the target of an autiommune response, induced in one of the ways outlined in Essential Concept 2–9. T-cell-associated recognition (Essential Concept 1–13) of a particular MHC determinant could be unusual, resulting in an inappropriately high or low response to cells that bear associated antigens. MHC structures could serve as sites for attachment and entry of potentially pathogenic viruses. If the MHC is important for nonimmunologic cell interactions during development, then some MHC determinants might cause inappropriate development.

    Conceivably some of the extensive polymorphism of MHC determinants could be the result of their associations with diseases, which constitute a powerful selective force in evolution.

C.   Medical practice and research have given us a well-defined taxonomy of diseases, with detailed phenomenological descriptions of each disease. In contrast, most nonhuman animal diseases have received little or no study. Thus it is likely that the function and significance of the MHC genes will be elucidated at least partly from clues provided by investigation of human disease.

Appendix: Techniques for Immunoassay and Immunodiagnosis

A2–1 Antigen–antibody reactions can be measured by the formation of insoluble complexes

A.   Precipitation of antigen-antibody complexes from solution (the *precipitin* reaction) can be used to estimate the amount of antigen or antibody in a test sample. Multivalent antigens may interact with multivalent antibodies to form large insoluble lattices (Figure 2–15a) or small soluble complexes (Figure 2–15b,c). When large antigen–anti-

(a)

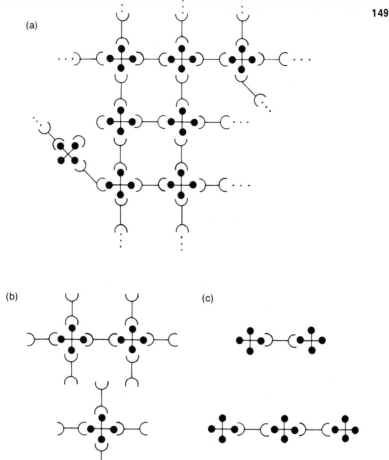

(b)

(c)

Figure 2–15 Complexes of antibody with antigen. Antigenic determinants are represented as solid circles and the antibody binding sites that recognize them as open semicircles. (a) Lattice formulation near the equivalence point. (b) Soluble complexes in the presence of excess antibody. (c) Soluble complexes in the presence of excess antigen. [Adapted from I. Roitt, *Essential Immunology,* 2nd ed., Blackwell, London, 1974, p. 6]

body complexes precipitate out of solution, the amount of antigen and antibody precipitated can be measured.

    1. Complexes precipitate most completely at roughly equal concentrations of antigen and antibody. Excess antibody allows single antigen molecules to be coated by several antibodies, and thus prevents lattice formation (Figure 2–15b). Excess antigen causes saturation of all antibody combining sites with different antigen molecules, again preventing lattice formation (Figure 2–15c). In the precipitin assay a fixed quantity of antiserum is reacted with increasing concentrations of antigen, and the amounts of antibody or antigen in the precipitate are measured either

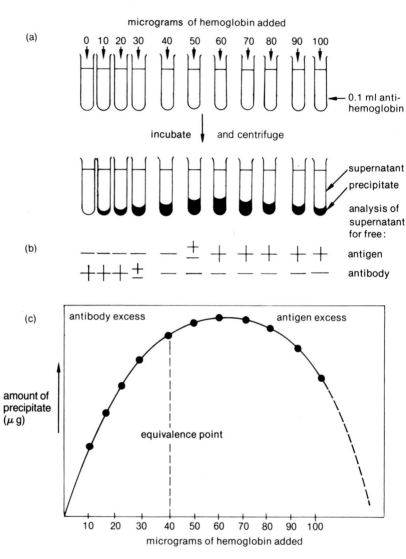

Figure 2-16 A precipitin curve for the reaction of hemoglobin with anti-hemoglobin. (a) Mixing of 0.1-ml aliquots of anti-hemoglobin with increasing amounts of hemoglobin. (b) Separation of immune precipitate and supernatant fraction by centrifugation. (c) Precipitin curve plot as amount of precipitate versus amount of antigen added. See text for details. [Adapted from I. Roitt, *Essential Immunology*, 2nd ed., Blackwell, London, 1974, p. 5]

chemically, by various assays for protein or carbohydrate, radio-chemically, if either reactant is labeled with a radioisotope, or biologically, if the antigen exhibits, for example, a toxic or enzymatic activity that can be measured in the soluble fraction before and after precipitation.

2.   Figure 2–16 shows a typical *precipitin curve* that might be obtained with standard solutions of antigen and antibody. In the example shown, 0.1-ml samples of antihemoglobin antiserum are added to increasing amounts of pure hemoglobin in a series of tubes (Figure 2–16a). These mixtures are incubated, and the resulting precipitates are collected by centrifugation and assayed. The supernatant fractions are assayed for presence of residual antibody and antigen (Figure 2–16b). The amounts of precipitates then are plotted against the amounts of antigen added (Figure 2–16c). The tube in which neither antigen nor antibody is found in the supernatant fraction defines the *equivalence point* of the precipitin curve. This point generally does not correspond to the point of maximum precipitation, which usually occurs at a slight weight excess of antigen.

Once such a standard curve is prepared, precipitin assays can be used to estimate amounts of the antigen in test samples of unknown concentration. Using the standard antiserum in this example, equivalence will be reached when the test sample added contains 40 μg of hemoglobin. Similar assays may be used to compare other serum samples to the standard antiserum; if dilutions of a test serum are added to tubes that each contain 40 μg of hemoglobin, the equivalence point will define the dilution of test serum in which the antibody concentration is the same as in the standard serum.

B.   Antigen–antibody precipitates also can be conveniently formed and observed by allowing one reactant to diffuse into a gelatinous medium, such as agar, that contains the other. In the widely used *Ouchterlony double-diffusion* technique, antigen and antibody samples are placed in small wells cut into an agar slab. The molecules of each diffuse out of their respective wells into the agar at a rate inversely proportional to their molecular weights, if the molecules have no affinity for the agar itself. If an antigen reacts with an antibody, then a line of precipitation (*precipitin* line) will form where the two reactants diffuse together.

1.   A diagram of such a test is shown in Figure 2–17. The antibody is a rabbit antibody against the κ light chain of mouse immuno-globulin. The κ light chain is a common element of the three immunoglobulin classes IgG, IgA, and IgM (Essential Concept 3–2). IgG and IgM, with molecular weights of 160,000 and 900,000,

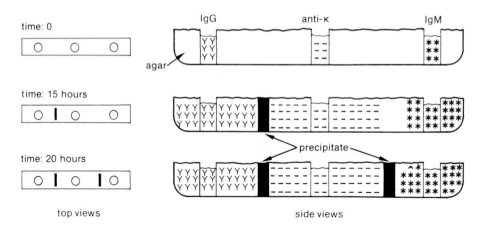

Figure 2–17 Ouchterlony double diffusion in an agar slab. The center well contains antibody against mouse κ chains. The outer wells contain IgM and IgG as antigens, both of which have κ chains which will complex with the antibody. See text for details.

respectively, are used as test antigens in the experiment. The IgG and the anti-κ antibodies diffuse toward one another at equal rates and form a precipitate near the point at which the antibody and IgG fronts meet. The anti-κ front continues to diffuse and a second precipitate forms when the anti-κ antibody meets the more slowly diffusing IgM.

2. If serial dilutions of an antigen, for example IgG, are tested against anti-κ antibody in this system, the distance between the antigen well and the precipitin line will vary with antigen concentration. Because the diffusion gradient of anti-κ is constant, the location of the precipitin line will be determined by the diffusion gradient of the antigen, which will depend upon its concentration in the well. Accordingly, this assay can be used to compare antigen concentrations in different samples.

3. The Ouchterlony technique can be used to determine whether two antigens are different or identical, or whether they share some but not all antigenic determinants. Three such experiments are shown in Figure 2–18.

In Experiment (a) anti-κ antibody forms a single continuous precipitin line equidistant from both antigen wells, thereby showing that the two antigen samples cannot be distinguished by this antiserum. This result is called a *reaction of identity*.

In Experiment (b) the antibody well contains a mixture of antibodies against IgG heavy chains (anti-γ) and IgM heavy chains (anti-μ). Because anti-μ precipitates IgM but not IgG, the anti-

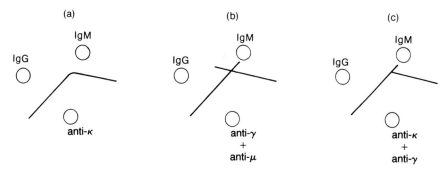

Figure 2–18 An Ouchterlony double diffusion analysis of related antigens. (a) Reaction of identity. (b) Reaction of nonidentity. (c) Reaction of partial identity (see text for details).

bodies migrate through the IgG precipitin line and precipitate IgM on the other side. The reverse is true for the anti-γ antibodies, which precipitate IgG but not IgM. The resulting pattern of crossed precipitin lines indicates that the antibody recognizes different determinants on the two antigens. This result is termed a *reaction of nonidentity*.

In Experiment (c) the antibody well contains a mixture of anti-κ and anti-γ antibodies. The anti-κ precipitates both IgG and IgM, forming a continuous precipitin line. The anti-γ, however, migrates through the IgM zone to precipitate IgG behind it, thereby forming a spur. This result indicates that the antibody recognizes determinants in the left antigen well that are not present in the right well. This result is termed a *reaction of partial identity*.

C.   The related technique of *immunoelectrophoresis* provides improved resolution for complex samples by combining electrophoresis of antigens in one dimension with subsequent double diffusion of antibodies and separated antigens in a second dimension. The experimental system is diagrammed in Figure 2–19. In this example the mixture of antigens to be analyzed is a whole serum.

   1.   Separation of serum components by gel electrophoresis alone is shown in Figure 2–19a. A serum sample is placed in the well near one end of a suitably buffered gel slab, and an electrical current is applied across the gel. The various serum components migrate through the gel at rates proportional to their charge/mass ratios. Four major classes of proteins are resolved as distinct components: albumins migrate most rapidly, followed by α-, β-, and γ-globulins. The amount of protein at each point in the gel can be determined by staining and measurement of light absorption (Figure 2–19b). All immunoglobulins are found in the γ- or β-globulin fractions.

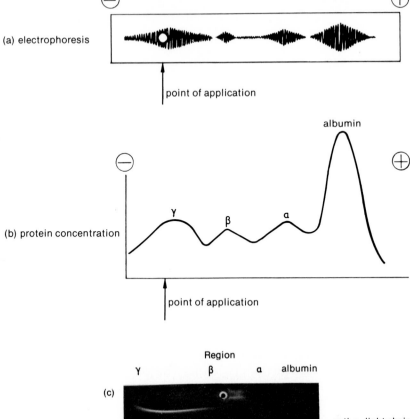

(a) electrophoresis

point of application

albumin

(b) protein concentration

γ

β

α

point of application

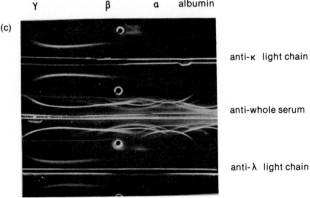

Region

γ   β   α   albumin

(c)

anti-κ light chain

anti-whole serum

anti-λ light chain

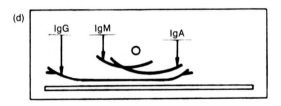

(d)

IgG   IgM   IgA

← **Figure 2–19** Immunoelectrophoresis in an agar slab. (a) A protein sample is placed in a hole in an agarose gel, and is placed in an electric field. The relative migration of various proteins is illustrated. (b) A quantitative assessment of the amount of protein that migrates across the gel. Four categories of proteins are noted: albumin, α-globulins, β-globulins, and γ-globulins. Most antibodies are γ-globulins. (c) Following electrophoresis, antibodies to serum protein are placed in the horizontal slot, and the antibodies and separated serum protein antigens diffuse toward each other to form precipitin lines. Anti-whole serum, placed in the center slot, forms a large number of precipitin lines with various serum components. Anti-κ serum, placed in the top slot, reveals only γ-globulins that contain κ light chains. Notice that only a single line is formed, demonstrating complete absorption of anti-κ by the first immunoglobulin it meets. Anti-λ serum, placed in the bottom slot, detects γ-globulins that contain λ chains. (d) An idealized anti-whole serum pattern, showing the relative positions of IgG, IgM, and IgA.

2. An immunoelectrophoresis experiment is illustrated in Figure 2–19c. Four samples of serum are placed in wells near the left side of a large gel slab and are subjected to electrophoresis in parallel. Slots then are cut into the gel parallel to the direction of electrophoresis and filled with various test antibody preparations. The antibodies and the separated antigenic components diffuse toward each other through the gel and form precipitin lines that indicate which of the antigenic serum components are reactive with the various antibodies. An idealized drawing of the precipitin lines that would be obtained with IgM, IgG, and IgA as antigens with anti-whole serum antibody is shown in Figure 2–19d. The analysis of such patterns is considered further in Problem 3–5.

D. Antigen-antibody complex formation can be measured by quantitatively precipitating immunoglobulins under conditions that will not precipitate free antigen, and then determining the amount of bound antigen in the precipitate.

1. The *Farr assay* employs 50% ammonium sulfate, which precipitates most immunoglobulins but not haptens and many proteins. Figure 2–20a shows the results of a typical Farr assay with antiserum against the hapten *digoxin,* a drug that commonly is used to regulate the heart action of cardiac disease patients. For convenience the hapten is labeled radioactively. Tests with a constant amount of the hapten in increasing dilutions of antiserum define the antibody concentration sufficient to precipitate 50% of the hapten under these conditions. Once such a standard curve is available, it can be used to compare the anti-digoxin antibody titer of other serum samples relative to that of the standard.

Precipitation also can be carried out with an immunoglobulin-specific antibody from another species (*heterologous anti-immu-*

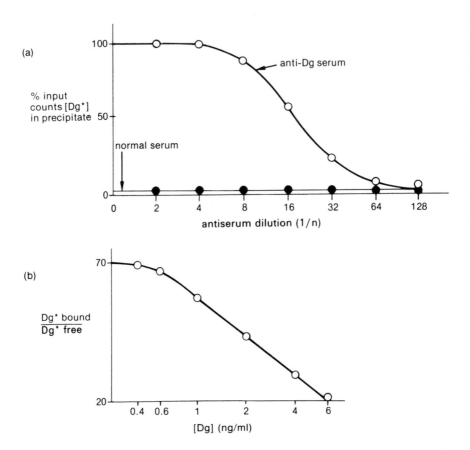

Figure 2–20 (a) The measurement of antibody–hapten complex formation using the Farr assay. A standard amount of labeled digoxin (Dg*) is added to each of a series of two-fold dilutions of anti-digoxin antiserum. After several hours, free antibody and antibody–hapten complex are precipitated by bringing the solution to 50% saturation with ammonium sulfate. The percentage of radioactivity in the precipitate then is plotted against serum dilution. (b) A competitive radioimmunoassay using the Farr technique. The serum dilution that gives approximately 70% precipitation in (a) is added to a series of tubes that contain the standard amount of labeled digoxin and varying concentrations (0.4 to 6 ng/ml) of unlabeled digoxin. A standard curve is prepared by plotting the ratio of bound to free labeled digoxin against nanograms of unlabeled digoxin added. This standard curve then can be used to determine the concentration of unlabeled digoxin in samples of patient's serum. Current radioimmunoassays for digoxin take advantage of the fact that dextran-coated charcoal particles will bind free but not antibody-bound digoxin.

noglobulin). For example, if the specific antibody used for antigen–antibody complex formation is from a rabbit, it can be precipitated by a goat antibody specific for rabbit immunoglobulin, added at a concentration that gives maximum precipitation.

2. The preceding techniques also can be used to measure competitive binding for *quantitative radioimmunoassay* of a known antigen in the presence of many other components. An example is the clinically important method used to monitor serum levels of digoxin. Monitoring is crucial because the drug is highly toxic at levels not far above the therapeutic serum concentration. For the assay, radiolabeled digoxin is incubated with sufficient digoxin-specific antibody to precipitate 70–90% of the radioactivity in the Farr assay. A standard curve then is prepared by adding known amounts of unlabeled digoxin to the incubation mixture and measuring the decrease of radioactivity in the precipitate due to competition between labeled and unlabeled antigen for the antibody binding sites (Figure 2–20b). Samples of serum from patients receiving digoxin then can be added to the assay mixture, and their digoxin content can be estimated from the observed decrease in bound radioactivity, using the standard curve.

3. Immunoprecipitation can be used not only analytically, but also as a highly specific preparative technique. Antibody specific for one component in a complex mixture can be used to precipitate the component either directly, using ammonium sulfate, or indirectly, using an appropriate heterologous anti-immunoglobulin. The purified component then can be eluted from the precipitate, often by treatment with a competing hapten, a protein denaturant, or a buffer of low pH.

A2–2 The strength of interaction between antigens and antibodies can be measured

A. The affinity of antibody binding sites for cognate monovalent antigens can vary widely. Binding can be described by Equation A2–1,

$$\text{Ag} + \text{Ab} \underset{k_2}{\overset{k_1}{\rightleftharpoons}} \text{Ag–Ab} \qquad \text{(A2–1)}$$

in which Ag, Ab, and Ag–Ab represent unbound antigenic determinants, antibody-binding sites, and bound antigenic determinants, respectively, and k_1 and k_2 are rate constants for the association and dissociation reactions, respectively. The antigen–antibody *affinity* in such a reaction can be measured as the ratio of complexed to free reactants at

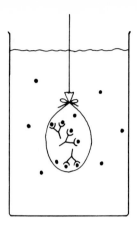

Figure 2-21 Equilibrium dialysis. A concentrated solution of antibodies ( ) against a hapten (•) is placed in a sac of dialysis tubing, which is permeable to the hapten but not to the antibodies, and the sac is suspended in a known volume of hapten solution. When the system reaches equilibrium, the concentration of free hapten will be the same throughout, but the sac will contain bound hapten as well. The difference in total hapten concentration inside and outside the sac can be measured and used to calculate the average affinity of the antibodies for the hapten (see text).

equilibrium. The affinity constant, K, is defined by Equation A2-2,

$$K = \frac{[\text{Ag-Ab}]}{[\text{Ag}]\,[\text{Ab}]} \qquad (A2-2)$$

K also is equal to k_1/k_2. Because K is an *association* constant, its value will be high for high-affinity complexes and low for low-affinity complexes. Typical K values vary from 10^5 to 10^{11} liters per mole.

1. Like any equilibrium constant, K is related to the standard free energy change of the binding reaction at pH 7 ($\Delta G_0'$) in kilocalories per mole, by Equation A2-3,

$$\Delta G_0' = RT \ln K \qquad (A2-3)$$

in which R is the gas constant (0.00198 kilocalorie per mole per degree) and T is the absolute temperature, 298°K.

2. The affinity of an antibody binding site for a monovalent hapten can be measured by *equilibrium dialysis* (Figure 2-21). A concentrated solution of antibody in a dialysis sac, which is permeable to hapten but not to antibodies, is placed in a known volume of buffer that contains hapten at a concentration in the range of $1/K$. At equilibrium, the concentrations of bound plus free hapten inside the sac [I] and free hapten outside the sac [O] will depend upon the concentration and average affinity of the antibodies inside the sac.

Using equilibrium dialysis, one can determine both the average association constant, K, and the antibody valence, n, from the relationship described by Equation A2–4,

$$\frac{r}{c} = Kn - Kr \qquad\qquad (A2\text{–}4)$$

in which r is the ratio of moles of hapten bound per mole of antibody and c is the concentration of unbound hapten ($= [O]$). The moles of hapten bound are determined by subtracting $[O]$ from $[I]$. Since Kn is a constant, a plot of r/c versus r for different hapten concentrations will approximate a straight line with slope $-K$, so that the association constant K can be determined as the negative of the slope, and the antibody valence as the r intercept at infinite hapten concentration.

B.   Binding of antibody to a typical multivalent antigen is not as easily defined as binding to a monovalent hapten. Because several different affinities may be involved, the term avidity is used to designate the strength of multivalent antigen binding. The kinetics of such binding are complex, because binding of one antigenic determinant affects the rates of binding of others on the same molecule. The net avidity of an antibody–multivalent antigen interaction is a complex function of the valences of both reactants and the affinities of the various determinants involved.

A2–3   Binding of antibodies to cell-surface antigens can be detected in several ways

A.   Cells can be agglutinated by cross-linking with antibodies. Cell agglutination is the basis for several widely used assays.

    1.   An agglutination assay is used commonly for the typing of human blood. Human red blood cells may carry the cell-surface antigens A and B, which define the well-known blood groups, AB, A, B, and O (Essential Concept 4–2). If, for example, antibody specific for blood group A antigens is reacted with red cells that carry Group A antigens, the resulting agglutination visibly alters the normal settling pattern of the cells in a test tube or in a well of a test tray (Figure 2–22). If the cells do not carry Group A antigens, then no agglutination is observed. Type A and type B blood cells are identified as being agglutinated only by specific anti-A- and anti-B-antibodies, respectively. Type AB cells are agglutinated by both specific antibodies, and type O cells by neither. Thus all four blood types can be identified by these simple tests. Knowledge of blood types allows transfusions to be made only with serologically compatible blood, thereby avoiding induction of agglutinating antibodies in the recipient.

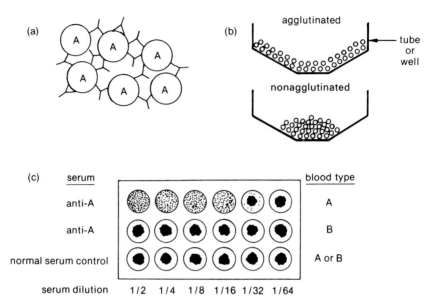

Figure 2–22 The red-cell agglutination assay for typing of human blood groups. (a) At the microscopic level, divalent anti-A antibodies cross-link red cells that carry A antigen to form a lattice of agglutinated cells. (b) Agglutination affects the settling pattern of cells in a test tube or in the well of a test tray. (c) This effect can be exploited to type blood cells for A antigen using a tray test with several dilutions of anti-A serum.

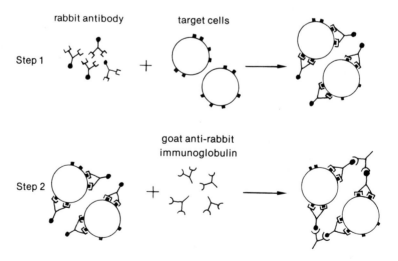

Figure 2–23 The use of a heterologous anti-immunoglobulin to agglutinate cells complexed with a non-agglutinating antibody. Some antibodies that bind to the cell surface are ineffective in promoting agglutination (Step 1). If antibodies directed against the first antibodies then are added to the system, agglutination occurs (Step 2). This technique, called the Coombs test, often is used in clinical laboratories to detect cell-surface antigens.

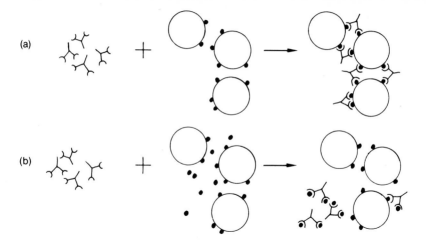

Figure 2–24 Competitive inhibition between cell-bound and free antigens. (a) Cells are agglutinated by antibodies against a cell-bound antigen. (b) Cells are not agglutinated when competing free antigen is present.

2. The cell-agglutination technique can be used to assay antibodies specific for antigens that either are normally present on a cell surface or can be coupled artificially to a cell surface. Coupling can be accomplished by treating red cells to promote electrostatic binding of proteins to their surfaces, or by chemically cross-linking antigens to red cells. Appropriate dilutions of the unknown antibody sample are incubated with the antigen-bearing test cells, and the antibody concentration (titer) is determined by comparing the resulting agglutination responses to those obtained with a standard antibody sample of known titer.

3. The sensitivity of the agglutination reaction with antibody can be increased markedly by incubation with a heterologous anti-immunoglobulin. This technique, known as the Coombs test, is particularly useful when agglutination by the first test antibody is inefficient; nonagglutinated cells that have bound the first antibody will be agglutinated by the second (Figure 2–23).

4. Competitive inhibition of cell-agglutination reactions can be used to assay free antigens identical to those on the surface of a target cell. For example, if an agglutination reaction is set up with an amount of antibody just sufficient to agglutinate visibly, then minute amounts of competing free antigen in test samples can be detected by preincubating with the antibody and then testing for inhibition of agglutination (Figure 2–24).

B. Cells that carry antibodies bound to cell-surface antigens may be lysed by complement. The ability of the terminal steps in the complement sequence (Essential Concept 1–9C) to lyse target cells is the basis for a number of widely used assays for antigen–antibody reactions. Guinea pig serum is a commonly used source of complement.

1. Complement-mediated lysis of target cells, usually red blood cells, can be measured in a variety of ways. Lysis can be followed directly by decrease in optical density of a cell suspension, or by release of cell components that normally are confined internally, such as hemoglobin, enzymes, or a previously introduced isotope such as ^{51}Cr. Alternatively, loss of membrane integrity can be followed by failure to exclude vital dyes such as trypan blue or eosin, or by failure to concentrate compounds such as fluorescein diacetate that are converted to fluorescent derivatives (fluorescein in this example) by intracellular enzymes.

2. Complement-mediated lysis can be used as an assay for humoral antibodies specific for antigens on the surface of target cells. As in the agglutination assays, these antigens either may be intrinsic membrane components or may be coupled artificially to target cells. In the assay, a sample to be tested for antibody is incubated with antigen-bearing target cells; complement then is added, and cell lysis or membrane disruption is measured (Figure 2–25, Step 1). If antibody is limiting, the degree of lysis will be a function of the sample's antibody concentration, which can be determined by comparison with a previously prepared standard curve that indicates degree of lysis as a function of known antibody concentration.

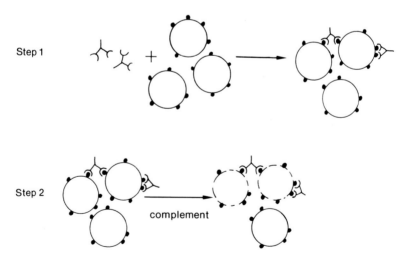

Step 1

Step 2

complement

Figure 2–25 Complement-mediated cell lysis as an assay for antibody binding to cell-surface antigens. Target cells are preincubated with limiting amounts of antibody (Step 1) and then treated with complement (Step 2), which lyses only cells to which antibody has bound.

The foregoing procedure can detect only antibodies of the complement-activating classes of immunoglobulins: IgM and most IgG subclasses. Nonactivating antibodies can be detected by including an additional step. Following incubation with the test antibody sample, the cells are further incubated with a heterologous anti-immunoglobulin of a complement-activating class prior to addition of complement. Cell-bound test antibodies will in turn bind the heterologous anti-immunoglobulin to produce complexes that will trigger complement-mediated cell lysis (Figure 2–25, Step 2).

3. Complement-mediated lysis also can be used as an assay for lymphoid cells that produce antibodies specific to a cell-surface antigen (the *Jerne plaque assay*). An excess of red blood cells bearing the target antigen is mixed with a suspension of the lymphoid cells to be assayed, plated as a monolayer on a suitable surface, and incubated to allow plasma cells to release their immunoglobulins (Figure 2–26a). The monolayer then is overlaid with complement, which creates a zone of red cell lysis (plaque) around any plasma cell that has secreted specific antibody (Figure 2–26b,c). The number of antibody-producing cells in the suspension thus will be indicated by the number of plaques observed in the monolayer. Cells producing antibodies that do not activate complement also can be assayed, by treating the monolayer of red cells and lymphoid cells with an appropriate heterologous anti-immunoglobulin prior to addition of complement. Specificity of the assay may be validated by demonstrating that preincubation of the lymphoid cell suspension with a free form of the target antigen prevents subsequent plaque formation, and relative estimates of antigen–antibody avidity may be obtained by adding varying amounts of a competing soluble antigen to the test dish.

4. Any complex of a soluble antigen with a complement-activating antibody can be assayed by the technique of *complement fixation*. This assay is based on the principle that complement that has been activated (fixed) by soluble antigen–antibody complexes will be unavailable for subsequent complement-mediated cell lysis. A limiting amount of complement, known to cause lysis of a certain number of red blood cells treated with anti-red-blood-cell antibody, is incubated with the test antigen and a sample of the antibody preparation to be assayed. The mixture then is added to a suspension of antibody-treated red blood cells, and its capacity to cause lysis is assayed. Given appropriate controls to show that the test antigen alone does not affect complement activity, reduced red blood cell lysis indicates the presence of antibody specific for test antigen in the sample assayed (Figure 2–27). The titer of this antibody can

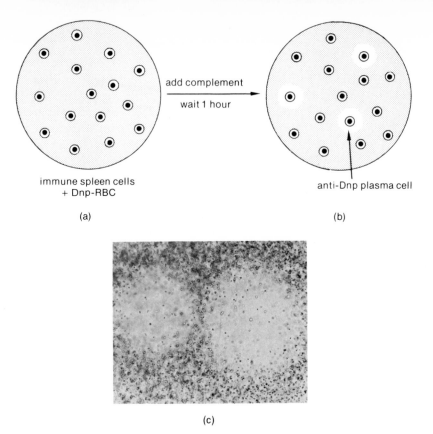

immune spleen cells
+ Dnp-RBC

add complement

wait 1 hour

anti-Dnp plasma cell

(a)

(b)

(c)

Figure 2–26 The Jerne plaque assay for antibody-producing cells. In the example shown, spleen cells from a mouse immunized with Dnp coupled to a carrier protein are mixed with melted agar and enough red blood cells bearing coupled Dnp groups to give a continuous lawn of cells when poured onto an agar plate. Anti-Dnp-specific plasma cells among the spleen cells continue to produce anti-Dnp antibodies, which bind to surrounding red blood cells (a). When complement is added, these cells lyse to form a plaque, which indicates the presence of an anti-Dnp-specific plasma cell (b). A photomicrograph of two plaques is shown in (c). The assay provides a convenient method for quantitating the antigen-specific plasma cells produced in an immune response.

be determined quantitatively by comparison with an appropriate standard curve prepared using specific antibody of known titer.

5.   An important clinical procedure is the assay of complement levels in human serum by determining the ability of serum samples to mediate lysis of red blood cells treated with specific antibodies. A sudden drop in serum complement activity usually indicates complement activation *in vivo,* presumably as the result of antigen–antibody reactions. In patients with some immunological diseases, a fall in complement activity usually heralds an immunologic crisis.

C.   Cellular antigens can be detected directly using specific antibodies with attached fluorescent, radioactive, enzymatic, or electron-opaque markers. This approach is valuable both for determining the locations of antigenic structural components in basic research on cell and tissue ultrastructure, and for identifying characteristic disease-related antigens in clinical diagnosis.

  1. Fluorescent compounds (fluorochromes), such as fluorescein and rhodamine, can be coupled chemically to antibodies without affecting antigen binding. When activated by illumination with light of an appropriate wavelength, the antibody-bound fluorochrome absorbs light energy, attains an excited state, and then returns to its ground state by emitting light at a characteristic longer wavelength. Fluorescein is excited at 490 nm and emits at 517 nm to give a yellow-green fluorescence. Rhodamine is excited at 515 nm and emits at 546 nm to give a red fluorescence. A fluorescence microscope equipped with the appropriate excitatory light source and filters allows visualization of

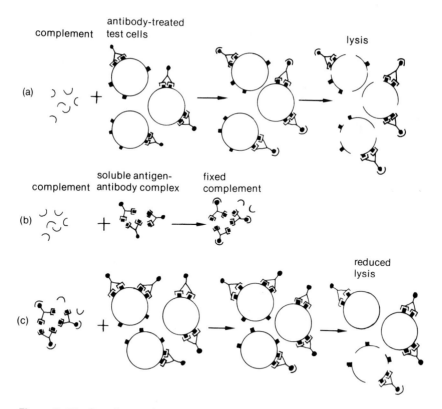

Figure 2–27 Complement fixation by soluble antigen–antibody complexes. (a) Complement lyses antibody-treated test cells. (b) Complement preincubated with soluble antigen–antibody complexes binds to the complexes. (c) Fewer complement molecules are available in the preincubated preparation to lyse antibody-treated test cells.

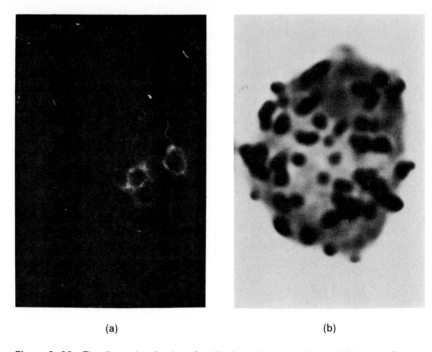

(a)   (b)

Figure 2–28   The direct visualization of antibody–antigen complexes. (a) Immunofluorescence identification of T lymphocytes in a lymph node B-cell region. [Photograph by G. Gutman.] (b) Autoradiography of a lymphocyte with ^{125}I-bound antibody. [Photograph by G. Edelman.]

fluorochrome-labeled antibodies bound specifically to cells and tissues (Figure 2–28a). The presence of two different antigens can be monitored simultaneously using two specific antibodies labeled with fluorochromes that fluoresce at different wavelengths. This technique may be used in urgent diagnosis of pathogenic organisms from an infected focus.

2.   Antibodies also can be labeled radioisotopically without destroying their abilities to bind antigen. A common technique is chemical- or enzyme-catalyzed iodination of tyrosine side chains on the antibody molecule, using either of two radioactive isotopes of iodine, ^{125}I or ^{131}I. Both these isotopes are γ-emitters, whose presence can be detected in a gamma counter. Both isotopes also emit short-range ionizing particles (Auger electrons and β particles, respectively) which can be detected photographically by *radioautography*, taking advantage of the capacity of the emitted ionizing radiation to expose a photographic emulsion locally. If antigen-bearing cells are exposed to a specific labeled antibody and then washed to remove unbound molecules, gamma counting allows precise quantitation of the amount of antibody

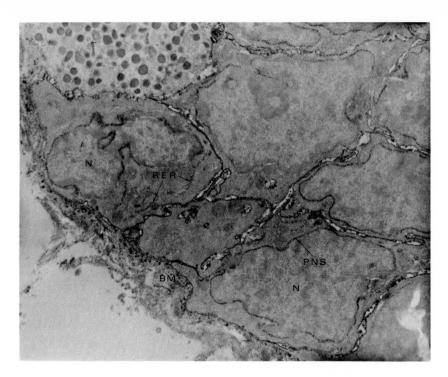

Figure 2–29 Horseradish peroxidase-coupled antibody to human secretory component (SC) reveals the subcellular locations of SC molecules to be the perinuclear space (PNS), the plasma membrane, and the rough endoplasmic reticulum (RER) of human small intestinal epithelial cells (N, nucleus; BM, basement membrane). [Courtesy of W. R. Brown, Y. Isobe, and P. Nakane.]

taken up by the cell population. Radioautography provides additional information. If the treated cells are spread on a suitable surface, covered with a photographic emulsion, and stored in the dark to allow exposure to the emitted ionizing radiation, then silver grains will appear on the developed film as an "autograph" that indicates the locations of bound antibodies. In this manner the distribution and number of antibody molecules bound to individual cells in the population can be determined (Figure 2–28b). The same technique can be used to determine the locations of specific antigenic structures in a tissue.

3. Enzymes that catalyze the formation of a microscopically visible product can be coupled to antibodies using bifunctional cross-linking reagents, without destroying the activity of the enzyme or the antibody. For example, horseradish peroxidase coupled to a specific antibody and bound to a specific cell or tissue site will convert added hydrogen peroxide to oxygen free radicals. These radicals in turn react with a chromogenic precursor (3, 3′-diaminobenzidine or 4-chloro-1-naphthol) to form an insoluble colored precipitate (Figure 2–29).

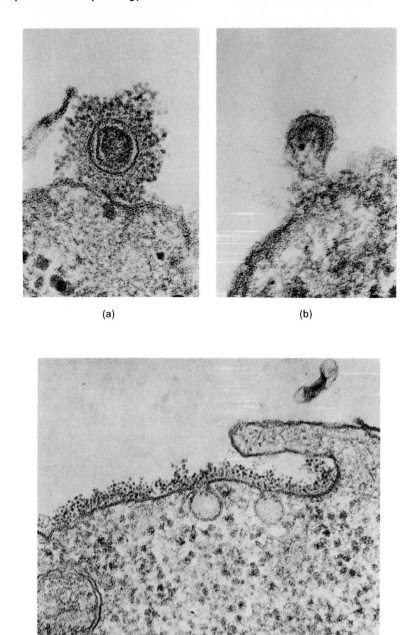

(a)   (b)

(c)

Figure 2–30 Ferritin-coupled antibody to mouse leukemia virus antigens is used to demonstrate that (a) a mouse virus carries these antigens; (b) a cat virus does not; (c) these antigens may be expressed on regions of a cell membrane. [From L. Oshiro, J. A. Levy, J. L. Riggs, and E. H. Lennette, *J. Gen. Virol.* **35,** 317 (1977). © 1977 by Cambridge University Press.]

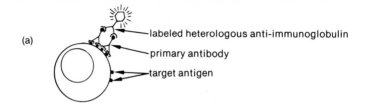

(a)
- labeled heterologous anti-immunoglobulin
- primary antibody
- target antigen

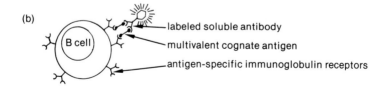

(b)
B cell
- labeled soluble antibody
- multivalent cognate antigen
- antigen-specific immunoglobulin receptors

Figure 2–31 Extension of immunolabeling techniques by (a) the indirect method, and (b) the sandwich method.

4. Antibodies can be made visible in the electron microscope by coupling to electron-dense or morphologically distinguishable particles. Antibodies coupled to ferritin, an iron storage protein from spleen that consists of a protein shell with a ferric hydroxide core, are seen in the electron microscope as small dense spots (Figure 2–30). Antibodies also can be linked to hemocyanin, a large oxygen-carrying protein complex from crustacean hemolymph, to latex microspheres, or to small viruses, all of which can be visualized by their characteristic morphology in electron micrographs.

5. Each of the preceding four techniques can be extended by a modification called the *indirect method,* which allows detection of unlabeled antibodies bound to a specific antigen by subsequent reaction with a labeled heterologous anti-immunoglobulin (Figure 2–31a). Another modification, called the *sandwich method,* can be used to detect a specific antibody on the surface of plasma cells by incubating them first with a cognate multivalent antigen, and then with labeled soluble antibody specific for the same antigen (Figure 2–31b).

Selected Bibliography

Textbooks for detailed reading

Freedman, S. O., and Gold, P., *Clinical Immunology,* 2nd ed., Harper and Row, Hagerstown, Md., 1976.

Fudenberg, H. H., Stites, D. P., Caldwell, J. L., and Wells, J. V., *Basic and Clinical Immunology,* Lange Medical Publications, Los Altos, Calif., 1976.

Sell, S., *Immunology, Immunopathology, and Immunity*, 2nd ed., Harper and Row, Hagerstown, Md., 1975. Clinical immunology and immunopathology are rapidly becoming independent disciplines. Each of the above texts covers these expanding fields in extensive clinical and histopathologic detail. These texts are useful as well-written, current reference books, and are probably most valuable for students of clinical medicine and practicing physicians.

Host defense mechanisms and phagocytosis

Davis, B. D., Dulbecco, R., Eisen, H. N., Ginsberg, H. S., and Wood, W. B., Jr., *Microbiology* (Chapter 22), Harper and Row, Hagerstown, Md., 1973. The classic view of host defense mechanisms at several levels.

Mortensen, R. F., Osmand, A. P., Lint, T. F., and Gewurz, H., "Interaction of C-reactive protein with lymphocytes and monocytes: complement-dependent adherence and phagocytosis," *J. Immunol.* **117,** 774 (1976). C-reactive protein is an important example of a nonspecific host defense that interacts with the specific immune system. This reference is the most recent in an impressive series by these authors.

Newhouse, M., Sanchis, J., and Bienenstock, J., "Lung defense mechanisms," *N. Eng. J. Med.* **295,** 990, 1045 (1976). The lung as a model for detailed examination of specific and nonspecific host defense mechanisms.

Stossel, T. P., "Phagocytosis," *N. Eng. J. Med.* **390,** 717, 774, 833 (1974). Normal and abnormal phagocytosis, with a special emphasis on human disorders.

Immunological deficiency diseases

Cooper, M. D., Faulk, W. P., Fudenberg, H. H., Good, R. A., Hitzig, W., Kunkel, H. G., Roitt, I. M., Rosen, F. M., Seligmann, M., Soothill, J. F., and Wedgewood, R. J., "Second international workshop on primary immunodeficiency diseases in man," *Clin. Immunol. Immunopathol.* **2,** 416 (1974). A compendium of current dogma, as delivered by a World Health Organization panel.

Fuks, Z., Strober, S., and Kaplan, H. S., "Interaction between serum factors and T lymphocytes in Hodgkin's disease," *N. Eng. J. Med.* **295,** 1273 (1976). An example of how modern cellular immunology has revealed specific mechanisms of immunodeficiency in adults.

Geha, R. S., Shneeberger, E., Merler, E., and Rosen, F., "Heterogeneity of 'acquired' or common variable agammaglobulinemia," *N. Eng. J. Med.* **295,** 1273 (1976).

Good, R. A., Varco, R. L., Aust, J. B., and Zak, J., "Transplantation studies in patients with agammaglobulinemia," *Ann. N. Y. Acad. Sci.* **64,** 882 (1957). (See Porter for description.)

Hitzig, W. H., "Congenital immunodeficiency diseases: pathophysiology, clinical appearance and treatment," *Pathobiol. Annu.* **6,** 163 (1976). A recent review, focusing on clinical manifestations.

Porter, H. M., "The demonstration of delayed-type reactivity in congenital agammaglobulinemia," *Ibid.* **64,** 932 (1957). An early view of the immune defect in agammaglobulinemia.

Strober, S., "T and B cells in immunological diseases," *Am. J. Clin. Pathol.* **68** Suppl. 671 (1977). A recent review on human lymphocyte subpopulations in health and disease.

Zuckerman, S. H., and Douglas, S. D., "The lymphocyte membrane: markers, receptors, and determinants," *Pathobiol. Annu.* **6,** 119 (1976).

Autoimmunity

Burnet, F. M., *Autoimmunity and Autoimmune Disease,* F. A. Davis, Phila., 1972. A scholarly and speculative approach to the problem of autoimmunity.

Lindstrom, J. M., Engel, A. G., Seybold, M. E., Lennon, V. A., and Lamberg, E. H., "Pathological mechanisms in experimental autoimmune myasthenia gravis," *J. Exp. Med.* **144,** 739 (1976). An exciting new line of investigation for an old and well-documented disease.

Louis, J. A., and Weigle, W. O., "A model of immunologic unresponsiveness and its relevance to autoimmunity," *Pathobiol. Annu.* **6,** 259 (1976). The latest in a series of perceptive experiments and hypotheses by Weigle on the mechanisms involved in self-nonself discrimination.

Möller, G., (Ed.), "Autoimmunity and self-nonself discrimination," *Transplant Rev.* **31** (1976). Animal and cellular models of autoimmunity and regulation of the immune response are discussed in 13 excellent short reviews.

T-cell immunity and transplantation

Bach, F. H., and van Rood, J. J., "The major histocompatibility complex—genetics and biology," *N. Eng. J. Med.* **295,** 806–892, 927 (1976). A major review of current knowledge of the genetics of transplantation.

Billingham, R., and Silvers, W., *The Immunobiology of Transplantation,* Prentice-Hall Inc., Englewood Cliffs, N.J., 1971. A short, lucid presentation of the biological basis of tissue and organ transplantation.

Immune-complex disease and antibody-mediated immunological injury

Cochrane, C. G., and Koffler, D., "Immune-complex disease in experimental animals and man," *Adv. Immunol.* **16,** 185 (1973).

Dixon, F. J. (Eds. Good, R. A., and Fisher, D. W.), *Immunobiology* (Chapter 22, Mechanisms of immunologic injury), Sinauer Associates, Inc., Stamford, Conn., 1971. Two articles on the biological aspects of antibody mediated, complement-dependent immunological injury.

Marx, J. L., "Autoimmune disease: new evidence about lupus," *Science* 192, 1089 (1976). Current research in autoimmunity, as described by a lay science writer.

Pisciotta, A. V., "Drug-induced leukopenia and aplastic anemia," *Clin. Pharmacol. and Ther.* **12,** 13 (1976). The larger problem of drug-induced damage of the hematopoietic system is considered in this article, placing in context those reactions which appear to be antibody-mediated.

Wilson, C. B., and Dixon, F. J., "Immunopathology and glomerulonephritis," *Ann. Rev. Med.* **25,** 83 (1974).

IgE-mediated clinical allergy

McDevitt, H. O., "Genetic considerations in atopic and other dermatologic conditions," *J. Invest. Dermatol.* **67,** 320 (1976). A thorough consideration of the basis for and implications of HLA-linked allergic disorders. Included is a general discussion of HLA-linked diseases.

Norman, P. S., "The clinical significance of IgE," *Hospital Practice* **8,** 41 (August 1975). A current view of the molecules, cells, and mediators responsible for allergy.

Appendix references

Berson, S. A., and Yalow, R. S. (Eds. Good, R. A., and Fisher, D. W.), *Immunobiology* (Chapter 30, Radioimmunoassay: a status report), Sinauer Associates, Inc., Stamford, Conn., 1971. A clear, simple exposition of the principles and practice of radioimmunoassay by its developers.

Eisen, H. N., *Immunology*, Harper and Row, Hagerstown, Md., 1974. Although a general text, it is still the clearest explanation of antigen-antibody interactions.

Garvey, J. S., Cremer, N. E., and Sussdorf, D. H., *Methods in Immunology* (3rd ed.), Addison-Wesley, Reading, Mass., 1977. A methodology text which is usable by amateurs. This is the third edition of a classic "cookbook" for immunology.

Hijmans, W., and Schaeffer, M. (Eds.), "Fifth international conference on immunofluorescence and related staining techniques," *Ann. N.Y. Acad. Sci.* **254** (1975). Proceedings of a conference which ranges widely over the techniques and applications of visual techniques for detecting "marked" antibodies.

Kabat, E. A., *Structural Concepts in Immunology and Immunochemistry* (2nd ed.), Holt, Rinehart, and Winston, New York, 1978. A thorough monograph for advanced students.

Problems

2-1   Indicate whether each of the following statements is true or false. Explain the error in each statement you consider to be false.

(a)   Chronic granulomatous disease is a phagocytic cell dysfunction caused by defective membrane receptors for IgG and IgM Fc regions.

(b)   Recurrent pneumonia in patients with *cystic fibrosis* (a disease in which thickened mucous secretions prevent normal mucous flow) is a good example of failure of innate immunity mechanisms.

(c)   The blood of children with Bruton's disease (X-linked agammaglobulinemia) usually lacks mature B cells.

(d)   Antagonists of mast-cell degranulation can inhibit the development of kidney disease in systemic lupus erythematosis (SLE).

(e)   T cells first appear in humans prior to the sixth month of gestation.

(f)   Contact sensitivity is a skin reaction that can be transferred passively with reaginic (IgE) antibody.

(g)   Evidence that structural genes for immunoglobulin H chains are on the X chromosome was first demonstrated by the genetic analysis of Bruton's disease.

(h)   Lymphocytic choriomeningitis virus is nonlethal in thymus-deprived hosts.

(i)   The immunopathological injury formerly associated with rabies virus vaccination involved the activation of an autoimmune process.

(j)   The activating agent in (i) was a passenger virus present in the primary host cells.

(k)   The effector cells in (i) were in the T-cell series.

(l)   Clinically, patients treated with antilymphocyte serum (ALS) would be expected to show a rapid decrease in circulating long-lived antibodies: for example, antibodies to polio virus.

(m)   Patients who lack the enzyme adenosine deaminase have a selective deficit in development of plasma cells (plasmacytopoiesis).

(n)   The most common cause of immunological deficiency in man is medical care.

(o)   The predisposition for ankylosing spondylitis is genetically linked to the major blood-group-antigen locus, ABO.

2-2   Supply the missing word or words in each of the following statements.

(a)   The lack of an appropriate immune response to infection in the case of severe combined immunodeficiency is due to the failure in development of _____ and _____ cells.

(b)   Rheumatoid arthritis is associated with serum antibodies, usually of the _____ class, which react against _____.

(c)   Patients with hayfever have abnormal concentrations of _____ antibodies, which, upon combination with their cognate antigen, activate _____.

(d)   Linear deposition of antigen–antibody complexes on the glomerular basement membrane is detected by fluorescent anti-IgG antibody in _____.

(e)   Patients with the disease described in (d) may have such patterns also in basement membranes of _____.

(f)   As a pharmacologist, you wish to prepare a cytotoxic agent to be used as a preventative for people with bee sting sensitivity. The purpose of your agent will be to eliminate _____ cells.

(g)   Hyperacute rejection of organ allografts involves infiltration of _____.

(h)   _____ is a disease of complement regulation. The disease involves recurrent, local episodes of acute inflammation, which may be fatal when they affect the larynx.

(i)   Patients with _____ have disorders of balance and movement as well as immune deficiency.

(j)   Rheumatic fever is an example of autoimmune disease induced by _____.

(k)   Skin lesions caused by poison oak involve an immune hypersensitivity of the _____ system.

(l)   Patients who develop progressive vaccinia viral infections following vaccination for smallpox most likely suffer from a disease that affects _____ lymphocytes.

(m)   C3 deficiency results in a decreased resistance to _____ infections.

(n)   Systemic lupus erythematosis results in immunological injury to several organs because of the production of _____.

(o)   Systemic anaphylaxis is a life-threatening consequence of immune hypersensitivity, and should be treated with _____ and _____.

(p)   _____ are generally oily substances that serve as tissue depots and otherwise nonspecifically stimulate the immune response when injected with immunizing antigens.

2-3   Proteins, although highly immunogenic, also are highly complex and difficult to purify without modern chromatographic techniques. Pioneering immunologists, who needed well-defined antigens to study the nature

Table 2–4
Precipitin reactions of anti-glucoglobulin antiserum (Problem 2–3)

Concentration of antibodies	Hapten–carrier antigen		
	Glucoglobulin (horse)	Gluco+albumin (egg)	Galacto+albumin (egg)
1:1000	++±	++	–
1:5000	++++	++++	–
1:10,000	++++	++++	–
1:20,000	+++±	+++	–
1:40,000	+++	+	–
1:50,000	+	±	–
1:100,000	±	–	–

[From O. Avery and W. Goebel, *J. Exp. Med.* **50,** 531 (1930). © 1930 by the Rockefeller University Press.]

of antigen–antibody interactions, turned to hapten–carrier conjugates that elicit antibody specific for determinants on both the carrier and the hapten. By attaching the same hapten to several noncross-reactive carriers, one can study the interaction of antibodies with determinants of known conformation.

In one experiment, glucose and galactose were used as haptens. Derivatives of each were coupled to horse globulin or egg albumin. Rabbits were immunized with the glucoglobulin conjugate. The resulting antiserum was tested for its ability to precipitate various conjugates, as given in Table 2–4. In this semi-quantitative assay, the results are recorded as either −, +, ++, +++, or ++++ (− indicating no reaction, ++++ indicating the greatest antigen–antibody precipitate). Although inexact, this system is surprisingly reproducible in the hands of a careful immunologist, and the difference between ++ and ++++ reactions is significant.

(a)   How do glucose and galactose differ in their chemical structures? What, then, does Table 2–4 show about the specificity of the antibodies?

(b)   If free glucose is added to the rabbit antiserum, no precipitate forms. How could you determine experimentally whether the glucose binds to the antibodies? Why is there no precipitate when glucose is added?

(c)   Assume that a specific site on the antibody molecule combines with a specific complementary determinant on the antigen. What are the limits on the number of combining sites per antibody molecule, or determinants per antigen, if a precipitation reaction is to occur?

(d)   In Table 2–4, the amount of precipitate increases with increasing antibody concentration, but suddenly decreases significantly when the 1:1000 dilution of antibody is tested. Can you suggest an explanation for a decrease in the total precipitate when the concentration of antibody is high?

(e)   Assume that you are working in an isolated community hospital. The clinical chemistry lab informs you that it can no longer make chemical analyses of blood sugar, while on the other phone the emergency room assistant tells you that three diabetics found at home in coma are about to arrive. You must determine whether the diabetics are in coma because of too much insulin (low blood glucose) or too little insulin (high blood glucose and acids). You have available only glucose and the reagents defined in Table 2–4. What can you do?

(f)   How could you proceed if you had radiolabeled glucose?

2–4   Figure 2–32 illustrates a technique known as rocket electrophoresis, in which antigen migrates under the influence of an electric field into a gel that contains antibody. Explain why the positions of precipitin lines vary with antigen concentration as shown in the figure.

2–5   Suppose that an animal is immunized with bovine serum albumin to which 2,4-dinitrophenol has been conjugated (Dnp–BSA). Immune serum is obtained and placed in the center well of an Ouchterlony plate, with antigens in the outer wells as shown in Figure 2–33. Explain the precipitin pattern obtained.

2–6   Suppose that as a physician you carry out the following experiments. You isolate a substance, called Z, from the plasma of a patient with a particular disease. You prepare an antiserum to Z (anti-Z) by injecting the substance repeatedly into a rabbit. You isolate similar substances— call them W, X, and Y—from three other patients suspected of having a disease similar to that of the patient from whom Z was prepared. You prepare an Ouchterlony plate and place the anti-Z antibody in

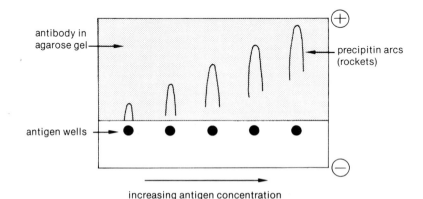

Figure 2–32 Rocket electrophoresis (Problem 2–4). Antigen migrates electrophoretically into a gel that contains antibody. The distance from the starting well to the front of the rocket-shaped arc is a function of antigen concentration. [Adapted from I. Roitt, *Essential Immunology,* 2nd ed., Blackwell, London (1974), p. 105.]

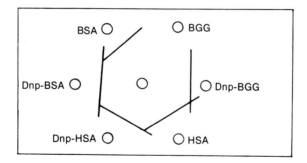

Figure 2–33 The precipitin pattern in an Ouchterlony test (Problem 2–5). BSA, bovine serum albumin; BGG, bovine gamma globulin; HSA, human serum albumin; Dnp–BSA, Dnp–BGG, and Dnp–HSA designate the same proteins carrying covalently linked haptenic dinitrophenyl groups. The center well contains anti-Dnp–BSA.

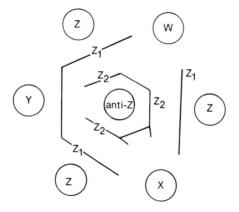

Figure 2–34 The precipitin pattern in an Ouchterlony test (Problem 2–6).

the center well. You arrange antigen preparations W, X, Y, and Z in the antigen wells, as shown in Figure 2–34.

(a) What is the minimum number of antigens present in Z?

(b) How similar are these antigens? Compare preparations W, X, and Y to preparation Z in detail.

(c) Would you conclude that your patients have similar diseases?

2–7 A serum sample is taken from an individual who has just recovered from an unknown disease. This serum neither agglutinates nor precipitates a suspension of bacteria thought to cause the disease or a suspension of membrane fragments from these bacteria. When passively immunized with a transfusion of this serum, patients suffering from this disease recover much more rapidly than those who receive no treatment.

(a) How could you show that immunoglobulins, and not some other serum proteins, are responsible for the therapeutic effect of the serum? (b)   How could you determine whether the immunoglobulins in the serum bind to the bacteria thought to cause the disease?

2–8   A clinical investigator and colleagues at the National Institutes of Health studied several patients with common variable hypogammaglobulinemia. These patients presented an intriguing contrast to autoimmune patients. They had greatly reduced levels of serum immunoglobulins (less than 2 mg/ml IgG compared to about 12 mg/ml normally, and less than 0.1 mg/ml IgM plus IgA compared to 4–5 mg/ml normally), but they had variable numbers of Ig+ B cells, ranging from normal to significantly

Table 2–5
Effects of pokeweed mitogen (PWM) on immunoglobulin biosynthesis by peripheral blood lymphocytes from normal and hypogammaglobulinemic individuals (Problem 2–8)

	IgG[a]	IgA[a]	IgM[a]
Control individuals:			
without PWM	212	303	537
with PWM	1641	1698	3715
Hypogammaglobulinemia patients:			
with or without PWM	<100	<100	<100

[a]Expressed as geometric mean immunoglobulin synthesis in nanograms for seven-day culture of 2×10^6 lymphocytes.
[Adapted from T. Waldmann, et al., Lancet **2,** 609 (1974).]

Table 2–6
Immunoglobulin synthesis by normal lymphocytes co-cultured with lymphocytes from Patient 2 with common variable hypogammaglobulinemia (Problem 2–8)

	IgG		IgA		IgM	
	Amount[a]	% inhi-bition	Amount[a]	% inhi-bition	Amount[a]	% inhi-bition
Normal A alone	1640		640		2860	
Patient 2 alone	0		0		26	
Co-culture 2 + A	0	100	14	98	400	86
Normal B alone	1920		2120		11200	
Patient 2 alone	0		12		0	
Co-culture 2 + B	60	97	80	96	0	100
Normal C alone	1120		760		4600	
Patient 2 alone	0		12		0	
Co-culture 2 + C	70	94	130	83	448	90

[a]Expressed as ng synthesized per culture in the presence of pokeweed mitogen during a seven-day period.
[From T. Waldmann, et al., Lancet **2,** 609 (1974).]

reduced. The patients ranged in age from 16–54 years. The clinical investigation team isolated peripheral blood lymphocytes from each patient and cultured them *in vitro* for seven days in the presence of pokeweed mitogen, which is active on human B cells. The amount of immunoglobulin secreted was measured by sensitive radioimmunoassays. Table 2–5 summarizes data from normal control individuals and from the patients. Table 2–6 shows the results when lymphocytes from one patient were cultured together with lymphocytes from three different normal individuals.

(a)   What do you conclude from these data?

(b)   The clinical investigation team then treated some lymphocytes from Patient 2 with an anti-immunoglobulin antiserum plus complement and cultured the remaining cells with normal lymphocytes. The results were equivalent to those shown in Table 2–6. What do you conclude from this observation?

(c)   Cells from five patients inhibited over 85% of the immunoglobulin production in mixed cultures. However, cells from three other patients with common variable hypogammaglobulinemia had no inhibitory effects whatsoever. Briefly outline the life history of B cells from stem cells to secreting plasma cells, and indicate each major point at which development might be blocked.

2–9   Consider the following series of experiments on graft transplantation among mice from four inbred strains (A/J, BALB/c, C57BL, and SJL). Skin was grafted from A/J female mice onto A/J, BALB/c, and C57BL females, and the results shown in Table 2–7a were obtained. Six weeks later some of the original mice received another skin graft, and the results shown in Table 2–7b were obtained. The remainder of the mice that had received the first skin grafts from A/J donors were sacrificed. The serum from the BALB/c mice was pooled, as were the cells. The effect of immune cells was studied by giving new BALB/c mice skin grafts with or without immune BALB/c cells injected intravenously three days before grafting (Table 2–7c). The effect of immune serum injected intravenously also was studied (Table 2–7d).

(a)   Is graft rejection an immune phenomenon? What would be the evidence for such an assertion?

(b)   Is graft rejection mediated by the cellular, or the humoral, system? What is the evidence for your choice?

(c)   Briefly outline an experiment that independently would support your answer to Part (b).

(d)   Does serum from immune mice strengthen, or weaken, the immune response? Suggest an explanation for the serum-transfer results in Table 2–7d.

(e)   How does the host's immune system distinguish foreign grafts from syngeneic grafts?

Table 2–7
Skin-graft experiments (Problem 2–9)

(a) The survival of skin grafts from donor A/J females to other inbred mice

Recipient	Number of grafts	Number of rejections	Mean survival time of graft
A/J	20	0	—
BALB/c	40	40	14 days
C57BL	40	40	11 days

(b) The survival of second grafts in inbred mice

Skin-graft donor	Skin-graft recipient	Number of grafts	Number of rejections	Mean survival time of graft
A/J	A/J	10	0	—
A/J	BALB/c	10	10	8 days
A/J	C57BL	10	10	8 days
SJL	A/J	10	10	11 days
SJL	BALB/c	10	10	11 days
SJL	C57BL	10	10	11 days

(c) The effect of injected immune cells upon graft rejection

Skin-graft donor	Skin-graft recipient	Cells	Number of grafts	Number of rejections	Mean survival time of graft
BALB/c	BALB/c	—	5	0	—
A/J	BALB/c	—	5	5	14 days
A/J	BALB/c	+	5	5	8 days
SJL	BALB/c	+	5	5	14 days

(d) The effect of injected immune serum on graft rejection

Skin-graft donor	Skin-graft recipient	Serum injected	Number of grafts	Number of rejections	Mean survival time of graft
A/J	BALB/c	—	10	10	14 days
A/J	BALB/c	+	10	10	17 days
SJL	BALB/c	+	10	10	14 days

2–10 A variety of pathologic conditions can cause extensive kidney damage, often leading to irreversible renal failure. Until recently, little could be done in such cases. At best, a patient's blood could be filtered mechanically by hemodialysis from time to time. In the 1960's, however, development of kidney transplantation greatly improved the quality of life for many such patients. Figure 2–35 shows the survival rates of transplanted kidneys taken from various sources.
(a)   What general pattern do you perceive? Why should kidneys from unrelated individuals fare so poorly?
(b)   Would you expect the immune system to detect or react against

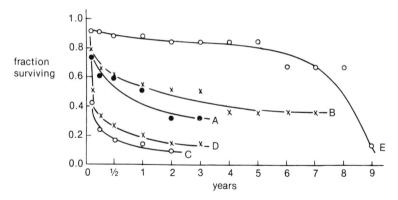

Figure 2–35 Survival data for renal transplants in humans based on 672 primary transplants (Problem 2–10). A, parental donor; B, sibling donor; C unrelated donor; D, cadaver donor; E, monozygotic twin donor. [From B. A. Barnes, *Transplantation* **3**, 812 (1965). © 1965 by The Williams & Wilkins Co., Baltimore.]

variants of cytoplasmic or nuclear constituents? Where must variants be located to be detected?

(c)   Actually, in most of the cases represented in Figure 2–35, the transplant recipient also received immunosuppressive drugs (such as corticosteroids). What do you think Curves C and D would have looked like if the patients had not received this treatment? Curve E? What are the dangers inherent in prolonged treatment with immunosuppressive drugs?

2–11   Organ transplantation among humans has required the use of immunosuppressants to block the graft-rejection process. Some immunosuppressants act primarily as inhibitors of cell division (e.g., antimetabolites that are analogues of the nucleotide bases); others act primarily by destroying lymphocytes (lymphocytolytic agents such as the adrenal steroids); and others are both lymphocytolytic and antiproliferative (e.g., x rays and DNA alkylating agents). Immunosuppression also can be achieved with antilymphocyte serum (ALS). Each of these immunosuppressants lacks one critical feature that the ideal immunosuppressant should have. What is this feature?

2–12   A colleague of yours proposes to treat a 45-year-old patient who requires a kidney transplant by whole body irradiation, replacement of his hematolymphoid system cells with marrow cells from the patient's 22-year-old son, and then transplantation of a kidney to the patient from his son, who has agreed to the operation. Your colleague reasons that the operation should succeed for his human patient as it has been shown to succeed in inbred mice that receive transplants from an F_1 offspring (Figure 2–7). Would you advise him to proceed with the operation or not? Give your argument.

2-13   Suppose that you are a young transplant surgeon repaying your medical
school loans by two years of medical service in an isolated community
hospital that lacks a doctor as well as money and transportation facilities.
You soon find that, due to inbreeding, the community has a high incidence
of congenital renal failure, and that the resulting childhood mortality
approaches 10% of individuals up to age 21. To counteract the high
mortality rate the average family has 12 children; thus most mothers
are highly multiparous (have had multiple pregnancies). You decide
to treat the disease by transplanting kidneys from normal children to
their defective siblings.

(a)   You know that the major human transplantation (HLA) antigens can be defined by agglutination of human leukocytes using serum
from multiparous women, who have become immune to paternal HLA
antigens. This test can be adapted to determine identity or nonidentity
of the paternally inherited HLA haplotype among sibling children. Mixed
lymphocyte reactions (MLR) between siblings can be used as a further
test of HLA identity. How would you apply these tests and interpret
the results to most efficiently identify the best donor sibling for a
diseased child?

(b)   Having defined the best match, you now seek an immunosuppressant. Lacking money and transportation facilities, you remove the thymus
from a young patient who has just died, mash it up, and inject it
into a horse to make anti-T-cell serum (ALS). Two weeks later, the
horse serum will agglutinate thymocytes at serum dilutions of up to
1:10,000. You transplant a kidney into your first recipient and inject
5 ml of the ALS. Within 6 hours the patient's red blood cell (RBC)
count falls from 5×10^6 RBC/mm^3 of blood to 1.5×10^6 RBC/mm^3.
What has happened, and what should you do?

(c)   Following a blood transfusion, the patient develops an infection
of *Staphylococcus albus* at the surgical incision site. Knowing that
S. albus usually is nonpathogenic, you check the differential white
blood count, and find that the patient's total leukocyte count has fallen
from 10,000 cells/mm^3 to <100 cells/mm^3. What has happened now?

(d)   Following appropriate therapy, the patient heals at the incision
site, but by two days post transplant it is clear that the transplanted
kidney is failing. You do a kidney biopsy, and see an infiltration of
the glomeruli by polymorphonuclear leukocytes (PMN's). What would
be the most likely cause of PMN infiltration? How could you make
the correct diagnosis?

(e)   Treatment of the kidney biopsy as suggested in the answer to
Part (d) reveals unbroken green lines outlining the glomerular tufts.
Why is the kidney failing? Assuming that another matched sibling is
available for a second transplant, what could you do to improve the
chances of success?

(f)   After you finally have made successful transplants in a few children, a smallpox infection threatens the community, and you find that no one has been vaccinated. Should you vaccinate everyone in the town?

2–14   Muscles are stimulated to contract when the nerve endings at neuro-muscular junctions release acetylcholine (ACh). This transmitter binds to acetylcholine receptor (AChR) proteins in muscle cell membranes to depolarize the membrane and initiate muscular contractions. A group of clinical researchers injected rats with from 1.1 to 350 picomoles of purified electric eel AChR protein suspended in complete Freund's adjuvant (see Problem 1–9). This immunization elicited a set of physical symptoms that included weight loss, generalized muscular weakness, a characteristic hunched posture with chin and elbows on the floor, and jerky movements of the head and forelimbs when attempting ambulation. The animals were graded, as shown in Table 2–8, on the following simple scale: 0, no definite weakness; +, weak grip with fatigability; ++, hunched posture with head down, movements uncoor-dinated; +++, severe generalized weakness, no grip, tremulous, mori-bund. Figure 2–36 shows a rabbit injected with AChR before (left) and after (right) reversal of neuromuscular blockade by a drug that markedly increases ACh levels.
(a)   Can you explain all the symptoms (including weight loss) by a single underlying cause?
(b)   What further studies could you do on the sera of these rats to test your explanation?

Table 2–8
A syndrome in rats after a single challenge with eel AChR (Problem 2–14)

Dose (pico-moles)	Number of animals with the syndrome			Maximum severity[c]		
	Total[a]	Early[b]	Late[b]	+	++	+++
350	21/23	21	15	2	2	17
110	10/10	9	9	0	2	8
55	2/2	2	2	0	1	1
35	8/9	6	6	1	1	6
11	6/11	5	4	3	2	1
3.5	7/9	6	4	2	5	0
1.1	0/10	0	0	0	0	0
0	0/10	0	0	0	0	0

[a]Number with syndrome/number injected.
[b]Rats were observed for up to 80 days. Early: before Day 16; late: generally after Day 20.
[c]See text.
[From V. A. Lennon, J. M. Lindstrom, and M. E. Seybold, *J. Exp. Med.* **141**, 1365 (1975). © 1975 by the Rockefeller University Press.]

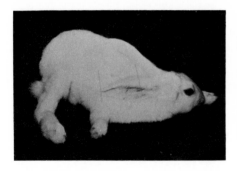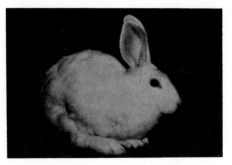

Figure 2–36   The effect of acetylcholinesterase inhibitors on paralysis (Problem 2–14). The left photograph shows a rabbit 5 days after the third injection of acetylcholine receptor. The right photograph shows the same animal one minute after receiving 0.3 mg of edrophonium intravenously. [From J. Patrick and J. Lindstrom, *Science* **180**, 871, (1973). Copyright 1973 by the American Association for the Advancement of Science.]

(c)   The adjuvant was absolutely required to induce the clinical syndrome. Can you suggest a reasonable explanation for this requirement?
(d)   Thymectomized rats do not develop this syndrome. In view of this finding, what models would you propose to explain the results of AChR immunization?
(e)   A human disease called *myasthenia gravis* is characterized by weakness and fatigability of voluntary skeletal muscles, particularly of the head, neck, upper limbs, and respiratory apparatus. The number of acetylcholine binding sites is reduced in biopsied nerve-muscle junctions in these patients. Furthermore, immunosuppressive therapy often is beneficial to these patients. What do you infer from these data? Might this disease have an autoimmune etiology? What further studies would you carry out to test this possibility?
(f)   Serum or purified immunoglobulins from myasthenia gravis patients and controls were added to purified AChR, and ^{125}I-labeled α-bungarotoxin (a molecule that binds specifically to AChR) was added to assay availability of binding sites. The results are shown in Table 2–9. What conclusions can you draw from these data?
(g)   Blood lymphocytes from myasthenia gravis patients and controls were incubated with purified AChR (or with medium alone) for five days, and then tested for AChR-stimulated DNA synthesis by measuring the incorporation of ^{3}H-thymidine into cellular DNA. The ratio of $\dfrac{\text{cpm (AChR)}}{\text{cpm (medium)}}$ is termed the stimulation index for a population of lymphocytes, and usually a stimulation index of >2 is significant. It is assumed that only T cells from immune hosts respond. The data are presented in Figures 2–37 and 2–38. What conclusions can be drawn from these data? Give three hypotheses to explain why these patients

Table 2–9

Serum and IgG from myasthenia gravis patients and controls assayed for ability to inhibit binding of ^{125}I-labeled bungarotoxin to extracted muscle AChR (Problem 2–14)

Patient	Tensilon test[a]	Binding of ^{125}I-bungarotoxin to AChR preincubated with:	
		Serum[b]	IgG[b]
J.F.	+	0.56 ± 0.06	0.56 ± 0.06
C.S.	+	0.97 ± 0.006	1.01 ± 0.06
D.S.	+	0.57 ± 0.06	0.58 ± 0.03
B.J.	+	1.03 ± 0.01	1.02 ± 0.11
R.Y.	−	0.75 ± 0.04	0.88
Controls		1.00 ± 0.03	1.00 ± 0.03

[a]+ indicates transient disappearance of muscle weakness following injection of Tensilon, a drug that increases ACh levels.
[b]Mean ± standard deviation (when more than one determination is made), normalized to mean of control values.
[From R. Almon, C. Andrew, and S. Appel, *Science* **186,** 55 (1975). Copyright 1975 by the American Association for the Advancement of Science.]

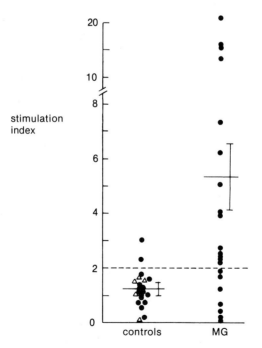

Figure 2–37 Stimulation indexes in response to acetylcholine receptor in 21 controls and 21 patients with myasthenia gravis (MG) [Problem 2–14] The triangles represent controls with an unrelated muscular disorder (amyotrophic lateral sclerosis). The mean and standard error of the mean are indicated for the two populations. Stimulation-index values greater than 2.0 are considered positive responses. [From D. P. Richman, J. Patrick, and B. G. W. Arnason, *N. Eng. J. Med.* **294,** 694 (1976). Reprinted by permission from the *New England Journal of Medicine* **294,** 694 (1976).]

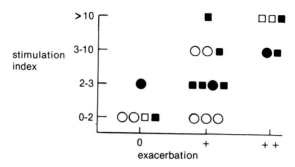

Figure 2–38 The cellular immune response to acetylcholine receptor in myasthenia gravis as a function of the activity of the disease (Problem 2–14). 0 represents stable disease, in an exacerbation serious enough to lead to hospitalization, and + + severe exacerbation requiring respiratory assistance. Squares denote males, and circles females; open symbols represent patients younger than, and closed symbols patients older than 50 years of age. [From D. P. Richman, J. Patrick, and B. G. W. Arnason, *N. Eng. J. Med.* **294,** 694 (1976). Reprinted by permission from the *New England Journal of Medicine* **294,** 694 (1976).]

may have a decreased frequency of ^{125}I-α-bungarotoxin muscle receptors.
(h)   Suppose that one could induce myasthenia gravis-like symptoms in mice by the injection of anti-AChR antibodies, and that the syndrome, although controllable with drugs, lasted at least several months. Could the syndrome be due to receptor blockade by injected antibodies?
(i)   Suppose that the mice in Part (h) gave data such as that described for humans in Parts (f) and (g). Propose several lines of *in vivo* and *in vitro* analysis by which you could elucidate the immunopathological mechanisms of this disease.

2-15   Your patient is a newborn child with multiple minor congenital anomalies involving the lips and ears. There is no history of congenital defects in two siblings. You incubate a cord blood sample with phytohemagglutinin for cytogenetic analysis, but obtain insufficient mitoses for analysis. The child begins to have tetanic seizures, although without evidence of intrauterine or postnatal infection. Blood analysis is unremarkable except for a low serum calcium, low white blood count, and an increased ratio of polymorphonuclear leukocytes to lymphocytes. Intravenous fluid and calcium relieve the tetany.
(a)   Do you expect to find any abnormalities in level or function of serum-IgA secretory component? If so, why?
(b)   A mild cold virus infection is endemic in the pediatric neonatology staff. Your patient develops a severe tracheobronchitis. You begin to suspect that fluid and calcium did not cure everything. You order a repeat cytogenetic analysis to confirm your suspicions. How should you order that the analysis be carried out?
(c)   You are required to do an emergency tracheostomy to save the infant's life. The tracheostomy is successful and you are about to suture the incision, when it occurs to you to remove a paratracheal lymph

node for biopsy. What might you expect to see in histological sections of this tissue?

(d)   What is your diagnosis and suggestion for therapy?

(e)   As a physician with a modern training in human genetics, what advice will you give to the parents regarding future pregnancies?

2–16   A high proportion of patients with *partial lipodystrophy* (symmetrical loss of fat from the face, arms, and trunk in a dermatomal distribution) suffer from a form of glomerulonephritis. Recently [*N. Eng. J. Med.* **294**, 461, 495 (1976)] a group of investigators from Hammersmith Hospital in London reported that these patients have normal serum levels of complement components 1 and 4, but abnormally low serum levels of C3; furthermore, C3 disappears rapidly upon injection into these patients. The relationship between the lipodystrophy and the glomerulonephritis is obscure. Biopsies of the kidney in these patients reveal granular deposits of C3 with no detectable immunoglobulin in the glomeruli.

(a)   What do you think is involved in activating and mediating the glomerulonephritis? Think in terms of causative processes, factors, and cells.

(b)   Can you think of a laboratory test that will confirm your activation hypothesis?

(c)   Would you classify this disease as an autoimmune disorder? As an immune hypersensitivity disease? As an allergic disorder?

2–17   Chronic arthritis may occur as a complication of intestinal-bypass surgery for morbid obesity. A recent report [*N. Eng. J. Med.* **294**, 121 (1976)] records an analysis of five arthritic postoperative patients. Their serum levels of complement components C3 and C4 were abnormally low, but they had no rheumatoid factor (IgM anti-IgG). Components of the alternate complement pathway were present in their serum in activated forms. In addition, they had circulating serum complexes containing IgM, IgG, C3, C4, and C5. The IgG antibody in these complexes was directed against bacteria that usually inhabit the gastrointestinal tract. The complexes were found in the serum preceding episodes of arthritis, but were absent after remission.

(a)   Propose a model for the pathogenesis of this disorder.

(b)   How would you propose to treat this disorder?

2–18   The patient is a 15-year-old boy with a lifelong history of diarrhea and gastrointestinal-tract infections with the fungus *Candida albicans*. *Candida albicans* usually is nonpathogenic, but in cases of immune deficiency, it becomes an opportunistic pathogen. This patient was sent to the clinical investigation team mentioned in Problem 2–8. Suspecting an immunologic deficiency disease, these investigators tested his levels of serum immunoglobulins, blood lymphocytes, and salivary IgA, with the results shown in Table 2–10.

Table 2–10

Levels of serum immunoglobulin, immunoglobulin-bearing lymphocytes, and salivary IgA in normal adults and a 15-year-old patient (Problem 2–18)

	Serum immunoglobulin (mg/ml)			Immunoglobulin-bearing blood lymphocytes (%[b])				Salivary IgA (mg/ml)
	IgG	IgM	IgA	IgG	IgA	IgM	IgD	IgA
Normal adults:								
mean	12.7	1.3	2.7	8.7	4.2	6.0	7.5	7.2
range[a]	(10–15)	(0.8–2.0)	(1.3–3.8)	(5.8–12.6)	(2.0–6.2)	(2.3–10.0)	(4.0–10.8)	(3.8–10.0)
Patient:								
Test 1[c]	11.3	1.2	1.2	8.0	13.0	8.0	14.0	0.2
Test 2[c]				11.0	10.8	13.0		
IgA-deficient patients:								
mean	—	—	—	—	—	—	—	0.3
range[a]	—	—	—	—	—	—	—	(0.1–0.4)

[a] Figures in parentheses represent mean ± standard deviation.
[b] Expressed as percent of total peripheral blood lymphocytes.
[c] Tests 1 and 2 represent two independent determinations on the patient.
[From D. P. Richman, J. Patrick, and B. G. W. Arnason, *N. Eng. J. Med.* **294**, 694 (1976). Reprinted by permission from the *New England Journal of Medicine* **294**, 694 (1976).]

Table 2–11

Salivary concentrations of free secretory component in normal controls, IgA-deficient patients, and the patient under study (Problem 2–18)

Individuals tested	Secretory component (µg/ml)
Normal controls:	
mean	220
± standard deviation	(40–400)
Patient	<10
IgA-deficient patients	170–>1000[a]

[a] Range observed among ten patients tested. Six of these patients showed > 1000 µg/ml.
[Data from W. Strober, R. Krakauer, H. L. Klaeveman, H. Y. Reynolds, and D. L. Nelson, *N. Eng. J. Med.* **294**, 351 (1976). Used by permission from the *New England Journal of Medicine* **294**, 351 (1976).]

(a) What do you conclude from these data?

(b) Propose a model for his disease, and a test to confirm or rule out your model.

(c) From the results of the test shown in Table 2–11, what do you conclude is the basic defect in this patient? Propose a therapy.

(d) The investigative team prescribed oral bovine colostrum, and the patient has been well and thriving since. How does this therapy work?

Answers

2-1 (a) False. In chronic granulomatous disease Fc receptors are intact; lysosomal enzyme functions are defective.
(b) True
(c) True
(d) False. SLE kidney disease is caused by complement-fixing immune complexes, not by the IgE system.
(e) True
(f) False. Contact sensitivity is a manifestation of cellular immunity.
(g) False. H-chain structural genes are not X-linked. Bruton's disease is an X-linked defect in the development of B cells.
(h) True
(i) True
(j) False. The activating agent was brain protein that bore cross-reacting antigens similar to those of human nervous tissue.
(k) True
(l) False. ALS affects circulating T cells predominantly, although it may affect circulating B cells if the serum is not completely specific due to improper absorption. ALS treatment does not remove long-lived antibodies.
(m) False. These patients have a combined T-cell and B-cell immune system defect.
(n) True
(o) False. It is linked to the human MHC, the HLA locus.

2-2 (a) T, B
(b) IgM, IgG immunoglobulins
(c) IgE, mast cells
(d) Goodpasture's syndrome
(e) pulmonary (lung) alveoli
(f) mast (or B_e)
(g) polymorphonuclear leukocytes
(h) Hereditary angioneurotic edema
(i) ataxia-telangiectasia
(j) cross-reacting antigen
(k) T-cell (or cellular-immunity)
(l) T
(m) bacterial
(n) immune complexes
(o) epinephrine, antihistamines
(p) Adjuvants

2-3 (a) Glucose and galactose are epimers, that is, stereoisomers that differ only in the orientation of the OH group on Carbon 4. The total lack of cross-reactivity illustrates the exquisite specificity of the immune response.
(b) You could show that radiolabeled glucose migrates with the antibody molecules through Sephadex columns or acrylamide gels, whereas radiolabeled galactose, the nonspecific hapten, does not. Essentially, each glucose molecule is a single antigenic determinant,

which can bind to a single antigen-binding site. Therefore, in the presence of glucose, no cross-linking can occur to form macromolecular aggregates or precipitates.

(c)   Both the antibodies and antigens must be at least bivalent for cross-linking and precipitation to occur. Even then, precipitation will not necessarily occur. There are certain so-called nonprecipitating antibodies, which for unknown reasons will not precipitate under any conditions. The IgM molecule has ten antigen-binding sites; IgA has two, four, or six antigen-binding sites; and all other immunoglobulins have two antigen-binding sites per molecule. There is no upper limit on the number of sites per antigenic molecule.

(d)   In a large excess of antigen, a high proportion of antigen molecules will have only one antibody molecule bound to them. Soluble antigen–antibody complexes are formed (Ag–Ab–Ag), rather than macromolecular aggregates. Consequently the total amount of precipitate decreases.

(e)   With the reagents in Table 2–4, you can set up a hapten-competition assay to measure free glucose concentrations, as follows. Using gluco-globulin at 1:20,000, find the highest dilution of antiserum that gives precipitation. Then add measured concentrations of glucose to tubes containing these concentrations of antigen and antiserum, and determine the concentrations of free glucose that reduce precipitation to +++, ++, +, and −. You now have a standard set of measurements, which you can compare with assays of patient serum and urine as sources of free glucose. You hope that the patients will still be alive by the time you get the results.

(f)   If you had radiolabeled glucose (and a counter for detecting it), you could determine glucose concentrations with a Farr assay, which is more rapid and more sensitive. You first would determine the concentration of antiserum that will coprecipitate 70% of added labeled glucose in the presence of 50% ammonium sulfate, and then would proceed with competition assays using standards and unknowns as in Part (e).

2–4   Precipitin lines will become visible only in a region of antigen–antibody equivalence. As each antigen sample electrophoretically migrates into the gel, it forms a gradient of decreasing antigen concentration from the sample well to the migrating front. The concentration near the front decreases as the front moves away from the well and the gradient becomes longer. Precipitin lines form at the point where the concentration at the front reaches the zone of equivalence. Because the antibody concentration is constant, this point will increase in distance from the well as antigen concentration in the well is increased. Ahead of the "rocket," antibody is in excess, and in its trail, antigen is in excess.

2–5   The antiserum contains antibodies directed against the antigenic determinants on the native BSA and against the Dnp hapten. The anti-Dnp antibodies react with the Dnp hapten on the Dnp–BGG, Dnp–BSA, and Dnp–HSA. Because some of the antigenic determinants on BSA also are present on HSA, some of the anti-BSA antibodies can cross-react with HSA. The result is a line of partial identity. The Dnp–BSA spur indicates precipitation of Dnp–BSA molecules by antibodies specific for BSA unique determinants. None of the antibodies that could react with HSA fail to react with BSA, so that there is only one spur. Similarly, reactions of partial identity are seen in comparing BSA and HSA with Dnp–BSA and Dnp–HSA, respectively. None of the anti-BSA antibodies cross-react with BGG, therefore there is no precipitin line with this antigen. Both HSA and Dnp–BGG are precipitated, but by different antibodies, so that there are overlapping spurs and no line of identity.

2–6   (a)   Substance Z contains at least two separate antigenic components, as indicated by the presence of two precipitin lines, which can be called Z_1 and Z_2.
(b)   W contains a component that appears antigenically identical to component Z_2; that is, W shows a reaction of identity with Z_2.

X contains a component that shares at least one antigenic determinant with component Z_2, but Z_2 contains at least one antigenic determinant that is nonidentical to those of X. The evidence for partial identity of X and Z_2 is the merging of the X line with the Z_2 line, but the Z_2 line has a spur that overlaps the X line.

Y contains a component that appears antigenically identical to component Z_1; that is, Y shows a reaction of identity with Z_1.
(c)   Your information will not permit you to draw any conclusions. All you know is that the substances from the diseased patients have at least one similar antigen. Analysis of a similar control preparation from a healthy individual may indicate whether these substances are related to the disease process.

2–7   (a)   To show that immunoglobulins are responsible, you could treat the immune serum with a heterologous anti-immunoglobulin, for example rabbit anti-human-immunoglobulin, and demonstrate that the serum loses its protective effect as the immunoglobulins are removed. Alternatively, you could purify the immunoglobulin fraction (by ammonium sulfate precipitation, chromatography, starch gel electrophoresis, etc.), and show that the isolated immunoglobulin fraction gives as good or better protection than the whole serum.
(b)   To demonstrate that the antibody binds to the bacteria you could show that treatment of the serum with bacteria will absorb out the protective agent. One such experimental approach would be to attach bacteria to an insoluble matrix and pass the protective serum over a column of this material, called an *immunoabsorbent column*. If the antibodies bind to the bacteria, they should be removed, and the absorbed serum eluted from the column should have lost its protective power.

Another approach would be to use an appropriate heterologous anti-immunoglobulin labeled with a flourescent dye (e.g., fluorescein). Bacteria would be incubated in the immune serum, washed, and then incubated with the fluorescent-labeled heterologous antibody. If the bacteria are stained specifically by the fluorescent antibody, then human immunoglobulins must be bound to the surface of the cells. The appropriate control to demonstrate specific binding is to incubate the bacteria first in a nonimmune human serum, and then to wash and add the fluorescent antibody. If the bacteria are stained under these conditions, then either the fluorescent antibodies or human immuno-globulins are being absorbed onto the bacteria in some nonspecific manner that would invalidate your results.

2–8   (a)   In the presence of the mitogen, normal cells synthesize considerable amounts of immunoglobulin. Even without mitogen they secrete some immunoglobulin. However, even with mitogen, the hypogammaglobu-linemia patients' cells secrete virtually no immunoglobulin. Furthermore, the patients' cells suppress immunoglobulin secretion by normal cells. Therefore these patients seem to suffer from hyperactive suppressor cells.

(b)   The suppressor cells either do not carry surface immunoglobulin or are not sensitive to lysis by anti-immunoglobulin and complement for some other reason. (The authors concluded that the suppressor cells were T cells, but provided no direct evidence for that conclusion.)

(c)   The generation of small lymphocytes from large lymphocytes could be blocked, or the small lymphocytes could fail to mature properly. Either eventuality would cause complete absence of sIg$^+$ cells, as well as agammaglobulinemia. Mature lymphocytes could have an internal biochemical block that would prevent stimulation subsequent to antigen binding, or they may have a block at any point along the pathway of blast transformation and immunoglobulin synthesis: for example, in mRNA transport from the nucleus, in the addition of carbohydrate, or in the secretory process. Alternatively, inhibition by other cells could prevent immunoglobulin synthesis or secretion. Clinicians have identified diseases that can be traced to blocks at almost every one of these points.

2–9   (a)   Graft rejection is an immune phenomenon. This phenomenon shows an accelerated second response: the BALB/c and C57BL mice reject the second A/J skin graft faster than they did the first graft. In addition, the second response shows specificity: a previous A/J skin graft does not accelerate rejection of a SJL graft. Finally, this phenomenon involves a distinction between self and non-self: A/J mice never reject an A/J skin graft.

(b)   Graft rejection is mediated by the cellular system. Mice that received immune cells showed an accelerated response when grafted for the first time with A/J skin. They rejected their first grafts in 8 days, whereas mice that did not receive immune cells took 14 days to reject their first grafts (Table 2–7c,d). The ability to reject grafts can be transferred by cells, but not by serum.

(c)   If the cellular system is primarily responsible for graft rejection, then animals deficient in T cells should show an impaired ability to reject grafts. Therefore you could test neonatally thymectomized mice or nude mice (which congenitally lack a thymus) for their ability to reject grafts from a different mouse strain.

(d)   Injection of immune serum lengthens the mean survival time of the graft (Table 2–7d); that is, it weakens the immune response to the graft. Destruction of grafted tissue presumably requires intimate contact between host lymphocytes and the grafted cells. Humoral antibodies that are specific for antigenic determinants on the surface of the grafted tissue cells may bind tightly to the surface of grafted cells and prevent host lymphocytes from recognizing or binding to the grafted cells. Any of the other mechanisms operative in antibody inhibition of the immune response also could be involved. Such humoral antibodies are termed *blocking* antibodies because they block the cellular immune response. They provide an example of how the humoral immune system can interfere with the functioning of the cellular immune system. Blocking antibodies may play an important role in the impairment of cellular immunity against cancer cells (Chapter 5).

(e)   Graft rejection is caused by the presence of histocompatibility antigens on the surface of cells in the donor graft that are different from those found on the host cells. This process is easily studied in inbred strains of mice because of the genetic identity of individuals within the strain. In mice the H-2 locus codes for the cell-surface antigens that play the most important role in the graft rejection process. Mice that differ at this locus will reject transplants from one another rapidly.

2–10   (a)   The survival of the kidney transplant depends upon the biological similarity between donor and recipient: the closer the genotypes, the higher the survival rate. Clearly, there must be heritable differences in human kidney cells, and these differences are detected by the immune system.

(b)   Although cytoplasmic and nuclear components may be released from dying target cells and may trigger an immune response, they should be inaccessible to the effector mechanisms of the immune system. Cell-surface molecules, however, would be detected easily. The major histocompatibility locus in humans is termed the HLA locus. Like the H-2 locus of mice, it codes for cell-surface molecules that trigger the graft-rejection process.

(c)   Curve E would have been relatively unaffected, but Curves C and D probably would have reached the abscissa within 1 to 4 weeks. However, prolonged immunosuppression renders the recipient vulnerable to severe and often fatal infections (e.g., pneumonia) that normally are controlled by the immune system. In addition, immunosuppressed patients seem to have a markedly increased incidence of cancer.

2–11   None of these immunosuppressants exhibits specificity. Each kills rapidly dividing cells or lymphocytes indiscriminately. Theoretically, the ideal immunosuppressant would remove just those lymphocytes that could react with the foreign cell-surface antigens of the transplant. To find a method for imposing such specific tolerance is one of the major goals of transplantation biology.

2–12   Inbred mice are homozygous for MHC determinants. Consequently, when mice of two inbred strains are crossed, their F_1 progeny express all the MHC antigens that are expressed in either parent. Thus if T cells of any F_1 individual are transferred to either parent in a marrow transplant, they will not recognize or react to any parental antigens as non-self determinants. By contrast, because humans are invariably heterozygous for MHC antigens, a given F_1 individual will receive only half the MHC determinants of either parent. In a bone-marrow transplant, the remainder of the parental determinants will be recognized as non-self by any F_1 T cells that are injected, and a multisystem graft-versus-host immune response will ensue. Since such a response is usually fatal to the recipient, your colleague would be well advised not to proceed with his operation as planned.

2–13   (a)   In a family with many children, the multiparous mother is highly likely to have antibodies to the products of both paternal HLA haplotypes because, assuming no crossing-over within the MHC, each child has an equal probability of expressing either one of the two paternal haplotypes. Therefore blood leukocytes from all children will agglutinate in maternal serum. Siblings can be matched for paternal haplotype by using leukocytes from the diseased child to absorb the maternal serum exhaustively at its agglutination end point. The absorbed serum then may be tested for ability to agglutinate leukocytes from other siblings. Those whose cells are still agglutinated must express the other paternal haplotype, whereas those whose cells are not agglutinated express the same paternal haplotype as the diseased child.

A transplant donor, however, also must be matched for maternally inherited HLA antigens, again because each child has an equal probability of inheriting either maternal haplotype. Identity of maternal HLA antigens can be determined using a mixed lymphocyte reaction in which blood lymphocytes from the intended recipient are incubated separately with lymphocytes from each of the siblings that were found to express the same paternal haplotype in the preceding test. After five days the number of lymphocytes that are undergoing blast transformation are counted in each of the cultures. Lack of any blast transformation indicates HLA identity.

(b)   The horse presumably made antibodies to surface antigens that are shared by RBC's and thymocytes. While you give the patient a blood transfusion, you could prove this assumption by showing that absorption of the ALS with an equal volume of RBC's removes its RBC agglutinating activity, without lowering the thymocyte agglutinating power.

(c)   The horse also made antibodies against antigens that are shared by all leukocytes, but are not present on RBC's. The acute bacterial infection almost certainly is due to a lack of polymorphonuclear leukocytes (PMN's). To treat this condition you could "plasmaphorese" the patient (remove the plasma from blood samples, returning the packed cells) to reduce the blood level of antibody, transfuse him with a PMN concentrate, and give back RBC, PMN, and a preparation of ALS that had been adsorbed with these cells and B cells.

(d)   The PMN's could infiltrate because of local infection or local complement activation by anti-kidney antibodies. The former would be unlikely to affect only glomeruli. To test for the latter you could use fluorescein-tagged antihorse-immunoglobulin or anti-human-C3 on the kidney biopsy.

(e)   The tests show local deposition of antibody and C3 on the glomerular basement membrane. This result indicates that your ALS contains anti-basement-membrane antibodies, which presumably were induced by basement membranes contained in the thymus mash, and which now are causing an acute inflammatory reaction that is leading to failure of the transplant. You should remove the transplant, absorb the ALS with the failing kidney, and put in another HLA-matched donor kidney along with the absorbed ALS.

(f)   You should vaccinate everyone in town *except* the transplant recipients. Although the live vaccinia virus used for smallpox vaccinations normally is nonpathogenic, it will cause a severe generalized infection and, probably, death of these recipients, due to their T-cell deficit caused by your immunosuppressive treatment. Consequently these individuals must be kept in isolation and *not* vaccinated.

2–14   (a)   The immunization protocol elicits antibodies specific for the acetylcholine receptor, which is likely to carry cross-reacting antigens in electric eel and rat. These antibodies probably bind at neuromuscular junctions and impair voluntary muscle stimulation. The muscular weakness, hunched posture, and jerky movements all could be traced to impairment of head and forelimb muscles. Weight loss would follow from failure to eat due to impairment of head and neck muscles and inability to move to the food supply.

(b)   You could confirm the presence of self-reactive antibodies and determine the precise effect of the antibodies on the neuromuscular system.

(c)   Clearly, organisms normally do not make such antibodies. A strong adjuvant is needed to break the natural tolerance to the self-antigens of the AChR protein.

(d)   The syndrome may represent a direct manifestation of T effector cells. Alternatively, if AChR were a thymus-dependent antigen in terms of B-cell triggering, humoral antibody could cause the syndrome.

(e)   Myasthenia gravis could be due to autoantibodies against acetylcholine receptors. Again, you could test sera for antibodies specific to human neuromuscular junctions. You might also test these sera against purified AChR from electric eels.

(f)   Some patients with myasthenia gravis have serum immunoglobulins that partially block subsequent binding of α-bungarotoxin to AChR. In additional tests of such patients, about half showed definite or possible inhibition. The immunoglobulin binding could cause neuromuscular blockade *in vivo,* thereby accounting for both the disease process and the finding that the concentration of muscle binding sites is reduced in these patients.

(g)   Patients with myasthenia gravis also show evidence of cellular immunity specific for AChR, and the degree of hypersensitivity correlates directly with the severity of the disease process. Thus T-cell immunity is implicated in this disease process, and the reduced frequency of muscle AChR is these patients may be due to (i) the cytotoxic and/or inflammatory effects of effector T cells, (ii) competitive inhibition of receptor sites by T cells or cell-free T-cell receptors, or (iii) competitive inhibition of receptor sites by specific antibody.

(h)   This syndrome could be due to receptor blockade only in its initial phases, because the half-life of most antibodies in mice is hours to days, not months. The complexes of anti-AChR with AChR in this instance must induce a prolonged immune response to the AChR.

(i)   The mice show evidence of both T- and B-cell immunity to AChR. To demonstrate the immunopathogenic effector function, you would have to test the effects of various subclasses of immunoglobulins and lymphocytes on *in vitro* receptor binding and on muscle stimulation by ACh. You also could fractionate immunoglobulins and cells for passive or adaptive transfer of the disease to normal, syngeneic hosts. Particularly useful for the cell-transfer studies would be fractionation procedures allowing enrichment or depletion of cells bearing surface Ig, C3 receptors, Fc receptors, Thy-1, Ly-1, Ly-2, and Ly-3. In each case, you would have to demonstrate that the putative effect of each transferred agent was a direct action of that agent, rather than induction of a secondary process.

2–15 (a) There is no reason to suspect any abnormalities in levels of secretory component. If you wished to check these levels, you should assay saliva rather than serum.

(b) Because you suspect that the patient has a T-cell deficit, you should order separate assays of blood lymphocytes with phyothemagglutinin (which stimulates T cells only) and pokeweed mitogen (which stimulates both T and B cells) to test your suspicion.

(c) In the histological sections you should see intact primary follicles and medullary development of plasma cells, but total lymphocyte depletion of the diffuse cortex.

(d) Your diagnosis should be DiGeorge syndrome (thymic aplasia). You must either keep the child in a germ-free isolator for life or investigate the possibilities of thymus transplant. If you consider a transplant, you must take into account the problem of GVHR. Also, you must supply calcium or parathyroid hormones for life.

(e) The parents need not worry about future pregnancies, because this syndrome results from a nongenetic congenital defect, perhaps due to intrauterine trauma, toxin, or infection.

2–16 (a) The glomerulonephritis involves activation of the alternate complement pathway, either by endogenous release of activators or by a subclinical infection with endotoxin-producing bacteria. The latter alternative seems unlikely in the absence of a specific antibody response. The activated C3 is depositing in the glomeruli, and is there activating an acute inflammatory response that involves vasoactive peptides and infiltration of polymorphonuclear leukocytes.

(b) If the activating agents are in the blood, then serum from these patients should fix complement spontaneously, thereby lowering the complement titer of a standard serum.

(c) There is no reason to believe that this inflammatory disorder involves any of the specific elements of the immune system.

2–17 (a) It is likely that recurrent release of gastrointestinal bacteria into the bloodstream is occurring due to an imperfection in the surgical procedure. These bacteria are inducing a specific immune response. The arthritis probably is due to immune complex-activated, complement-dependent acute inflammation.

(b) You should treat the symptoms with anti-inflammatory agents, and attempt to find the locus of infection in order to eliminate recurrence. If you can find no locus of infection, you must entertain the possibility that the immune response is directed against cross-reacting endogenous antigens, and try to identify them or plan immunosuppressive therapy.

2–18 (a) The boy's serum immunoglobulin levels are normal. Likewise his levels of B-cell subclasses are normal, with a possibly significant increase in B_α and B_δ cells. There is no evidence here of immune deficiency.

(b)   The patient is deficient in salivary IgA. Either IgA or IgA-synthesizing cells do not reach the submucosal tissues, or there is a defect in production or function of secretory component. You might test the latter possibility by developing an immunoassay that would not be sensitive to IgA, but would measure for secretory component (SC) specifically. The investigating team developed a radioimmunoassay for this purpose.

(c)   The patient suffers from a defect in production of functional SC. The defect could be either failure of synthesis, or production of an altered component that neither binds to IgA nor is secreted. Any therapy must either restore epithelial production of functional SC, or replace gastrointestinal IgA. IgA is in highest concentrations in colostrum and milk.

(d)   Presumably bovine colostrum contains IgA, some of which is anti-*Candida*, or is directed against substances that promote *Candida* infection. How IgA protects epithelial surfaces other than by combining with antigenic microorganisms is still unknown.

3 ANTIBODIES

The antibody molecule has evolved to perform two distinct functions—antigen recognition and elimination. Antibody molecules can interact with a virtually unlimited number of antigens, yet antibodies destroy or eliminate antigens by a small number of effector mechanisms. To carry out its dual function the antibody molecule has evolved discrete globular domains. One of these domains binds antigen, and the others mediate effector functions. Thus the functional duality of the antibody molecule is reflected in its three-dimensional structure. The organization of antibody gene families also reflects this functional duality. These gene families must be capable of storing or generating information for hundreds of thousands to possibly millions of different antibody molecules. This chapter considers the structure and function of antibody molecules as well as the organization and evolution of their gene families.

Essential Concepts

3-1 Immunoglobulin structure is known from studies of myeloma proteins

A. The serum of a normal vertebrate contains a large variety of proteins, including the five classes of immunoglobulins (Figure 3–1). The immunoglobulins in turn include the organism's circulating antibody population. The basic structures and gross chemical properties of immunoglobulins are very similar, but their combining specificities vary widely, thereby reflecting the spectrum of antigens that the individual has encountered during its lifetime.

The immunoglobulins are so similar and yet normally so heterogeneous that isolation of an individual molecular species for detailed chemical study is difficult. Fortunately, homogeneous immunoglobulins can be obtained by taking advantage of an abnormal condition, a cancer of antibody-producing cells called *multiple myeloma*. In an individual

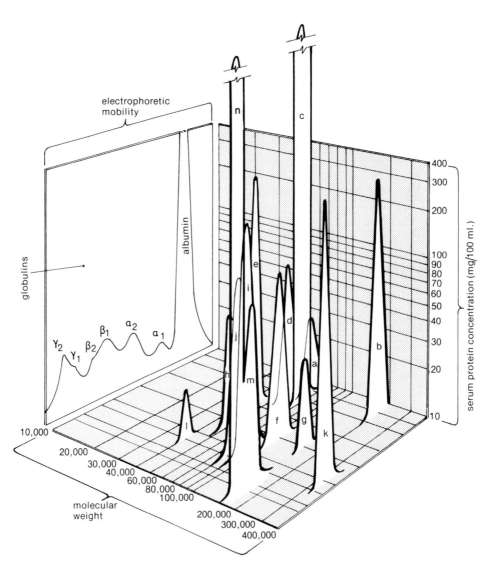

Figure 3–1 Some human serum proteins characterized by molecular weights, electrophoretic mobilities at pH 8.6, and concentrations in the blood serum. For purposes of comparison, the mobilities and concentrations of the globulins (α, β, γ) and albumin are shown at the rear. Proteins are identified by the following letters: a, prealbumin; b, α_1 lipoprotein; c, albumin; d, α_1 acid glycoprotein; e, α_1 antitrypsin; f, haptoglobulin; g, ceruloplasm; h, α_2 HS glycoprotein; i, transferrin; j, hemopexin; k, fibrinogen; l, β_2 glycoprotein; m, IgA; n, IgG. Serum complement components are displayed in a similar manner in Figure 1–37.

afflicted with this disease, neoplastic transformation generally occurs in a single plasma cell or its immediate precursor, so that the resulting tumor secretes a homogeneous immunoglobulin (*myeloma protein*). This protein can comprise 95% of the serum immunoglobulin, and therefore is easy to isolate in pure form. The myeloma protein from any afflicted individual generally is different from the myeloma proteins of all other individuals. Myeloma tumors have been observed in many mammalian species, including man, rat, mouse, horse, and dog.

B. Myeloma proteins are indistinguishable from normal immunoglobulins by all available criteria. All the types of polypeptide chains and genetic markers seen in normal immunoglobulins have been found in myeloma proteins. Extensive amino acid sequences are identical in normal and myeloma immunoglobulins. Some myeloma proteins bind known antigenic determinants. For example, about 5% of the myeloma proteins from a particular inbred strain of mice react with cell-surface determinants of enteric bacteria, such as phosphorylcholine and simple sugars. Presumably, myeloma tumors develop from lymphocytes that have proliferated in response to specific antigens on intestinal bacteria. Some of these myeloma proteins have idiotypes that are identical to their normal counterparts induced by immunization with the appropriate hapten. This observation suggests that myeloma proteins have variable regions that are similar, if not identical, to those of normal antibody molecules.

C. The utility of myeloma proteins for study of immunoglobulin structure was increased by the discovery that myeloma tumors can be induced artificially in two laboratory strains of mice (BALB/c and NZB) by injection of mineral oil into the peritoneal cavity (Figure 3–2). Because these mice are highly inbred, the immunoglobulin genes of all individuals from each strain are similar if not identical. Induced tumors can be transplanted from one mouse to many other individuals of the same strain to increase the production of a particular myeloma globulin. Myeloma tumors can be frozen without loss of viability, and banks of thousands of mouse tumors now are maintained. Study of myeloma proteins has provided a detailed picture of the structure of antibodies.

3–2   Immunoglobulin molecules are composed of two kinds of polypeptides

A. Immunoglobulin molecules of the most common class, IgG, are made up of two identical light chains of molecular weight 23,000 and two identical heavy chains of molecular weight 53,000 (Figure 3–3). Each light chain is linked to a heavy chain by noncovalent associations

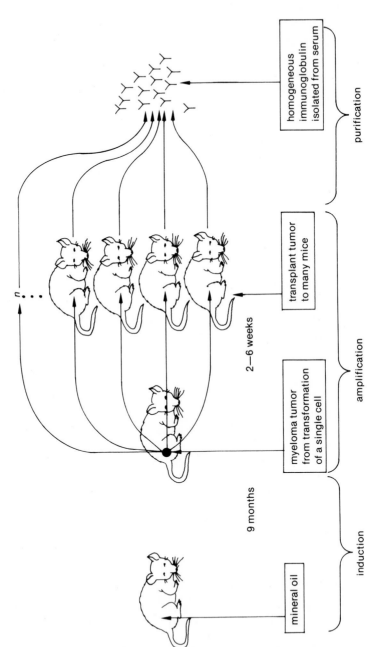

Figure 3–2 The induction and amplification of a mouse myeloma tumor.

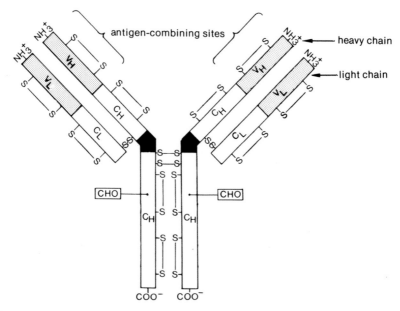

Figure 3–3 A schematic drawing of the human immunoglobulin molecule, showing its principal structural features. V and C indicate variable and constant regions, respectively, of the heavy (H) and light (L) chains, as explained in the text. Shaded segments indicate V regions; the remainder of each chain is C region –S–S– symbols represent the 12 intra-chain and 4 interchain disulfide bridges. Dark portions of the two heavy chains indicate the hinge region. CHO represents carbohydrate groups attached to the heavy chains.

and also by one covalent disulfide bridge. In the IgG molecule the two light chain–heavy chain pairs are linked together by disulfide bridges between the heavy chains. As shown in Figure 3–3, the molecule can be represented schematically in the form of a Y, with the amino (N–) termini of the four chains at the top and the carboxyl (C–) termini of the two heavy chains at the bottom. The portion of the molecule that includes the disulfide linkages between heavy chains where the three arms of the Y come together is called the hinge region. The arms of the Y are flexible. Twelve intrachain disulfide bridges are spaced periodically, two in each light chain and four in each heavy chain. Carbohydrate groups are attached through the side chains of asparagine residues in the two heavy chains at the positions shown in Figure 3–3. Thus immunoglobulins are glycoproteins.

B. A dimer of light chain–heavy chain pairs, $(L–H)_2$, is the basic structural subunit of other classes of immunoglobulin molecules as well as of IgG. The structures of other classes and subclasses differ in the positions and number of the disulfide bridges between heavy chains,

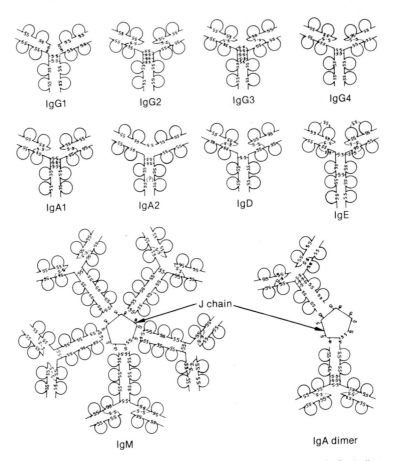

Figure 3–4 Subunit structures of various human immunoglobulins. –S–S– indicates a disulfide bridge. The question mark indicates that the interchain disulfide bridge structure is unknown. IgG1, IgG2, IgG3, and IgG4 are subclasses of IgG. IgA1 is the monomeric subclass of the IgA class. The J chain joins the higher polymeric forms of IgA as well as the five subunits of the IgM molecule. [Adapted from J. Gally in *The Antigens*, M. Sela (Ed.), Academic Press, New York, 1973, p. 209.]

and in the number of $(L–H)_2$ subunits in the molecule (Figure 3–4). IgD and IgE molecules, like IgG, are composed of one $(L–H)_2$ subunit. The IgA moelcule may have one, two, or three $(L–H)_2$ subunits. The serum IgM molecule has five $(L–H)_2$ subunits, that is, it is equivalent to an aggregate of five IgG-like molecules. The membrane-bound IgM molecule has one $(L–H)_2$ subunit. In the higher polymeric forms of IgA and in IgM, the $(L–H)_2$ subunits are held together by disulfide bridges through a polypeptide called the *J chain*. The heavy chains of the various classes of immunoglobulins differ in amino acid sequence and correspondingly in function (Essential Concept 3–6).

3-3   The light- and heavy-chain subunits of immunoglobulin molecules are differentiated into variable and constant regions

When the amino acid sequences of several myeloma light chains first were compared, a striking pattern emerged (Figure 3–5). In the N-terminal half of the chain the sequences were found to vary greatly from polypeptide to polypeptide. By contrast, in the C-terminal half of the chain the sequences of all the molecules were identical. Consequently these two segments of the molecule were designated the *variable* (V_L) and *constant* (C_L) regions of the light chain, respectively. The V_L region begins at the N-terminus and is approximately 110 amino acid residues in length. The C_L region makes up the remainder of the chain, and also is about 110 residues in length.

Heavy-chain sequences exhibit a similar pattern. A variable (V_H) region begins at the N-terminus and is approximately the same length as the V_L region of the light chain, about 110 residues. The heavy-chain constant (C_H) region for the IgG molecule is about three times this length, or about 330 residues.

Because the N-terminal portions of each L–H pair comprise the antigen-binding sites in an immunoglobulin molecule (Figure 3–3), the sequence heterogeneity of the V_L and V_H regions accounts for the great diversity of antigenic specificities among antibody molecules. The C_H regions make up the portion of the immunoglobulin molecule that carries out effector functions, which are common to all antibodies

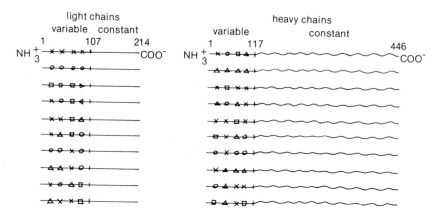

Figure 3–5 A schematic representation of the variable and constant regions for light and heavy chains from ten IgG molecules. NH_3^+ indicates the N-terminus and COO^- the C-terminus. ×, O, △, and □ indicate amino-acid-sequence-differences. Lines without these symbols indicate sequence identity among the proteins compared. The lengths of the V and C regions are indicated by residue number, beginning with Residue 1 at the N-terminus.

of a given class. Each immunoglobulin molecule has at least two identical antigen-binding sites. This bivalence permits antibodies to cross-link antigens with two or more antigenic determinants. The flexibility of the arms of the antibody molecule allows it to bind simultaneously antigenic determinants that are separated by various distances.

3-4 The antigen-binding site, formed by the light- and heavy-chain variable regions, can exhibit a broad range of specificities

A. X-ray crystallographic studies of two myeloma immunoglobulins that bind different haptens have shown that the active site is a crevice between the V_L and V_H regions (Figure 3–6), and that the dimensions of the crevice can vary significantly. The size and shape of the active site varies due to differences in the relationship of the V_L and V_H regions, and due to amino-acid-sequence variation in the V_L and V_H regions. Antibody specificity results from the molecular complementarity between determinant groups on the antigen molecule and amino acid residues in the active site.

B. The antigen-binding sites of antibodies resemble the active sites of enzymes in several ways. Both involve multiple, weak noncovalent associations, including electrostatic, hydrogen bonding, and van der

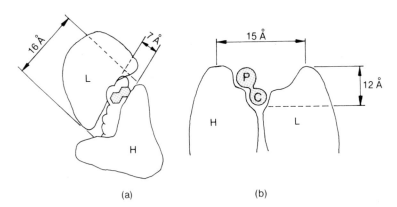

(a)   (b)

Figure 3–6 (a) A schematic top view of the shallow cleft between the heavy and light variable regions of the human myeloma protein NEW, which specifically binds the hapten, vitamin K_1OH (shaded). The dimensions of the binding site are 16 Å x 7 Å x 6 Å. [Redrawn from F. Richards *et al.*, *The Immune System: Genes, Receptors, Signals*, E. Sercarz, A. Williamson, and C. Fox (Eds.), Academic Press, New York, 1975, p. 53.] (b) A schematic side view of the interaction of the variable regions of mouse myeloma protein McPC603 with its specific hapten, phosphorylcholine (shaded). The dimensions of the binding site are 20 Å × 15 Å × 12 Å. [Redrawn from E. Padlan *et al.*, *The Immune System: Genes, Receptors, Signals*, E. Sercarz, A. Williamson, and C. Fox (Eds.), Academic Press, New York, 1975, p. 7.]

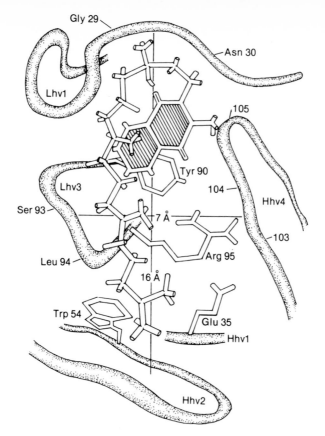

Figure 3–7 A schematic drawing of the hapten, vitamin K₁OH, bound to the combining site of a human IgG molecule. Lhv1, Lhv3, Hhv1, Hhv2, and Hhv4 designate the approximate locations of the hypervariable regions of the light and heavy chains, respectively. The quinone group (two fused six-membered rings) of the hapten is bound at the top in a shallow crevice (16 Å × 7 Å × 6 Å); the phytyl tail folds over the quinone and extends along most of the length of the active site. [From I. M. Amzel *et al., Proc. Natl. Acad. Sci. USA* **71,** 1427 (1974).]

Waals interactions, which combine to give strong binding. Both antibodies and enzymes exhibit binding (dissociation) constants that range from 10^{-4} to 10^{-10} M, corresponding to standard free energy changes of binding of from -6 to -15 kcal/mole. The binding sites of both are predominantly nonpolar niches. In addition, both antibodies and enzymes exhibit significant cross-reactivity with structurally related ligands.

C.   The walls of the antigen-binding site are composed of *hypervariable* (hv) segments of the V_L and V_H regions (Figure 3–7). These regions of extensive diversity initially were defined by comparing immunoglobulin chains from a given class after alignment for sequence homology. Such a comparison is shown in Figure 3–8, using the common one-letter abbreviations for amino acid residues. These abbreviations, and the

208

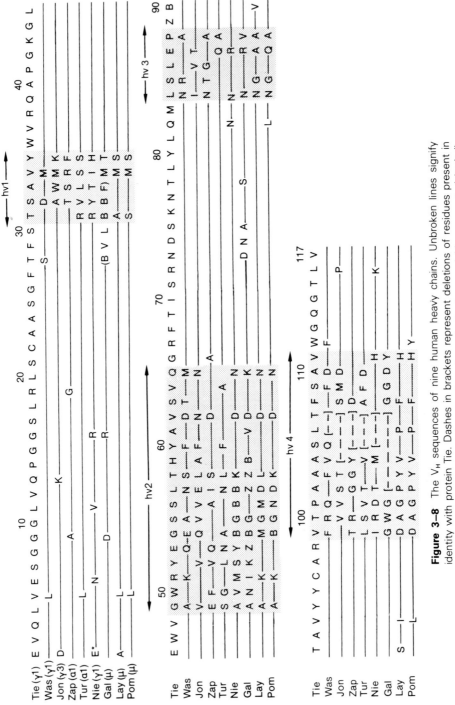

Figure 3–8 The V$_H$ sequences of nine human heavy chains. Unbroken lines signify identity with protein Tie. Dashes in brackets represent deletions of residues present in protein Tie. Sequence variations tend to cluster in the hypervariable segments (shaded). E* denotes pyrrolidine carboxylic acid. [From J. D. Capra and J. M. Kehoe, *Proc. Natl. Acad. Sci. USA* **71**, 4032 (1974).]

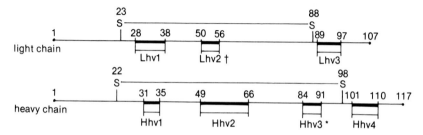

Figure 3–9 A linear map of hypervariable segments in the variable regions of light and heavy chains. Residue numbers indicate the approximate end points of these segments, and the position of the central disulfide bridges. * indicates a hypervariable segment that is not part of the antigen-binding crevice (see Figure 3–7). † indicates a hypervariable segment that sometimes is a part of the antigen-binding crevice.

Table 3–1
Amino acid abbreviations and codons[a]

Amino acid	Three-letter abbreviation	Single-letter abbreviation	mRNA codon
Alanine	Ala	A	GCX
Arginine	Arg	R	CGX, AGZ
Asparagine	Asn	N	AAY
Aspartic Acid	Asp	D	GAY
Either Asp or Asn	Asx	B	————
Cysteine	Cys	C	UGY
Glutamic acid	Glu	E	GAZ
Glutamine	Gln	Q	CAZ
Either Glu or Gln	Glx	Z	————
Glycine	Gly	G	GGX
Histidine	His	H	CAY
Isoleucine	Ile	I	AUY, AUA
Leucine	Leu	L	CUX, UUZ
Lysine	Lys	K	AAZ
Methionine	Met	M	AUG
Phenylalanine	Phe	F	UUY
Proline	Pro	P	CCY
Serine	Ser	S	UCX, AGY
Threonine	Thr	T	ACX
Tryptophan	Trp	W	UGG
Tyrosine	Tyr	Y	UAY
Valine	Val	V	GUX

[a] In the mRNA codon sequences, A, C, G, and U represent the four common ribonucleotides; X represents any one of the four nucleotides; Y represents either pyrimidine nucleotide; and Z represents either purine nucleotide.

alternative three-letter amino acid designations, are defined in Table 3–1, which also lists the codons in messenger RNA that correspond to each amino acid. The diversity in hypervariable segments includes sequence insertions and deletions as well as amino acid substitutions. Three hypervariable segments generally are present in V_L regions, and four in V_H regions (Figure 3–9).

Three lines of evidence indicate that hypervariable regions comprise the antigen-binding sites of most antibody molecules.

1.   The x-ray analyses of two myeloma proteins that bind simple haptens (Figures 3–6 and 3–7) show that five or six of the seven hypervariable regions constitute the walls of the antigen-binding crevice. Moreover, the three-dimensional structures of the V_L and V_H regions from all myeloma proteins analyzed so far, in species as diverse as mouse and man, are remarkably similar except for differences in the hypervariable segments. The structure formed by the nonhypervariable portion of the V region, termed the framework region, is highly conserved, that is, it is relatively invariant (Essential Concept 3–5B). This observation suggests that the same hypervariable segments may comprise the antigen-binding sites of all antibody molecules. One heavy-chain hypervariable region (hv3) is not part of the active site; the function of this region is unknown.

2.   Special antigens can be constructed to include a chemical group that can link covalently to the antibody molecule at or near the antigen-combining site. Such antigens are known as *affinity labels.* A wide variety of affinity labels have been reacted with specific antibodies and found to attach only to residues in the hypervariable regions, and not to other residues of the light or heavy chains.

3.   Special immunization procedures have permitted the induction of homogeneous antibody molecules. When the amino acid sequences of these homogeneous antibodies are compared, they also show hypervariable regions similar to those of myeloma immunoglobulins.

D.   The antigen-binding sites of antibodies differ from the substrate-binding sites of most enzymes in one fundamental way: two chains, rather than one, fold to make the antigen-binding site. Thus extensive binding-site diversity can be generated by the combinatorial properties of light chain–heavy chain association in antibody synthesis (Figure 3–10). For example, if any light chain can associate with any heavy chain to produce a functional antibody, then 1000 different light chains and 1000 different heavy chains can be combined in pairs to produce $10^3 \times 10^3 = 10^6$ different antibody molecules. The combinatorial diversity increases as the product of the numbers of different light and heavy chains available. Although it is not known whether every $(L–H)_2$ combination produces a functional antibody, two independent lines of evidence suggest that *combinatorial association* is an important mechanism for increasing antibody diversity.

1.   X-ray analyses permit identification of the residues that make

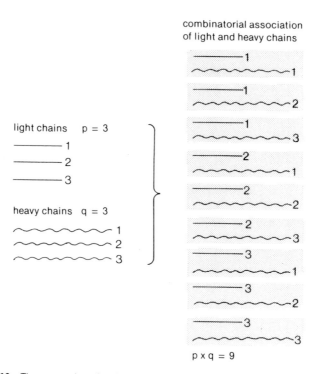

Figure 3–10 The generation of antigen-binding-site diversity by combinatorial association of three different light chains and three different heavy chains. The total number of different binding sites that can be generated from p light chains and q heavy chains is $p \times q$.

contact in the association of V_L with V_H regions. These contact residues are highly conserved in antibody molecules analyzed so far. This finding implies that most V_L regions should be able to associate with most V_H regions.

2. Hybrid cells can be formed by the fusion of two different myeloma cells or of a myeloma cell and a normally induced antibody-producing cell. A number of such hybrid cells have been shown to synthesize both parental and hybrid immunoglobulin molecules that include most of the possible L–H combinations (Figure 3–11). Thus most V_L and V_H regions appear capable of associating normally in an antibody-producing cell.

E. The diversity of antigen-binding capability is still further increased by a phenomenon called *multispecificity*, the ability of a single antibody molecule to combine with a spectrum of different antigens. Multispecificity is biologically significant. Because a particular antibody receptor can be triggered by different antigenic determinants, an organism can

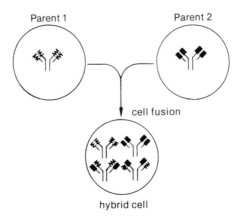

Figure 3–11 The fusion of two myeloma tumor cells to yield a hybrid cell that produces both parental and hybrid immunoglobulin molecules. ▬ and 〜 represent variable regions characteristic of the immunoglobulins produced by the two parental cell types.

respond to completely novel antigens, including synthetic compounds never before encountered by the species.

1.   Although a single antibody molecule has a unique three-dimensional structure, it can combine with the inducing antigenic determinants, determinants with similar structures (cross-reacting antigens), and perhaps even determinants with quite disparate structures. A stable antigen–antibody complex will result whenever there is a sufficient number of short-range interactions, regardless of the total fit. The antigen-combining site is large, and a lack of fit in one area can be compensated for by increased binding elsewhere. Disparate antigens may fit into the antigen-binding crevice in different ways (Figure 3–12). Each species of antibody has a different spectrum of determinants with which it can combine.

2.   Although individual antibodies are multispecific, the collection of antibodies induced in response to a particular antigen behaves in a highly specific manner, normally reacting only with the inducing antigen and very closely related structures. This apparent paradox can be explained as follows. Many different molecular species of antibody normally are induced in an immune response, and each will react with a different spectrum of antigens. Thus every antibody molecule will react with the inducing antigen, but each antibody will differ in the spectrum of disparate antigens it can bind. If each molecular species of antibody is present at the 1% level, the disparate reactions will be below the limits of detection for most routine immunologic assays (Table 3–2).

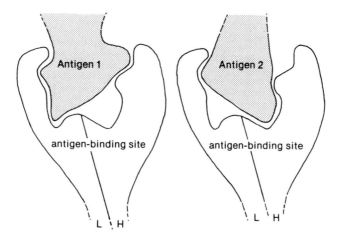

Figure 3–12 A schematic representation of multispecificity in a single antibody molecule.

Table 3–2
Hypothetical specificity profiles of individual antibody species raised against an immunogen, Hapten A[a]

	Antibody species					
	1	2	3	4	5 •••	n
Specificities	A	A	A	A	A	A
	A′	A′	A′		A′	A′
	A″		A″	A″		A″
	B	C	F	J		T
	E		G	W	H	L
	Q	M	R	X	P	Y
	V	S	N	K	Z	U
	•	•	•	•	•	•
	•	•	•	•	•	•
	•	•	•	•	•	•
	•	•	•	•	•	•

[a]Letters represent antigenic determinants that are recognized by the various antibody species. A′ and A″ represent determinants that are closely related in structure to Hapten A. The recognition specificities for disparate determinants generally are not common to different antibody species.

3-5   Homology units in immunoglobulins correspond to molecular domains with different functions

A.   On the basis of primary structure comparisons, light and heavy chains may be divided into two groups of *homology units* of similar amino acid sequence (Figure 3–13). Each of these units is about 110 residues in length and has a centrally placed disulfide bridge. One group consists of the V_L and V_H regions. The other group consists of the C_L region and three subsegments of the C_H region, designated C_H1, C_H2, and C_H3.

1.   The sequences of the two V-region homology units are similar, as are those of the four C-region homology units (Figure 3–14). Although the V- and C-region units have no apparent sequence homology to one another, some relationship is suggested by the observation that both homology units are roughly the same length, and that both have a centrally located intrachain disulfide bridge that spans about 60 residues. Homologous polypeptides presumably reflect genes that diverged from a common ancestor at some past time. Accordingly, these homology relationships suggest strongly that present-day light-chain and heavy-chain genes evolved by duplication and divergence from a single primordial gene that coded for a polypeptide of about 110 residues (see Essential Concept 3–13).

2.   X-ray crystallographic studies at about 3-Å resolution on immunoglobulins of different classes from different animal species

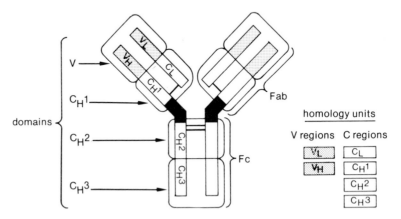

Figure 3–13   A diagrammatic representation of the homology units and domains of the IgG molecule. Pairs of homology units fold together to form four globular domains termed V, C_H1, C_H2, and C_H3, as indicated by boxes in the figure. Limited proteolytic attack at the hinge region (shaded segment of heavy chains) cleaves the molecule into Fab and Fc fragments.

			110										120	
Eu C_L	(Residues 109-214)	Thr	Val	Ala	Ala	Pro	Ser	Val	Phe	Ile	Phe	Pro	Pro	Ser
Eu C_H1	(Residues 119-220)	Ser	Thr	Lys	Gly	Pro	Ser	Val	Phe	—	—	Pro	Leu	Ala
Eu C_H2	(Residues 234-341)	Leu	Leu	Gly	Gly	Pro	Ser	Val	Phe	Leu	Phe	Pro	Pro	Lys
Eu C_H3	(Residues 342-446)	Gln	Pro	Arg	Glu	Pro	Gln	Val	Tyr	Thr	Leu	Pro	Pro	Ser

										130									
Asp	Glu	Gln	—	—	Leu	Lys	Ser	Gly	Thr	Ala	Ser	Val	Val	Cys	Leu	Leu	Asn	Asn	Phe
Pro	Ser	Ser	Lys	Ser	Thr	Ser	Gly	Gly	Thr	Ala	Ala	Leu	Gly	Cys	Leu	Val	Lys	Asp	Tyr
Pro	Lys	Asp	Thr	Leu	Met	Ile	Ser	Arg	Thr	Pro	Glu	Val	Thr	Cys	Val	Val	Val	Asp	Val
Arg	Glu	Glu	—	—	Met	Thr	Lys	Asn	Gln	Val	Ser	Leu	Thr	Cys	Leu	Val	Lys	Gly	Phe

140												150							
Tyr	Pro	Arg	Glu	Ala	Lys	Val	—	—	Gln	Trp	Lys	Val	Asp	Asn	Ala	Leu	Gln	Ser	Gly
Phe	Pro	Glu	Pro	Val	Thr	Val	—	—	Ser	Trp	Asn	Ser	—	Gly	Ala	Leu	Thr	Ser	Gly
Ser	His	Glu	Asp	Pro	Gln	Val	Lys	Phe	Asn	Trp	Tyr	Val	Asp	Gly	—	Val	Gln	Val	His
Tyr	Pro	Ser	Asp	Ile	Ala	Val	—	—	Glu	Trp	Glu	Ser	Asn	Asp	—	Gly	Glu	Pro	Glu

		160										170							
Asn	Ser	Gln	Glu	Ser	Val	Thr	Glu	Gln	Asp	Ser	Lys	Asp	Ser	Thr	Tyr	Ser	Leu	Ser	Ser
—	Val	His	Thr	Phe	Pro	Ala	Val	Leu	Gln	Ser	—	Ser	Gly	Leu	Tyr	Ser	Leu	Ser	Ser
Asn	Ala	Lys	Thr	Lys	Pro	Arg	Glu	Gln	Gln	Tyr	—	Asp	Ser	Thr	Tyr	Arg	Val	Val	Ser
Asn	Tyr	Lys	Thr	Thr	Pro	Pro	Val	Leu	Asp	Ser	—	Asp	Gly	Ser	Phe	Phe	Leu	Tyr	Ser

		180										190							
Thr	Leu	Thr	Leu	Ser	Lys	Ala	Asp	Tyr	Glu	Lys	His	Lys	Val	Tyr	Ala	Cys	Glu	Val	Thr
Val	Val	Thr	Val	Pro	Ser	Ser	Ser	Leu	Gly	Thr	Gln	—	Thr	Tyr	Ile	Cys	Asn	Val	Asn
Val	Leu	Thr	Val	Leu	His	Gln	Asn	Trp	Leu	Asp	Gly	Lys	Glu	Tyr	Lys	Cys	Lys	Val	Ser
Lys	Leu	Thr	Val	Asp	Lys	Ser	Arg	Trp	Gln	Glu	Gly	Asn	Val	Phe	Ser	Cys	Ser	Val	Met

		200													210				
His	Gln	Gly	Leu	Ser	Ser	Pro	Val	Thr	—	Lys	Ser	Phe	—	—	Asn	Arg	Gly	Glu	Cys
His	Lys	Pro	Ser	Asn	Thr	Lys	Val	—	Asp	Lys	Arg	Val	—	—	Glu	Pro	Lys	Ser	Cys
Asn	Lys	Ala	Leu	Pro	Ala	Pro	Ile	—	Glu	Lys	Thr	Ile	Ser	Lys	Ala	Lys	Gly		
His	Glu	Ala	Leu	His	Asn	His	Tyr	Thr	Gln	Lys	Ser	Leu	Ser	Leu	Ser	Pro	Gly		

Figure 3–14 Amino-acid-sequence homologies of the four constant-region homology units of the human myeloma protein Eu. Deletions indicated by dashes have been introduced to maximize the homology. Identical residues are lightly shaded; dark shadings indicate alternative identities at a given position. [From G. M. Edelman *et al., Proc. Natl. Acad. Sci. USA* **63,** 78 (1969).]

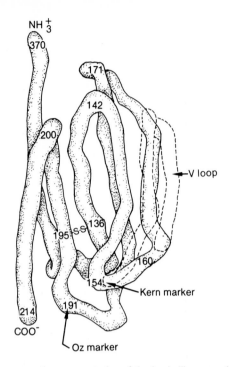

Figure 3–15 A diagrammatic representation of the basic "immunoglobulin fold" present in mammalian immunoglobulin molecules. Solid lines show the folding of the polypeptide chain in the constant regions C_L and C_H1. Dotted lines indicate the additional loop of polypeptide characteristic of the V_L and V_H regions. NH_3^+ and COO^- correspond to the N and C termini of these subunits, respectively. Numbers refer to positions at which residue substitutions are found in the C_L region. [From R. J. Poljak *et al.*, *Proc. Natl. Acad. Sci. USA* **70,** 3305 (1973).]

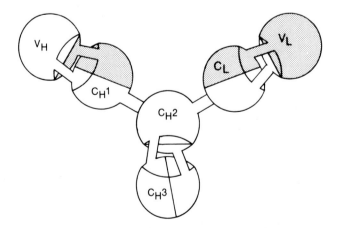

Figure 3–16 The domains of the human IgG molecule as determined by X-ray analysis at 6 Å. Shaded regions indicate that portion of each domain contributed by light chains. [Reproduced from R. J. Poljak *et al.*, *Nature* **235,** 137 (1972), figure 3.]

show that the V_L, V_H, C_L, and $C_H 1$ regions are strikingly similar in their three-dimensional conformation. These homology units each exhibit the characteristic "immunoglobulin fold" (Figure 3–15). The V regions differ from the C regions only by the presence of an extra polypeptide loop and by structural variation in the antigen-binding crevice. The three-dimensional structures of these homology units must have been highly conserved throughout vertebrate evolution, because the genes that code for the C_H regions of different immunoglobulin classes (e.g., IgG and IgA) probably diverged from one another hundreds of millions of years ago.

B. X-ray analysis shows that the immunoglobulin molecule is differentiated into discrete, compact, globular domains connected by short segments of more extended polypeptide chain (Figure 3–16). Each domain consists of a pair of corresponding homology units folded together. The V_L and V_H homology units form the V domain; the C_L and $C_H 1$ units form the $C_H 1$ domain; two $C_H 2$ units form the $C_H 2$ domain; and two $C_H 3$ units form the $C_H 3$ domain (Figure 3–13). Thus the basic $(L–H)_2$ immunoglobulin unit is composed of six globular domains: two V, two $C_H 1$, one $C_H 2$, and one $C_H 3$.

1. Proteolytic digestion under suboptimal conditions can cause limited cleavage of native immunoglobulin molecules between globular domains. Presumably the compactly folded domains are protected from proteolysis, whereas the regions of more extended polypeptide chain between homology units are accessible. Early experiments with cleavage showed that the IgG molecule can be broken into three fragments by cleavage of the hinge region of the heavy chain (Figure 3–13). Two of these fragments, designated Fab (for antigen-binding fragment), are identical. Each consists of one V and one $C_H 1$ domain, so that each carries one antigen-binding site (Figure 3–17). The third fragment, which turned out to be readily crystallizable and consequently is designated the Fc fragment, consists of the $C_H 2$ and $C_H 3$ domains.

2. Such fragmentation by mild proteolysis subsequently has allowed isolation of the combinations of globular domains listed in Table 3–3. These fragments have proved to be very useful in elucidating structure–function relationships in antibody molecules.

C. The antigen-binding functions and effector functions of immunoglobulins are carried out by different domains of the molecule. The V domains are responsible for antigen binding, whereas the C domains carry out the various effector functions (Essential Concept 1–9). These functions include the stimulation of B cells to undergo proliferation and differentiation, activation of the complement system, opsonization, transfer of IgG from mother to fetus across the placental barrier, transfer

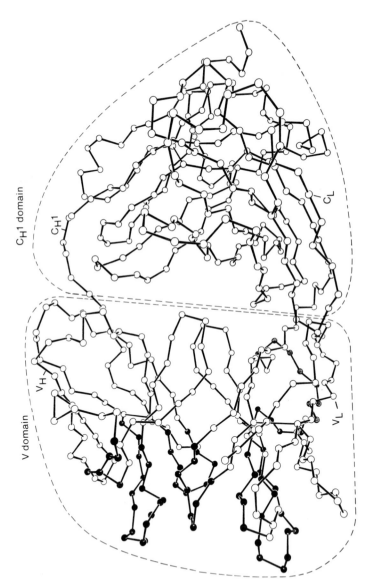

Figure 3–17 A drawing of the α-carbon backbone of the Fab' fragment of the mouse myeloma protein McPC603. The hypervariable regions associated with the antigen-binding site are indicated by black circles. The third hypervariable region, not associated with the antigen-binding site, is indicated by shaded circles. [From D. R. Davies et al., Contemp. Top. Mol. Immunol. **4,** 127 (1976).]

Table 3–3
Domains obtained from immunoglobulin molecules by mild proteolytic digestion

Domain	Name of fragment
[a]$V-C_H1$	Fab
C_H2-C_H3	Fc
$(V-C_H1)_2$	$(Fab')_2$
$V-C_H1-C_H2$	Fabc
C_H1	—
C_H3	Fc'
V	Fv
[b]V_L	—
[b]C_L	—

[a]The N-terminal half of the heavy chain, designated the Fd piece, can be isolated from the Fab fragment.
[b]Produced from proteolytic digestion of light chain.

of immunoglobulin into milk, sweat, tears, saliva, and gastrointestinal secretions, and fixation of certain classes of antibodies to mast cells. Some of these functions are triggered by antigen–antibody combination (B-cell stimulation, mast-cell degranulation, and complement fixation), whereas others are not (placental transfer, epithelial transfer, and mast-cell fixation). It is likely, although unproven, that each of the C domains contains the active site for at least one effector function. There is some evidence that the C_H2 domain of the IgG molecule plays a role in complement activation. The C_H3 domain will bind to lymphocyte and certain macrophage membranes, and is responsible for triggering activation of mature B cells after a specific antigen is bound by the V domain of an immunoglobulin surface-receptor molecule. Accordingly, the V domain must communicate with the C_H2 and C_H3 domains to trigger appropriate effector functions. Presumably this communication involves conformational changes that occur throughout the antibody molecule when an antigen is bound by the V domain. However, these conformational changes probably require binding of antigen to more than one V domain. Binding of univalent haptens does not activate complement or trigger B-cell activation. Apparently these effector functions are initiated by cross-linking the arms of a single antibody or by cross-linking two or more antibody molecules to each other.

3–6   The five classes of immunoglobulin molecules differ in the structures of their heavy-chain constant regions

A.   The five immunoglobulin classes are distinguished structurally by differences in their heavy-chain constant regions. Comparisons of C_H region amino acid sequences show that there are five major heavy-chain classes, designated α, γ, δ, ε, and μ. These heavy-chain classes define the corresponding immunoglobulin classes IgA, IgG, IgD, IgE, and IgM, respectively (Table 3–4). The C_H amino acid sequences of these classes are homologous, but they differ by more than 60% of their residues. Some classes can be divided into subclasses, defined by C_H regions that are distinct but more similar in amino acid sequence; for example, in humans the γ class can be divided into $\gamma1$, $\gamma2$, $\gamma3$, and $\gamma4$ subclasses. The genes that code for heavy chains are known collectively as the *heavy-chain (H) gene family*.

B.   In addition there are two major *types* of light chains based on C_L-region amino-acid-sequence comparisons. These two types, designated κ and λ, differ by about 60% in their C_L amino acid sequences (Table 3–5). Like some heavy-chain classes, the λ-type light chains may be further divided into subtypes defined by distinct but very similar

Table 3–4
Subunit structures of the five immunoglobulin classes in humans

Class	Heavy chain	Subclasses	Light chain	Molecular formula
IgG	γ	$\gamma1$, $\gamma2$ $\gamma3$, $\gamma4$	κ or λ	$(\gamma_2\kappa_2)$ $(\gamma_2\lambda_2)$
IgA	α	$\alpha1$, $\alpha2$	κ or λ	$(\alpha_2\kappa_2)_n^a$ $(\alpha_2\lambda_2)_n^a$
IgM	μ	none	κ or λ	$(\mu_2\kappa_2)_5$ $(\mu_2\lambda_2)_5$
IgD	δ	none	κ or λ	$(\delta_2\kappa_2)$ $(\delta_2\lambda_2)$
IgE	ϵ	none	κ or λ	$(\epsilon_2\kappa_2)$ $(\epsilon_2\lambda_2)$

[a] n may equal 1, 2, or 3.

Table 3–5
The amino-acid-difference matrix for various mammalian C regions[a]

	Human C_κ	Mouse C_κ	Rat C_κ	Human C_λ
Human C_κ				
Mouse C_κ	41			
Rat C_κ	38	28		
Human C_λ	60	65	61	
Mouse C_{λ_1}	56	68	61	39

[a]Numbers indicate the percentages of amino acid differences between the two chains compared. Differences between γ and κ chains (shaded squares), even from the same species, are more pronounced than γ–γ or κ–κ differences (unshaded squares).

C_L sequences. Immunoglobulin light chains from various mammals can be assigned readily to the λ and κ type, based on sequence homology (Figure 3–18). The genes that code for these light-chain types comprise the λ *gene family* and the κ *gene family,* respectively.

C.   The classes of immunoglobulins are defined by the classes of their constituent heavy-chain subunits only (Table 3–4). The class of an immunoglobulin molecule is independent of the class of light-chain subunits that it contains. A single immunoglobulin molecule always has identical light and identical heavy chains. However, immunoglobulin molecules of a given class may contain either λ or κ light chains. The subunit compositions of the five immunoglobulin classes are listed in Table 3–4.

D.   In general a given B-cell clone produces only one type of light chain, κ or λ, and one of the five classes of heavy chain. At certain stages in their differentiation, however, B cells may simultaneously produce two classes of heavy chains, and thus two classes of immuno-globulins. These stages may reflect switching of a clone from production of one heavy-chain class to another in the course of maturation (Essential Concept 1–7C). By contrast, no clone ever has been observed to produce more than a single type of light chain, as if the choice between expression of κ or λ gene families were made irreversibly very early in B-cell differentiation. Fully mature plasma cells invariably produce only a single species of heavy chain and a single species of light chain.

E.   Although all immunoglobulin molecules probably bind antigens in a similar fashion, the different classes serve different physiological functions (Essential Concepts 1–8 and 1–9). The functional differences of the five classes reflect the structural differences in their heavy-chain constant regions, which comprise the effector domains of all immuno-globulin molecules.

3–7   Two genes code for each immunoglobulin polypeptide chain

A.   Two properties of immunoglobulins discussed so far appear to present a paradox. Both light and heavy chains represent large families of similar proteins that exhibit diverse sequences in one region of the molecule and virtually identical sequences in the remainder. That is, the same C-region sequence may be found in association with any one of a large number of V-region sequences. In addition, a given variable domain with a particular idiotype and antigen-binding specificity may be associated with several of the five immunoglobulin classes, thereby indicating linkage of one V_H sequence with more than one class of C_H sequence. To explain these observations without postulating extensive coding redundancy among immunoglobulin genes, it was proposed several years ago that immunoglobulin V regions and C regions

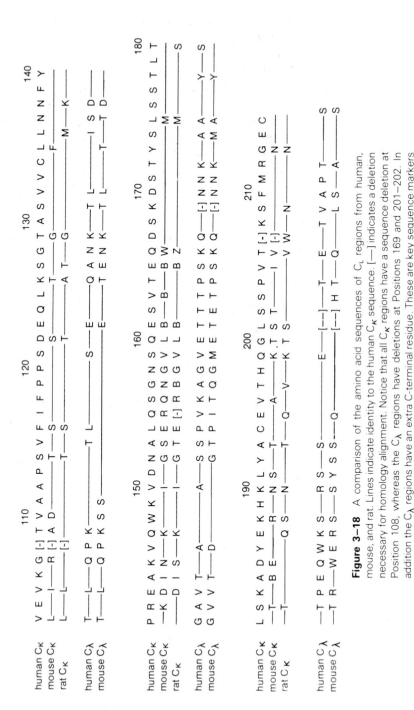

Figure 3–18 A comparison of the amino acid sequences of C_L regions from human, mouse, and rat. Lines indicate identity to the human C_κ sequence. [—] indicates a deletion necessary for homology alignment. Notice that all C_κ regions have a sequence deletion at Position 108, whereas the C_λ regions have deletions at Positions 169 and 201–202. In addition the C_λ regions have an extra C-terminal residue. These are key sequence markers that differentiate the two types of chains, in addition to the amino-acid-homology differences given in Table 3–5.

are coded by separate genes, which somehow are expressed together in various combinations to produce the observed immunoglobulin polypeptides. This novel hypothesis has become a central tenet of molecular immunology, and may turn out to be an important concept in understanding other aspects of metazoan development, as well as the immune system.

B.   The existence of separate V-region and C-region genes recently has been demonstrated directly in two experiments with nucleic acids from mouse cells. These experiments make use of several recently developed techniques of nucleic acid biochemistry.

1.   Experiments with embryonic DNA cleaved into small fragments by digestion with restriction endonucleases suggest that the V and C regions of the κ light chain are coded by two separate genes in the germ line. This suggestion is based on the finding that sequences complementary to κ light chain mRNA are found on two different DNA fragments (Figure 3–19). Furthermore, these sequences appear to undergo some type of covalent modification during the differentiation of antibody-producing cells. When fragments of DNA from myeloma cells are analyzed in the same manner, sequences complementary to the κ light chain mRNA are found on only one DNA fragment. These findings are consistent with the view that separate V and/or C genes are rearranged or translocated during differentiation. These experiments are described more fully in the legend to Figure 3–19.

2.   A V_λ gene has been isolated from embryonic mouse DNA and replicated by splicing it enzymatically into the DNA of a bacterial plasmid (a small, circular, autonomously replicating molecule), introducing the recombinant plasmid into a bacterium, and culturing the bacteria as a source from which recombinant plasmid DNA can be isolated in large quantities. By applying newly developed sequencing techniques to this DNA, the entire nucleotide sequence of the embryonic V_λ gene has been determined. This sequence unequivocally demonstrates that the C_λ gene is not adjacent to the V_λ gene in embryonic DNA (Figure 3–20). Additional experiments have demonstrated that the V_λ and C_λ genes are not adjacent in the differentiated myeloma DNA. The untranslated DNA between the leader and V_λ sequences and between the V_λ and C_λ sequences in differentiated antibody-producing cells is designated "intervening" DNA (Figures 3–20 and 3–20A). Intragenic intervening sequences also have been found in genes for ovalbumin, globin, and tRNA's. There is increasing evidence that intervening sequences are a general feature of eucaryotic genes.

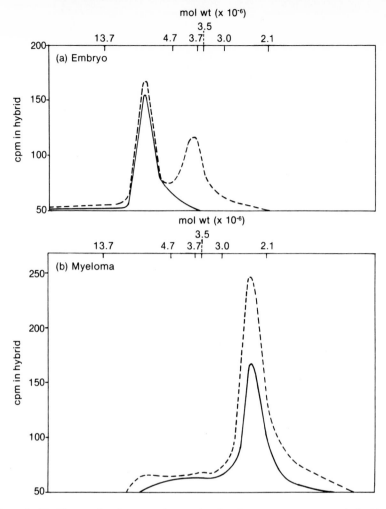

Figure 3–19 The results of an experiment showing that separate genes code for V_κ and C_κ regions in the germ line (see text). Messenger RNA (mRNA) molecules will *hybridize* to complementary DNA sequences to form base-repaired duplex structures, which can be detected by a variety of techniques. Thus a specific mRNA may be used as a probe to assay for the presence of the complementary sequence in a DNA preparation. For this experiment, mRNA specific for the κ light chain was isolated from a mouse myeloma tumor. One sample of the mRNA was kept intact as a probe for both V- and C-region sequences, and another sample was partially digested to serve as a probe for C-region sequences only. Samples of DNA were isolated from (a) mouse embryo cells and (b) myeloma tumor cells, cleaved with a restriction endonuclease, and subjected to electophoretic separation of different-sized fragments. The mRNA probes then were tested against the DNA fragments for hybridization. Dashed profiles indicate DNA fragments that hybridized with the complete immunoglobulin mRNA (V + C probe); solid profiles indicate DNA fragments that hybridized with the partially digested mRNA (C probe). In the embryo DNA preparation (a), the probe hybridized to a fragment of only one size, whereas the V + C probe hybridized to a fragment of this size and another of a different size; these results imply that V- and C-region sequences were present on different pieces of DNA. By contrast, in the myeloma cell DNA preparation both the C and V + C probes hybridized to a fragment of only one size. This result implies that the V- and C-region sequences in the myeloma preparation were present on the same or similar-sized pieces of DNA. [Adapted from S. Tonegawa *et al.*, *Cold Spring Harbor Symp. Quant. Biol.* **41**, 877 (1976).]

leader sequence

Met Ala Trp Thr Ser Leu Ile Leu Ser Leu Leu Ala Leu Cys Ser Gly
ATG GCC TGG ACT TCA CTT ATA CTC TCT CTG CTG TGC TCA GGT CAG CAG CCT TTC TAC ACT GCA GTG GGT ATG CAA CAA
TAC CGG ACC TGA AGT GAA TAT GAG AGA GAG GAC CGA GAG ACG AGT CCA GTC GTC GGA AAG ATG TGA CGT CAC CCA TAC GTT GTT

leader sequence

UGA Phe Ala Thr Asp Asp Trp Ile Ser Tyr Leu Phe Ala Gly Ala Ser Ser Glp Ala Val Val Thr Gln Glu Ser   1
TAC ACA TCT TGT CTC TGA TTT GCT ACT GAT GAC TGG ATT TCT TAC CTG TTT GCA GGA GCC AGT TCC CAG GCT GTT GTG ACT CAG GAA
ATG TGT AGA ACA GAG ACT AAA CGA TGA CTA CTG ACC TAA AGA ATG GAC AAA CGT CCT CGG TCA AGG GTC CGA CAA CAC TGA GTC CTT

Ala Leu Thr Thr Ser Pro Gly Gly Thr Val Ile Leu Thr Cys Arg Ser Ser Thr Gly Ala Val Thr Thr Ser Asn Tyr Ala Asn
                 10   20   30   hv1
TCT GCA CTC ACC ACA TCA CCT GGT GGA ACA GTC ATA CTC ACT TGT CGC TCA AGT ACT GGG GCT GTT ACA ACT AGT AAC TAT GCC
AGA CGT GAG TGG TGT AGT GGA CCA CCT TGT CAG TAT GAG TGA ACA GCG AGT TCA TGA CCC CGA CAA TGT TGA TCA TTG ATA CGG

Trp Val Gln Glu Lys Pro Asp His Leu Phe Thr Gly Leu Ile Gly Gly Thr Ser Asp Arg Ala Pro Gly Val Pro Val Arg Phe
                 40   50   60
hv2
AAC TGG GTT CAA GAA AAA CCA GAT CAT TTA TTC ACT GGT CTAATA GGT GGT ACA AGT GAT CGT GCC CCA GGT GTT CCT GTC AGA
TTG ACC CAA GTT CTT TTT GGT CTA GTA AAT AAG TGA CCA GAT TAT CCA CCA TGT TCA CTA GCA CGG GGT CCA CAA GGA CAG TCT

Ser Gly Ser Leu Ile Gly Asp Lys Ala Ala Leu Thr Ile Thr Gly Ala Gln Thr Glu Asp Asp Ala Met Tyr Phe Cys Ala Leu
                 70   80   90
hv3
TTC TCA GGC TCC CTG ATT GGA GAC AAG GCT GCC CTC ACC ATC ACA GGG GCA CAG ACT GAG GAT GAT GCA ATG TAT TTC TGT GCT
AAG AGT CCG AGG GAC TAA CCT CTG TTC CGA CGG GAG TGG TAG TGT CCC CGT GTC TGA CTC CTA CTA CGT TAC ATA AAG ACA CGA

Trp Tyr Ser Thr His Phe His Asn Asp Met Cys Arg   Trp Gly Ser Arg Trp   Tyr Ser Leu Thr Thr Ile Phe
                 100   110   120
VIC(1)   VIC(2)
CTA TGG TAC AGC ACC CAT TTC CAC AAT GAC ATG TGT AGG   GGA AGT TGT AGA TGG   TAC AGT CTC ACT ACC ATC
GAT ACC ATG TCG TGG GTA AAG GTG TTA CTG TAC ACA TCT   ACC CCT TCA ACA TCT   ATG TCA GAG TGA TGG TAG

Leu Thr Gly Gly Tyr Met Ser Leu Val Cys Ser Leu Leu Leu UAG
                 130
TTC TTA ACA GGT GGC TAC ATG TCC CTA GTC TGT TCT CTT TTA CTA TAG AGA AAT TTA TAA AAG CTG TTG TCT CGA GCA ACA AAA
AAG AAT TGT CCA CCG ATG TAC AGG GAT CAG ACA AGA GAA AAG GAT ATC TCT TTA AAT ATT TTC GAC AAC AGA GCT CGT TGT TTT

AGT TTT ATT CAA CAA ATT GTA TAA TTA TGC CTT GAT GAC AAG CTT TGT TTA TCA ACT TGG CAG AAC ATA GAA TC
TCA AAA TAA GTT GTT TAA CAT ATT ATT AAT ACG GAA CTA CTG TTC GAA ACA AAT AGT TGA ACC GTC TTG TAT CTT AG

Figure 3–20 The complete nucleotide sequence of an immunoglobulin light chain gene from mouse embryo DNA (λe). Directly above is given the protein sequence coded by this gene. Leader sequences exhibit homology for the leader sequence of λ chains synthesized in vitro. The three hypervariable regions are indicated by hv1, hv2, and hv3. VIC(1) indicates the point at which the λe sequence terminates its homology with λ protein sequences. VIC(2) indicates the point at which the junction between V- and C-regions occurs in λ polypeptide chains. [Courtesy of S. Tonegawa et al., Proc. Natl. Acad. Sci. USA **75**, 1485 (1978).]

3-8   Translocation of V and C genes could be the mechanism for differentiation of an antibody-producing cell

A.   Since V and C regions are coded by separate genes in the germ line, their information must be combined at some level to produce a complete immunoglobulin polypeptide. Theoretically, this combination could occur by joining of sequences at the DNA, the RNA, or the polypeptide level. Radioactive labeling experiments on antibody synthesis suggest that joining does *not* occur at the protein level (see Problem 3–14). Recent experiments with high-molecular-weight nuclear RNA from myeloma cells suggest that joining occurs at the RNA level. The initial transcript for κ chain V and C sequences is 40 S or 9000 nucleotides in length. This high-molecular-weight nuclear RNA undergoes several RNA processing events in which the intervening nucleotide sequences are removed and the transcript is shortened to 13 S or 1200 nucleotides (Figure 3–20A). The 13 S transcript, in which the V and C sequences now are adjacent, is transported to the cytoplasm for translation. Accordingly, in addition to translation and transcription there are two new levels at which control may be exerted in the expression of antibody genes: (1) during translocation of the V and C genes at the DNA level, and (2) during RNA processing (Figure 3–20A). Eucaryotic genes with intragenic intervening DNA sequences, such as the genes for ovalbumin and globin, also must employ RNA processing. It is not known whether expression of these genes also involves DNA translocation.

B.   Each plasma cell is differentiated to synthesize only a single molecular species of antibody. If V and C genes are translocated at the DNA level, this event could be the mechanism that commits a cell to the exclusive production of a particular immunoglobulin molecule. According to this hypothesis, the rearrangement of light-chain and

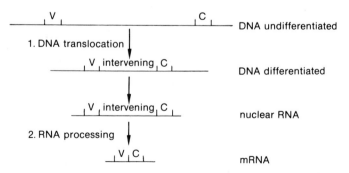

Figure 3–20A   A model of the translocation of antibody genes and the processing of antibody RNA transcripts (see text).

heavy-chain V genes and C genes would activate transcription of the resulting V–C genes.

C. Several lines of evidence suggest that a single V_H gene can become associated with two or more C_H genes during the differentiation of antibody-producing cells.

> **1.** During a normal immune response the predominant serum antibody class shifts from IgM to IgG ($C_\mu \rightarrow C_\gamma$), while retaining antigen-recognition specificity. Moreover, IgM and IgG antibodies produced in the course of the response may exhibit identical idiotypes. These observations suggest that the same V_H regions are associated with different immunoglobulin classes, and therefore with different C_H regions.

> **2.** Single lymphocytes may synthesize two or more classes of immunoglobulins with identical antigen-recognition specificity and idiotype. For example, some B cells carry both IgM and IgD molecules of identical idiotype as cell-surface receptors.

> **3.** A single B cell may produce daughter cells that differ in the class of immunoglobulin synthesized while maintaining antigenic specificity and idiotype.

> **4.** Analysis of both amino acid sequences and idiotypes have suggested that identical V_H regions can be exhibited by two classes of myeloma immunoglobulins derived from a single patient. These so-called *biclonal myelomas* presumably arise by neoplastic transformation of a lymphocyte, which subsequently differentiates to produce two daughter clones, each expressing the same V_H region associated with a different C_H region. The light chains of the two myeloma immunoglobulins appear to be identical.

D. Two general models have been proposed to account for the association of a single V_H gene with two or more C_H genes (Figure 3–21).

> **1.** The *simultaneous translocation* model postulates that copies of a replicated V_H gene may be joined to each of the classes of C_H genes in the heavy-chain family (Figure 3–21a). Differentiation then would involve successive activation of complete V_H–C_H genes by conventional mechanisms of gene regulation.

> **2.** The *successive translocation* model postulates that a single V_H gene may switch from one C_H gene to a second (or third) during the differentiation process (Figure 3–21b). Accordingly, each cell could transcribe only a single V_H–C_H gene at any given time.

> This model could be disproved by a demonstration that a single cell can synthesize two or more classes of immunoglobulin with the same V regions over a period of time longer than the lifetime of heavy-chain mRNA.

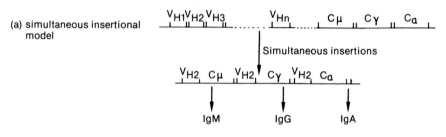

(a) simultaneous insertional model

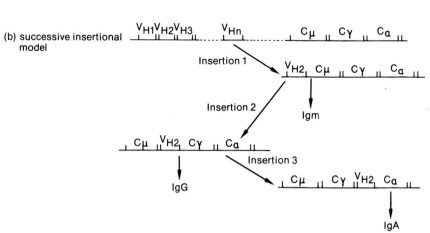

(b) successive insertional model

Figure 3–21 Two models for the joining of a V_H gene to various C_H genes (see text). [Adapted from C. Sledge *et al., Proc. Natl. Acad. Sci. USA* **73**, 923 (1976).]

E.   Several models have been suggested for V–C translocation at the DNA level (Figure 3–22).

1.   The *copy-insertion model* suggests that a given V gene may be copied and spliced near one or more C genes.

2.   The *excision-insertion model* requires that the V region be excised from the chromosome and later reintegrated near its C gene.

3.   The *deletion model* suggests that a V gene may be moved near a C gene by deleting some of the intervening genetic material. A looping-out process could successively associate a V gene with different C genes.

4.   The *inversion model* suggests that the V and C genes may be translocated through an inversion loop.

F.   The association of a single V_H gene (or copies of it) with two or more C_H genes during the differentiation of lymphocyte clones permits a particular antigen-binding site to be associated with a variety of different

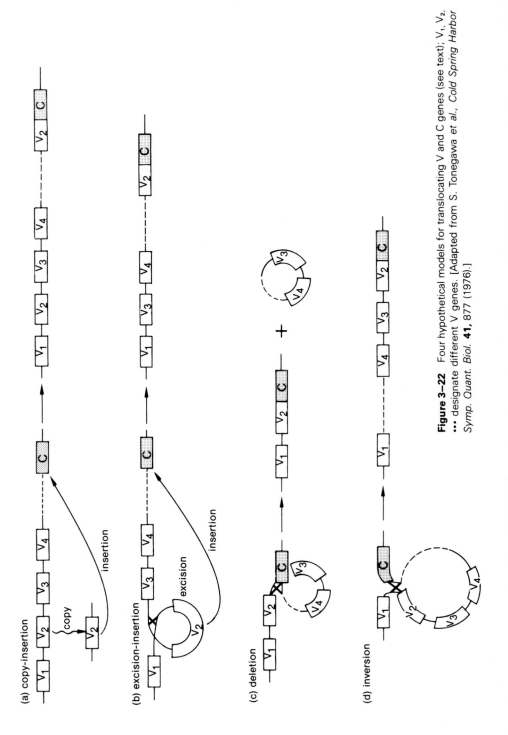

(a) copy-insertion

(b) excision-insertion

(c) deletion

(d) inversion

Figure 3–22 Four hypothetical models for translocating V and C genes (see text); V_1, V_2, ••• designate different V genes. [Adapted from S. Tonegawa et al., *Cold Spring Harbor Symp. Quant. Biol.* **41**, 877 (1976).]

effector functions (Figure 3–23). Theoretically, any given antigen-specific V domain may be joined to the appropriate C_H regions to fix complement (C_γ or C_μ), cross the placenta (C_γ), or be secreted across the mucous membranes (C_α). This process is termed *combinatorial translocation*. The immune system employs two combinatorial mechanisms in the generation of diverse antibodies: combinatorial translocation of V_H regions with different C_H regions, and combinatorial association of light chains with heavy chains.

G.   The antibody gene families exhibit a regulatory phenomenon known as *allelic exclusion*. In an animal heterozygous for genetic markers on light and heavy chains, a given lymphocyte clone expresses only one light-chain and one heavy-chain allele. This behavior contrasts to that of all other common mammalian proteins studied, such as allelic forms of hemoglobin, which are produced codominantly in the cells of a heterozygous individual. Although the molecular basis of allelic exclusion is unknown, it, too, could be a consequence of the V–C translocation mechanism. If the translocation event can occur on only one chromosome for light chains and on only one chromosome for heavy chains, then only one member of any pair of alleles could be expressed in a given clone after translocation had occurred. According to this view, the V–C translocation events would be decisive in the three choices that must be made during the differentiation of every antibody-producing cell: selection of one of the two light-chain families; selection of a particular V and C gene from the chosen light-chain family and from the heavy-chain family; and selection of the V–C light-chain and heavy-chain alleles that will be expressed.

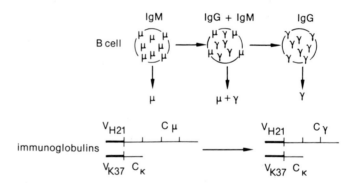

Figure 3–23 Events that occur during the maturation of the immune response, from the production of IgM to IgG antibody. A single cell is depicted going through three stages of antibody synthesis: μ synthesis, $\mu + \gamma$ synthesis, and γ synthesis. During this shift there is no change in the idiotype of the antibodies produced. Thus the same V domain may be associated with different C domains (combinatorial joining). There probably are several other stages in the differentiation of most antibody-producing cells (e.g., IgM to IgM +. IgD, etc.; see Essential Concept 1–8C).

3-9   Mammalian immunoglobulins are coded by three unlinked clusters of genes

A.   Genetic analysis of the immunoglobulins has been carried out in mice, rabbits, and humans, using serologic reagents to follow the inheritance of three types of antigenic markers on various immunoglobulin chains.

> **1.**   *Allotypes* are immunoglobulin variants (polymorphisms) that exhibit a Mendelian pattern of segregation. For example, three human C_κ-region variants, termed the *Inv* markers, differ by one or two amino acids out of 107 (Figure 3-24). Antibodies specific for each variant can be found in the serum of some mothers who have had infants of differing Inv type. These mothers have become immunized against the foreign fetal C_κ determinants. This process is known as *homologous* (same species) *immunization*. Serologic identification of the three Inv markers in family and population studies has shown that these polymorphisms behave like three alleles of a single structural gene.
>
> Allotypes also have been found on rabbit λ and κ chains and on many of the heavy-chain classes and subclasses from man, mouse, and rabbit (Table 3-6). The allotypic amino acid changes generally are localized to C regions (Table 3-7). Consequently, allotypes have permitted the genetic mapping of C genes.
>
> **2.**   *Isotypes* are the antigenic determinants that characterize each class and subclass of heavy chain and each type and subtype of light chain. Isotype-specific antibodies are prepared by immunizing one animal species with the immunoglobulin chains of a second, a process known as *heterologous immunization*. Homologous immunizations are useful for detecting the subtle differences between allotypes, because most of the immunoglobulin structure will be shared by donor and host. In contrast, heterologous

position

Inv	108	153	191	214
1		V	L	COO⁻
1,2		A	L	COO⁻
3		A	V	COO⁻

Figure 3–24   Genetic polymorphisms in human C_K regions. The amino acid sequence of these three human C_K regions is identical to that given in Figure 3–14 except for the substitutions indicated at Positions 153 and 191. These three C_K regions are coded by three alleles of a single structural gene (see text). [Adapted from A. G. Steinberg *et al.*, *Immunogenetics* **1,** 108 (1974).]

Table 3–6
Allotypes of human, mouse, and rabbit[a]

HUMAN	
Immunoglobulin family	Alleles
Kappa	Inv(1), Inv(1,2), Inv(3)
Lambda	none identified
Heavy	
G1	Gm1, Gm(non-1); *Footnote b*
	Gm3, Gm17; *Footnote b*
	Gm2, 18, 20; *Footnote c*
G2	Gm23, Gm(non-23); *Footnote b*
G3	Gm21, Gm(non-21); *Footnote b*
	Gm5, Gm(non-5); *Footnote b*
	Gm11, Gm(non-11)
	Gm6, 10, 14, 15, 16, 24, 25; *Footnote c*
G4	Gm(4a) Gm(4b); *Footnote b*
A1	none identified
A2	Am(1), Am(−1); *Footnote b*
D	none identified
M	none identified
E	none identified

MOUSE	
Kappa	none identified
Lambda	none identified
Heavy	
G1	$4^{a,c,d,e,f,g,h}$, 4^b; *Footnote d*
G2a	1^a, 1^b, 1^c, 1^d, 1^e, 1^f, 1^g, 1^f
G2b	$3^{a,c,h}$, 3^b, 3^d, 3^e, 3^f, 3^g
G3	none identified
A	$2^{a,h}$, 2^b, $2^{c,g}$, $2^{d,e}$, 2^f
D	5^a, 5^b
M	6^a, 6^b

RABBIT	
Kappa	b4, b5, b6, b9
Lambda	c7, c21
Heavy	
V_H	a1, a2, a3; *Footnote e*
	x32, x−
	y33, y−
C_μ	n81, n82
C_α	f71, f72, f73; *Footnote f*
	g74, g75
C_γ	d11, d12; *Footnote f*
	e14, e15

Table 3-7
Amino acid substitutions that correlate with allotypes

Species	Immunoglobulin family	Residue position	Alternate residues
Human	Kappa Inv (1), (1, 2), (3)	153, 191	(Figure 3–24)
	Heavy		
	Gm (1) ⎫ Gm (non-1) ⎬	355–358	RDEL REEM
	Gm (3) ⎫ Gm (17) ⎬	214	R K
	Gm (11) ⎫ Gm (non-11) ⎬	296	F Y
Rabbit	Kappa b4, b5, b6, b9	Multiple	Throughout C_κ (Figure 3–28)
	Heavy		
	al, a2, a3	Multiple	Throughout V_H
	d11 ⎫ d12 ⎬	225	M T
	d14 ⎫ d15 ⎬	309	T A

immunizations are necessary for detecting the major differences between isotypes, because members of the same species will exhibit the same isotypes.

All the isotypes characteristic of a given species are found in the serum of every individual in the species. Accordingly, each isotype must be encoded by a different gene that is present in every member of the species. For example, at least four human C_λ-region variants (Figure 3-25) are present in all humans.

Notes to Table 3-6

[a]Adapted from R. Mage et al. in The Antigens, M. Sela (Ed.), Academic Press, New York and London, 1973, p. 300.

[b]Allelic pairs that are known or suspected to be caused by amino acid substitutions at homologous positions in the polypeptide chain (see Table 3–7).

[c]Allelic alternatives whose structural basis is unknown.

[d]The alleles for the various immunoglobulin classes are found on various inbred strains of mice. Many of the serological markers that define these alleles have been localized to their respective C_H regions. None have been localized to V_H regions.

[e]The a, x, and y serological markers are found on three different kinds of V_H regions. x– and y– indicate that an antiserum has not been raised to the allelic alternatives of x32 and y33, respectively.

[f]The f and g markers are located at two different positions in the C_α region. C_α regions exhibiting many combinations of the f and g markers have been found in various populations of rabbits. The d and e markers of γ chains also are located at two different positions, and γ chains with three of the four combinations of these markers have been identified.

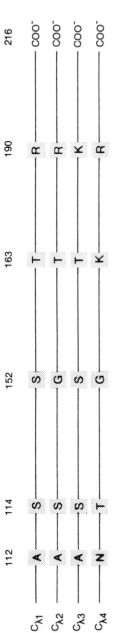

Figure 3–25 Amino-acid-sequence variations found in the C_λ regions of human immunoglobulins. Position 152 is designated the Kern marker. Position 190 is designated the Oz marker. For each of these variations there is an antiserum that can detect one variant but not the other. Hence for the Kern marker, glycine chains are designated + and serine chains −. Likewise, for the Oz marker, lysine chains are + and arginine chains −. Each of these four C_λ sequences is found in the serum of all humans. Thus this polymorphism represents isotypes coded by at least four C_λ genes present in every individual. [Adapted from J. Fett and H. Deutsch, *Immunochemistry* **12**, 643 (1975).]

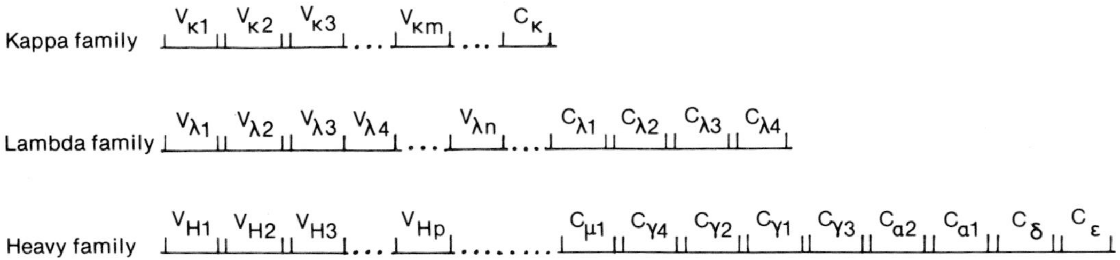

Figure 3–26 The proposed chromosomal organization of the antibody genes into three unlinked clusters in human germ cells. The number of V genes in each cluster is unknown, and the order of the C_λ and C_H genes is uncertain. [Adapted from G. Edelman and J. Gally, *Annu. Rev. Genet.* **6**, 1 (1972).]

Isotypes can reflect limited variation of a few residues, as in human λ chains, which therefore presumably arose by recent gene duplication. Isotypes also can reflect more extensive variation of many residues, as in μ and γ chains, which therefore presumably arose by more ancient gene duplication.

3. *Idiotypes* are the antigenic determinants that distinguish one V domain from all other V domains (Essential Concept 1–2C). Serologic reagents for idiotypes generally are obtained by homologous immunizations. In practice, anti-idiotypic antibodies can recognize antigenic determinants in or outside of the antigen-binding site. Anti-idiotypic antibodies may recognize a series of very closely related V domains. Idiotypes have been used for mapping of V genes.

B.   Genetic analysis of allotypes, isotypes, and idiotypes has led to several conclusions about the organization of antibody genes.

1.   Immunoglobulin polypeptides are coded by three unlinked clusters of autosomal genes (Figure 3–26). One cluster codes for heavy chains of all classes and subclasses; a second codes for κ light chains; and a third codes for λ light chains. These three gene clusters are called the H, κ, and λ gene families, respectively.

2.   Each of the three immunoglobulin gene families includes V genes and C genes. In rabbits, which exhibit both V_H and C_H allotypes (Table 3–6), it has been shown that recombination can give rise to new combinations of V_H and C_H genes. This demonstration further emphasizes the separation of V and C genes within the heavy-chain gene family. If V and C genes were intermingled, V_H and C_H markers would not be separable by recombination. In man the κ-gene family appears to have a single C gene, whereas the λ-gene family has at least four, and the heavy-chain gene family has at least ten (Figure 3–26). The number of V genes in each family is still a matter of controversy (Essential Concept 3–10).

3.   Genetic analysis of idiotypes in mice has demonstrated twelve V_H markers that segregate in a Mendelian fashion and are closely linked to the C_H allotypic markers. Recombinational analysis of some of these idiotypes has permitted determination of their map order and estimation of the genetic map distance across this region (Figure 3–27). The results indicate that multiple V_H genes are linked to the C_H gene cluster in the DNA of the mouse.

C.   Allotypes can be classified into two categories, designated simple and complex. Alternative forms of *simple allotypes* segregate in a Mendelian fashion in mating studies, and differ by only one or a few

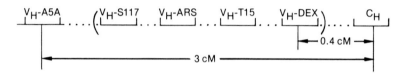

Figure 3–27 A genetic map of loci that determine V_H idiotypes of the mouse. T15 determines a phosphorylcholine-binding myeloma protein; A5A determines a homogeneous antibody response to group A streptococcal carbohydrate; DEX determines the response to α-1,3-dextran; ARS determines the response to *p*-azo-phenylarsonate; and C_H represents the locus of the corresponding C_H genes. The order of the V_H loci within the brackets is unknown. Between V_H–DEX and the C_H marker, the recombination frequency is 0.4%; between V_H–A5A and the C_H marker it is 3.0%. [Adapted from R. Riblet *et al.*, *Eur. J. Immunol.* **5**, 778 (1975).]

amino acid substitutions. Most immunoglobulin allotypes fall into this category (Table 3–6). Alternative forms of *complex allotypes* also generally segregate in a Mendelian fashion, but they differ by multiple amino acid residues. The Group *a* and Group *b* allotypes of the rabbit are complex allotypes (Table 3–7 and Figure 3–28).

The distinction between simple and complex allotypes is important because different genetic or evolutionary mechanisms must be invoked to account for their origins. Simple allotypes probably are coded by alternative alleles at a single genetic locus. Complex allotypes are more difficult to explain. Three genetic models have been proposed to account for their existence (Figure 3–29). Each model has different implications for the organization of antibody gene families that exhibit the phenomenon of complex allotypes.

1.   Complex allotypes could evolve by extensive divergence of alleles at a single genetic locus (Figure 3–29a). If so, intense selective pressure would have been required to fix many amino acid substitutions in a relatively short period of evolutionary time.

2.   Complex allotypes could evolve by gene duplication, mutational divergence, and subsequent crossing-over events that reduce the number of genes back to one (Figure 3–29b). In different populations or different inbred strains, different genes could remain.

3.   Complex allotypes could be coded by closely linked genes that have arisen by duplication and divergence, and that are governed by a control mechanism that permits only one of them to be expressed. The products of such genes would mimic a Mendelian pattern of segregation, although the genes would not be true alleles (Figure 3–29c).

```
           110                120                130              140
b4 Cκ   D P [ ] V A P T V L I F P P A A D Q V A T G T V T I V C V A N K Y F P
b9 Cκ   — P I — — — — — L — — — — — — — — — — S — — — — — — L T — Z — — — — F R —

           150                160                170
b4 Cκ   [ ] D V T V T W E V D G T T Q T T G T Q D S K T P Q D S A D C T Y N L S
b9 Cκ   D — I — — — — — — K — — — D E I — Q S — — I E N — T — — — S P E — — — — [ ]

           180             190              200             210
b4 Cκ   S T L L T S T Q Y N S H K E Y T C K V T Q G T T S V V Q S F N R G D C
b9 Cκ   — S — — K A — — — — — S [ ] — — — — — — Q — H N S A G — I — Z
```

Figure 3–28 The C_κ regions coded by two complex allotypes of rabbit κ chains, b4 and b9 (see Table 3–7). These C_κ regions differ by 33% of their amino acid sequence and by three sequence gaps. [From V. Farnsworth et al., Proc. Natl. Acad. Sci. USA **73**, 1293 (1975).]

(a) CLASSICAL ALLELIC MODEL

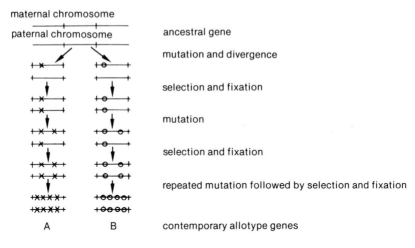

maternal chromosome

paternal chromosome   ancestral gene

                                           mutation and divergence

                                           selection and fixation

                                           mutation

                                           selection and fixation

                                           repeated mutation followed by selection and fixation

      A   B   contemporary allotype genes

(b) GENE DUPLICATION-DELETION MODEL

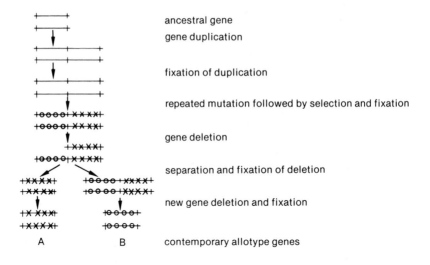

                                           ancestral gene
                                           gene duplication

                                           fixation of duplication

                                           repeated mutation followed by selection and fixation

                                           gene deletion

                                           separation and fixation of deletion

                                           new gene deletion and fixation

      A   B   contemporary allotype genes

(c) CONTROL MODEL

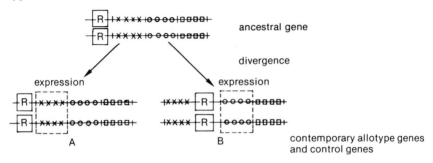

                                           ancestral gene

                                           divergence

      expression   expression

      A   B   contemporary allotype genes
                                           and control genes

← **Figure 3–29**   Three models for the evolution of complex allotypes (see text). X's and O's represent mutational differences in the divergence of two ancestral genes that exhibit Mendelian behavior in contemporary individuals, A and B, of a particular species. In (c) the dotted boxes indicate that different genes are expressed in different strains, and that this expression is regulated by a *cis*-dominant regulatory element, R. [Adapted from G. Gutman *et al.*, *Proc. Natl. Acad. Sci. USA* **72,** 5046 (1975).]

D.   Powerful new techniques of nucleic acid chemistry and genetic engineering are now available for studying the organization of the antibody gene families. Many of these techniques involve the isolation and purification of specific mRNA, which already has been achieved for mouse light chains.

   1.   Messenger RNA for mouse κ chains has the structure shown in Figure 3–30. There are untranslated regions at the 5′ and 3′ ends of the mRNA. There also is a 3′ tail of polyadenylic acid. In both of these characteristics the mRNA of κ chains resembles many other eucaryotic mRNA's.

   2.   Complementary RNA and DNA molecules can associate to form hybrid duplexes. Under appropriate conditions the rate of this reaction is dependent on the number of DNA copies of a particular mRNA sequence that are present in the genome. Consequently, measurement of the rate of hybridization between a particular κ-chain mRNA and somatic DNA can provide an estimate of the number of V genes in the genome that are identical or closely related in sequence to the mRNA. The results of such experiments are discussed in Essential Concept 3–10.

   3.   DNA copies of individual κ-chain mRNA's have been made by replication of the RNA, using the enzyme reverse transcriptase. Also, mammalian genes now can be isolated directly from the DNA, as was done for the mouse V_λ gene described earlier. The resulting synthetic or isolated genes can be inserted into bacterial plasmids and produced in quantity, as described in Essential Concept 3–7B2. More of these artificially-cloned anti-

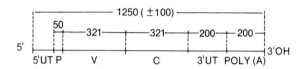

Figure 3–30   A model for the structure of κ mRNA from myeloma tumors of the BALB/c mouse. Numbers indicate lengths of various segments in nucleotides. UT indicates untranslated portion. P indicates a region that may code for an N-terminal precursor sequence that is cleaved prior to secretion. Poly(A) indicates polyadenylic acid. [Reproduced from C. Milstein, *et al.*, *Nature* **252,** 354 (1974), figure 6a.]

body genes will be subjected to DNA sequencing, which may yield new insights into the organization of antibody genes and the basis for antibody diversity.

3-10 The origin of antibody diversity is still debated

A.   The vertebrate immune system is capable of synthesizing perhaps 10^5 to 10^8 different antibody molecules, which collectively can recognize a virtually unlimited number of different antigens. How does an organism generate this vast antibody diversity? Many immunologists in the 1930's and 1940's favored the hypothesis that antigens could *instruct* the organism to make complementary antibodies by serving as templates around which antibody polypeptides might fold. However, the instructionist theories were ruled out in the early 1960's when it was shown that the three-dimensional structure of an antibody molecule is determined entirely by its amino acid sequence. This demonstration was accomplished by completely unfolding specific Fab fragments in a strong denaturing solvent, after reducing their disulfide bridges. Under appropriate renaturing conditions, a large percentage of these denatured antibody molecules subsequently refolded correctly *in the absence of antigen*, thereby reconstituting their specific antigen-binding sites. Following this demonstration, attempts to explain antibody diversity became focused on the origin of amino-acid-sequence diversity among the V_L and the V_H regions.

B.   Two general theories have been put forward to explain the observed amino-acid-sequence diversity of light-chain and heavy-chain variable regions.

> **1.**   The *germ-line theory* postulates that most, if not all, V-region genes are separately encoded in the germ line of the organism. These genes are assumed to have arisen by gene duplication, mutation, and selection during vertebrate evolution. According to this theory, the diversity of V-region genes exists prior to the differentiation of each individual, and antibody synthesis requires merely the activation of preexisting antibody genes in each lymphocyte.

> **2.**   The *somatic variation* theory postulates that V-region diversity develops from a relatively small number of germ-line genes, which diversify by mutational or recombinational processes during development of the immune system. According to this theory, V-region diversity is generated anew in each individual rather than passed from one generation to the next.

The germ-line theory proposes a separate germ-line V-gene for each V region the organism can synthesize. The extreme form of the somatic theory postulates only a single germ-line V-gene for each antibody family. As explained in the remainder of this ·section, the correct explanation for antibody diversity probably lies somewhere between these two extremes.

Both germ-line and somatic theories assume antigen-induced clonal expansion of lymphocytes that carry antigen-specific cell-surface receptors. Therefore both theories are compatible with induction of immune responses by clonal selection (Essential Concept 1–3).

C.   Each of the two general theories of antibody diversity has given rise to modified versions that currently are being investigated.

1.   The *germ-line* model cannot be ruled out by the argument that there is insufficient DNA in the germ line to encode the observed diversity of V regions. The total DNA in a human sperm cell could code for the equivalent of more than 10^7 V genes. If combinatorial association of light and heavy chains is generally applicable, then 10^3 V_L genes and 10^3 V_H genes could generate 10^6 different antibody molecules. The fraction of the genome required to code this information would be less than 0.02%, which appears reasonable for a function as important as B-cell immunity.

2.   The *somatic combinatorial* model suggests that two or more genes code for the V region of each antibody polypeptide. One specific formulation of this model postulates that each hyper-variable region is coded by a distinct gene and that the relatively constant remainder of the V region (framework portion) is coded by still another gene. During the differentiation of an antibody-producing cell, the hypervariable-region genes are inserted into the framework gene at appropriate positions to yield a complete V gene. The combinatorial properties of this model amplify enormously the number of antibody genes that can be produced from a limited number of framework and hypervariable-region genes. For example, 100 V_L framework genes and 100 each of the three V_L hypervariable-region genes could generate 100^4 or 10^8 different V_L genes. According to this model, antibody diversity arises from the evolutionary variability of germ-line hypervaria-ble-region and framework genes, and their combinatorial joining during somatic differentiation.

3.   The *ordinary-somatic-mutation model* suggests that the average antibody family has perhaps 100–200 germ-line V-region genes. Additional V-region diversity arises from the somatic mutations that occur ordinarily in the division of eucaryotic cells. The extensive antigen-independent proliferation of lymphoid cells during development of the immune system (Essential Concept 1–4) thus gives rise to a large variety of V-region genes in the lymphocyte population.

4. The *hypermutation model* postulates that V-region diversity arises from a few hundred germ-line V genes by a special mutational mechanism. Such a mechanism, for example, could involve a series of enzymes that specifically degrade and then repair one of the DNA strands at hypervariable regions, making frequent errors in the process. In this manner enormous sequence diversity could be generated in a relatively short time.

5. The *somatic recombination model* proposes that V-region diversity arises from a few hundred germ-line V genes, which undergo extensive somatic crossing-over between sister chromatids during proliferation and differentiation of lymphoid cells. This mechanism also would have the potential for generating virtually unlimited numbers of V genes in a relatively short time. This model is similar to the somatic combinatorial model, except that it allows recombination to occur anywhere throughout the V gene.

D.   One useful approach for evaluating these theories has been comparative analyses of amino-acid sequences from large numbers of myeloma and antibody V regions. Amino-acid-sequence data are now available for more than 700 different mouse and human myeloma V regions, each obtained from a different individual. To analyze this large amount of data, the approach of *genealogic analysis* is particularly useful in allowing the relationships between V regions to be displayed in a compact form.

1. The hypothetical genealogic tree shown in Figure 3–31 depicts the minimum number of genetic events required to generate the set of V_κ regions in an individual animal, for example a mouse, from a single ancestral V_κ gene. This mouse's V_κ-region sequences (reduced in number for clarity) are represented by the uppermost set of branches on Level E. Genetic events include gene duplications, single-base substitutions, and sequence insertions or deletions. Each V-gene duplication is represented by a branching of the tree. The number of single-base DNA substitutions that distinguish between two adjacent nodal sequences at the same level is the sum of the numbers on the two branches leading to them. For example, sequences $V_{\kappa A_1}$ and $V_{\kappa A_2}$ on Level A differ from the ancestral sequence V_κ by five substitutions each, and from each other by ten substitutions. Sequence deletions are indicated by [/]$_n$, where n indicates the numbers of the amino acids (or corresponding codons) deleted. On the terminal twigs of the tree (Level E) very similar sequences will be clustered together—for example, 8, 9, and 10—whereas dissimilar sequences will be widely separated.

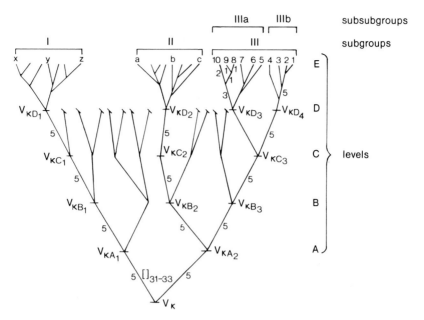

Figure 3–31 A hypothetical genealogic tree of V_κ regions from a single individual. A genealogic tree is constructed from a set of proteins (terminal twigs at Level E) by generating a series of ancestral or nodal sequences (Levels D, C, etc.) using a minimum number of base substitutions, sequence insertions or deletions, and gene duplications. [See L. E. Hood, J. H. Wilson, and W. B. Wood, *Molecular Biology of Eucaryotic Cells,* W. A. Benjamin, Inc., Menlo Park, Calif., 1975, appendix to Chapter 7.]

2. The genetic events required to generate the set of V regions at Level E in Figure 3–31 could occur either during the evolution of vertebrates (germ-line theory) or during the development of each individual (somatic theory), or partly during both. The different theories for antibody diversity place germ-line genes at different levels on the genealogic tree. The germ-line theory contends that the sequences at Level E represent germ-line genes, whereas somatic theories argue that sequences at some lower level represent germ-line genes.

3. Each individual produces its own set of V regions. A decision between germ-line and somatic theories could be made if the complete sets of V-region sequences from several closely related individuals could be compared. A finding that the sets were essentially identical would be strong support for the germ-line theory, whereas a finding that the sets differed significantly would support some form of somatic variation theory. Unfortunately, such a comparison is experimentally unfeasible. Instead, immu-

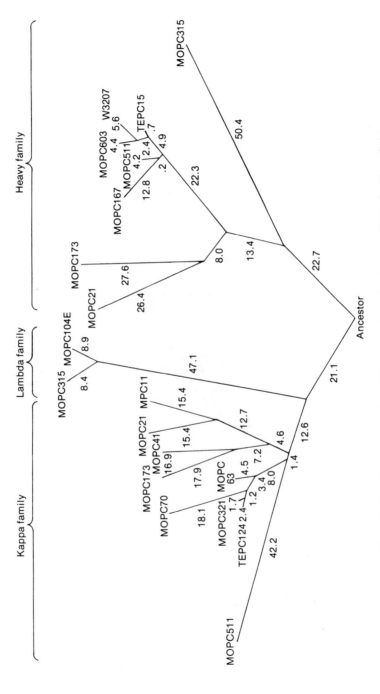

Figure 3–32. A genealogic tree of V regions from the three antibody families of the BALB/c mouse. [Courtesy of E. Loh.]

nologists can compare only randomly selected sequences, in the form of myeloma proteins or other homogeneous antibodies, from the sets of sequences produced by different individuals. Nevertheless, comparison of these sequences can yield information on the degree of similarity between individual trees.

4.   Comparison of sequences from myeloma proteins again can be made most conveniently by constructing genealogic trees. Figure 3–32 shows a tree made with actual data, in which the twigs represent V sequences from the sets of many genetically identical individuals. If these sets are identical, then the V_κ branch of this tree represents evolution of the V_κ family. Consequently, genealogic relationships should be observed not only between early ancestral sequences, but also between very similar sequences at the top level. If somatic variation is involved and the sets are not identical, then similar sequences at the top level should no longer be genealogically related, because somatic variations would be expected to take different paths in different individuals. The expected relationship between similar sequences derived by random somatic mutation from a germ-line gene in different individuals is compared with the genealogic relationship between evolutionarily derived germ-line sequences in Figure 3–33.

5.   Two important questions can be asked with regard to any proposed somatic mutational mechanism. First, how many somatic mutational events can occur in a particular V gene during the differentiation of each antibody-producing cell? This number determines the level at which the germ-line sequences must be

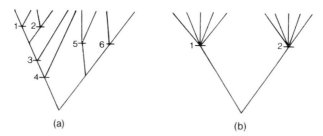

(a)   (b)

Figure 3–33 Two possible diversity patterns for a set of ten closely related V regions. (a) A genealogic pattern implies that individual organisms have very similar, if not identical, V-region genealogic trees. This model is consistent with any model, such as the germ-line model of diversity, that postulates mutation followed by selection. (b) A radiation pattern implies that individual organisms mutate their antibody V genes along different mutational pathways. This pattern is consistent with any of the somatic theories of diversity. The numbered nodal sequences indicate the minimum number of germ-line genes that must be postulated to avoid parallel mutations in each model.

placed on the genealogic tree. Models that postulate hypermutation place the germ-line level lower, whereas models that rely
on ordinary mutation rates must place the germ-line level higher
on the tree.

Second, how many identical or parallel mutations can occur
in the same V gene in separate individuals? For example, if
two individuals were to evolve the gene for V-region 1 by somatic
mutation of the germ-line V gene $V_{\kappa A2}$ in Figure 3–31, then 20
identical mutations of the $V_{\kappa A2}$ gene in these two individuals
would have had to occur; if the germ-line level were B, then
15 identical mutations would have had to occur, and so on. Because
it is difficult to explain multiple parallel V-gene mutations by
most of the somatic mechanisms proposed to date, the germ-line
level on the genealogical tree must be raised to avoid requiring
multiple parallel mutations.

E.   Genealogic analysis of actual amino-acid-sequence data has
imposed the following constraints on theories of antibody diversity.

1.   The V regions from all antibody families studied so far can
be arranged into a genealogic pattern (Figure 3–32). Random
somatic mutation, hypermutation, or somatic recombination
operating on one or a *few* V genes would not be expected to
give a genealogic pattern, because of differences in the mutational
pathways in different individuals. Therefore, V-region diversity
probably arises from multiple germ-line genes in most antibody
families.

2.   Several identical V-region sequences now have been found
in myeloma proteins from independently-arising mouse tumors.
In one set of experiments, 18 mouse V_λ regions were sequenced;
12 of the sequences appeared identical, whereas the remaining
six differed by one to three amino acid substitutions (Figure
3–34). This finding suggests that the sequence found 12 times
must be coded in the germ line, because of the unlikelihood
that somatic variation would frequently generate identical V_λ
genes in different individuals.

3.   Within a particular antibody family, the V regions may be
grouped into clusters of closely related sequences (Figure 3–32).
These clusters are termed *subgroups* (Figure 3–31). The V regions
within a subgroup often differ from those of other subgroups
by sequence insertions or deletions as well as by distinct sets
of amino acid substitutions (Figure 3–35). These differences
suggest that if somatic variation is involved in generating the
observed V-region sequences, then at least each subgroup must
be specified by a separate V gene, in order to avoid postulating
extensive parallel genetic alterations. Thus the number of defined

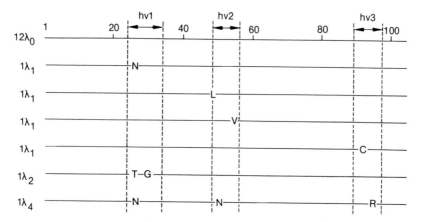

Figure 3–34   Amino-acid-sequence differences among 18 mouse V_λ regions of the V_λ subgroup. The variant residues are indicated using the one-letter amino acid code; otherwise these V_λ regions are identical. The three hypervariable regions are indicated by dotted lines. [Adapted from M. Cohn *et al.* in *The Immune System: Genes, Receptors, Signals,* E. E. Sercarz, A. R. Williamson, and C. F. Fox (Eds.), Academic Press, New York, 1975, p. 89.]

subgroups in a particular immunoglobulin-chain family probably represents a minimal estimate of the number of corresponding germ-line V genes.

4.   The germ-line versus somatic controversy should, then, focus on the question of whether diversity *within a subgroup* arises during evolution of the germ line or somatically during development. The amino-acid-sequence data do not provide a clear answer to this question.

In summary, the finding that V-region sequences can be arranged into genealogic trees suggests that most antibody families have multiple germ-line V genes. The demonstration of identical V-region sequences in different individuals suggests that at least some immunoglobulin V regions are coded directly by germ-line genes. The question that remains is whether somatic variation operates to further increase the diversity of germ-line V genes.

F.   The idiotypic analysis of certain myeloma proteins and homogeneous antibodies has placed additional constraints on theories of antibody diversity.

1.   Certain idiotypes behave like alleles that segregate in a Mendelian fashion in mating experiments. Once again, to avoid invoking parallel mutation in separate individuals, it must be postulated that these idiotypes represent germ-line V genes.

2.   Several different V_H idiotypes have been used as genetic markers and mapped to closely linked but separate genetic loci

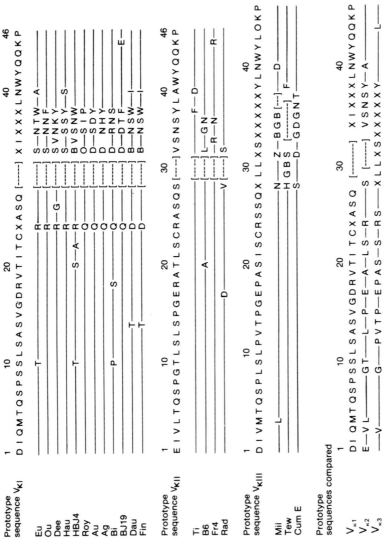

Figure 3–35 N-terminal sequences from human V_κ regions of different subgroups. The sequences have been arranged into three subgroups, designated $V_{\kappa 1}$, $V_{\kappa 2}$, $V_{\kappa 3}$. The corresponding prototype sequences represent the predominant residues at each position for each subgroup. In each subgroup the individual sequences are compared against the prototype and differences are indicated. [—] indicates a deleted residue. X indicates that no predominant residue can be determined. The first two or three letters of the patient's name are used to indicate the individual myeloma proteins. [Data from J. Gally in *The Antigens*, M. Sela (Ed.), Academic Press, New York, 1973, p. 236.]

(Figure 3–27). Recombinational analysis of these markers suggests that the chromosomal region they occupy extends over three map units. Although this technique gives only a rough estimate of actual DNA content, the results suggest that this region contains sufficient DNA for thousands of V_H genes and/or spacer genes.

G.   In principle, the number of germ-line genes within a subgroup can be estimated directly by studies at the nucleic acid level. In recent studies of this nature, specific light-chain mRNA has been isolated from a number of κ-secreting and λ-secreting myeloma tumors. These mRNA's or their complementary DNA copies (cDNA) have been hybridized to DNA from the myeloma tumor, from somatic tissue, and from the germ line. Under conditions of excess genomic DNA, the kinetics of hybridization can be related to the number of genes complementary to the mRNA or cDNA probe. In another study, referred to previously, a V-region gene has been isolated from embryonic DNA, and sequenced. The results of these experiments support the view that some V-region sequences are coded in germ-line genes, whereas others arise by somatic alteration of these genes. These studies have led to three conclusions.

1.   Individual mouse V_κ subgroups appear to be coded by distinct germ-line genes, based on hybridization kinetics.

2.   The mouse V_λ subgroup appears to be coded by 1–5 germ-line genes, again based on hybridization kinetics. This number is perhaps 10 times too small to account for the number of V_λ amino acid sequences thought to exist. The data in Figure 3–34 prove that there are at least seven such sequences, and statistical calculations based on the size of the sample examined predict that the actual number of V_λ sequences produced by the mouse is 30 to 40. This discrepancy, plus the interesting observation that all of the amino acid differences found between V_λ variants occurred in the hypervariable regions, suggest that most of these variants arise by some type of somatic mechanism.

3.   The DNA sequence of a V_λ gene isolated from mouse embryo DNA (λe) has been determined (Figure 3–20). From protein-sequence analysis the mouse appears to have two V_λ subgroups. The 18 mouse V_λ regions shown in Figure 3–34 fall into the $V_{\lambda I}$ subgroup. A single V_λ sequence (MOPC315) falls into a second subgroup, $V_{\lambda II}$. These two V_λ subgroups differ from one another by thirteen amino acid residues. The DNA sequence of the embryonic V_λ gene is like the $V_{\lambda I}$ sequence at four positions, like the $V_{\lambda II}$ sequence at nine positions, and like neither at one position (Figure 3–36). The embryonic sequence could represent a third germ-line V_λ gene. The nucleotide sequence analysis of other V genes will be enlightening in this regard.

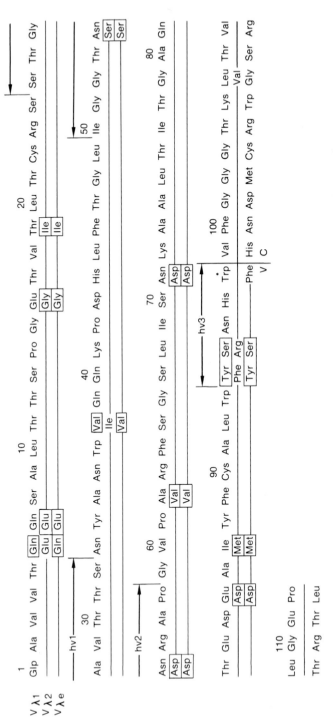

Figure 3–36 The variable-region amino acid sequences in the two λ subgroups from mouse (λ₁ and λ₂) and the amino acid sequence that would be coded by a λ gene (λe) isolated from embryonic DNA (Figure 3–20). Joined boxes indicate residue identities between the sequences at variable positions. Horizontal lines indicate identity to the λ₁ sequence. V/C indicates the position at which the Vλe sequence becomes nonhomologous to both the Vλ₁ and Vλ₂ sequences (see Figure 3–20). * indicates the position at which λe is different from both λ₁ and λ₂.

H.   In summary, all current theories of antibody diversity must include multiple germ-line V genes. However, both general theories may turn out to be partially correct, in that some V regions appear to be directly coded in the germ line, whereas some members of closely related V-region subgroups may arise by somatic mutation.

3-11   Four general mechanisms may contribute to the recognition of diverse antigens

In this chapter, four general properties of antibodies have been described to account for the ability of organisms to recognize and respond to a virtually unlimited number of antigenic determinants. These properties include mechanisms for generating diversity at the protein level as well as at the gene level. They can be summarized as follows.

1.   A large number of immunoglobulin-chain V regions are encoded by V genes in the germ line.

2.   Additional V-region diversity may arise during development of the individual by somatic alteration of V genes.

3.   The number of different antibody combining-site specificities that can be generated theoretically approaches the product of the number of V_L and V_H genes, as a result of the combinatorial association of light chains and heavy chains in the differentiation of antibody-producing cells.

4.   The diversity of antigens recognized by the antibody population is increased by antibody multispecificity, the ability of a given antibody-combining site to bind any one of several different antigenic determinants.

Although all four of these properties contribute to the diversity of antibody specificity, their relative importance for the organism's total antigen-recognition capability is not yet established.

3-12   Immunoglobulin gene families exhibit the properties of informational multigene systems

A.   Clues to the evolution and maintenance of the immune system can be obtained by comparing its genes to those of other multigene families. A multigene family is a group of genes that exhibit close linkage, sequence homology, and related or overlapping functions. Multigene families can be divided into three general categories by several criteria (Table 3-8).

1.   The *simple-sequence* families include the nucleotide sequences generally known as DNA satellites. These sequences represent 10^3–10^7 repetitions of a short fundamental sequence, generally

Table 3–8
The classification and properties of multigene families[a]

Category	Gene products	Multiplicity	Gene or protein homology	Information content	Examples of coincidental evolution	Examples of change in family size
Simple-sequence						
(1) satellites	none known	10^3–10^6	80–100%		different satellites of Drosophila	mouse satellite
Multiplicational						
(1) 18S–28s ribosomal RNA	RNA	100–600	97–100%	one unit	spacer regions of X. laevis and X. mulleri;	
(2) 5S ribosomal RNA	RNA	100–200	97–100%	one unit	spacer regions of X. laevis and X. mulleri	gene number in X. mulleri and X. laevis
(3) tRNA	RNA	6–400		one unit		
(4) histones	proteins	10–1200	87–99%	few units	histone mRNA's of two species of sea urchin	gene number in different sea urchin species
Informational						
(1) antibodies	proteins	100s	30–100%	many units	rabbit and mouse κ chains	V_λ and V_κ in mammals
(2) hemoglobins	proteins	210	<75–100%	few units	human and cow δ chains	human and rabbit β-like chains

[a]All properties pertain to single closely linked sets of genes.
[From L. Hood et al., Annu. Rev. Genet. **9**, 305 (1975).]

6–15 nucleotides in length. Such simple sequences generally are clustered around the centromeres of most eucaryotic chromosomes. They are not transcribed or translated, and their function in unknown.

2. A *multiplicational* family generally is composed of nearly identical genes that have been duplicated extensively at the DNA level, because they are required in large quantities during certain stages of the cell cycle or during certain stages of development. Examples are the genes for histones and ribosomal RNA's.

3. An *informational* family has individual gene members that can differ markedly in sequence from one another, although all are homologous and obviously share an ancient ancestry. The immunoglobulin genes constitute three informational multigene families.

B. Multigene families exhibit two common evolutionary features, *rapid change in family size* and *coincidental evolution*. These features will be considered with regard to the immunoglobulin families (Figure 3–37).

(a) change in family size

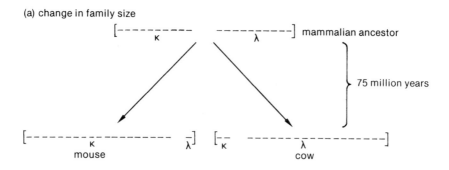

(b) coincidental evolution

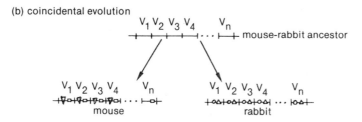

Figure 3–37 Two unusual evolutionary features of antibody genes and other multigene families. (a) A diagrammatic representation of the expansion and contraction of the κ- and λ-gene families in two mammals. (b) A diagrammatic representation of coincidental evolution during the divergence of the mouse and rabbit evolutionary lines. ▽, □, ○, and △ represent coincidental changes in the amino acid condons of the respective evolutionary lines. [From L. Hood, *Proc. Robert A. Welch Foundation Conf. on Chem. Res.* **18**, 153 (1974).]

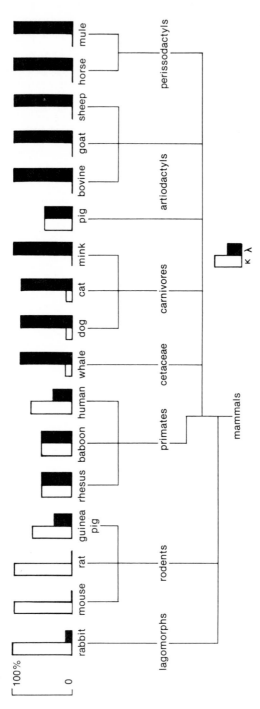

Figure 3–38 Frequency distribution of λ and κ light chains in sera of different mammals. [From L. Hood, J. A. Grant, and H. Sox in *Developmental Aspects of Antibody Formation and Structure*, J. Sterzl and I. Riha (Eds.), Academic Press, New York, 1970, vol. 1, p. 283.]

1. The conclusion that immunoglobulin gene families change rapidly in size is based on observed differences in the diversity of a particular immunoglobulin family in different species (Figure 3–37a). For example, human V_κ regions are considerably less diverse than their mouse counterparts, whereas human V_λ regions are considerably more diverse than their mouse counterparts. In addition, the λ/κ ratios in the sera of various mammals range from predominantly λ, in horse, cow, and dog, to predominantly κ, in rat and mouse (Figure 3–38). These observations suggest that the diversity of the light-chain families has changed markedly and differently in distinct mammalian evolutionary lines since their divergence. Presumably, these changes in diversity reflect changes in the number of germ-line V genes in the corresponding families. Because all mammals shared a common ancestor about 75 million years ago, the V_κ and V_λ families must have expanded or contracted differently in various evolutionary lines.

2. The V genes in a given immunoglobulin family have evolved so as to generate species-specific genealogic trees. This finding implies that clusters of related genes within a species tend to evolve similarly (*coincidentally*). Coincidental evolution is most dramatically illustrated by the presence of *species-associated residues* at certain positions in the amino acid sequences that distinguish the V regions of an immunoglobulin family in one species from the V regions of the corresponding family in a second species (Figures 3–37b and 3–39). The presence of species-associated residues suggests that the V genes evolved after divergence of the two species.

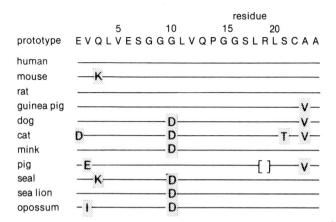

Figure 3–39 Species-associated residues (boxed) in pooled heavy chains from a variety of different mammals. [From J. M. Kehoe and J. Capra, *Contemp. Top. Molec. Immunol.*, **3**, 143 (1974).]

C.   Various genetic and evolutionary mechanisms have been proposed to explain how multigene families undergo rapid size changes and coincidental evolution. One attractive mechanism for explaining both evolutionary features is *homologous but unequal crossing-over.*

1.   Homologous but unequal crossing-over occurs when chromosomes carrying closely linked homologous genes mispair and recombine to yield one chromosome with an increased number of genes and another with a decreased number of genes (Figure 3–40). Such crossover events can lead to rapid change in family size if the chromosome with the expanded gene number or the chromosome with the contracted gene number becomes fixed in the population.

2.   Unequal crossing-over also may lead to coincidental evolution by a somewhat more subtle process, whereby one form of the gene increases in number at the expense of other genes in the family. Coincidental evolution occurs when a variant gene becomes fixed, that is, replaces all other genes in a particular evolutionary line. Figure 3–41 illustrates how fixation can occur by homologous but unequal crossing-over. If different species fix different variants, then apparent coincidental evolution will occur, as reflected in species-associated residues.

D.   Informational multigene families can be simple (5 or 6 genes) or complex. For example, the β-like hemoglobin genes of man are a simple family of linked genes that show sequence homology and

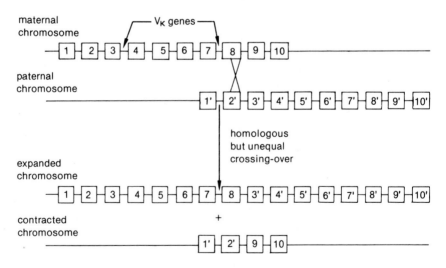

Figure 3–40 A model for homologous but unequal crossing-over. [From L. Hood *et al., Annu. Rev. Genet.* **9**, 305 (1975).]

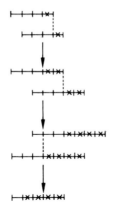

Figure 3—41 A model for gene fixation by repeated homologous but unequal crossing-over. [From L. Hood, et al., Annu. Rev. Genet. **9**, 305 (1975).]

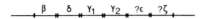

Figure 3—42 A map of the simple informational gene family that encodes the β-like hemoglobins of man. The linkage of the ζ and ϵ genes to the other β-like genes is uncertain. [From L. Hood et al., Annu. Rev. Genet. **9**, 305 (1975).]

related phenotypic functions (Figure 3–42). However, immunoglobulin gene families are complex: they constitute the only well documented examples of complex informational multigene families. The three immunoglobulin gene families make up a system that has evolved to express one unit of information on each lymphocyte (unit differentiation), and that can expand this information by clonal selection and amplification in response to specific antigenic stimuli from the environment. The molecular and genetic strategies of the immunoglobulin multigene system are summarized in Table 3–9.

E.   The informational multigene families may code for a variety of simple and complex traits in higher organisms, as illustrated by a partial list of potential informational multigene families in Table 3–10. If any of the potential complex families share some of the strategies listed in Table 3–7, then studies of the immunoglobulin genes will play an important role in understanding how these families handle information. In addition, because homogeneous and specific antibody gene products can be obtained in large quantities from animals throughout the spectrum of vertebrate evolution, study of the immune system affords the best available opportunity for defining the unusual genetic mechanisms that operate in the evolution of multigene systems.

Table 3–9

Possible strategies for handling of information in the immune system[a]

Information storage and generation

   Multiple different germ lines
   Somatic variation and selection
   Combinatorial joining of *V* and *C* genes
   Multispecificity

Information expression

   DNA translocation
      RNA processing
      Allelic exclusion
   Clonal selection and amplification
   Expression of subsets of genes
   Regulation by cell-surface molecules coded by other multigene families
   Positive or negative response to stimulus (induction and tolerance, help and
   suppression)

Information and evolution

   Homology units
   Domains
   Special evolutionary mechanism(s) leading to coincidental evolution and change
      in family size
   Duplication of multigene families to assume new functions, regulate the old family,
      or interact with the old family

[a][From L. Hood *et al., Annu. Rev. Genet.* **9,** 305 (1975).]

Table 3–10

Possible informational multigene systems

Structural proteins[a]	Developmental systems
Actin *	T allele
Keratins *	Transcriptional signals
Collagens *	Translational signals
Chorionic proteins *	Membrane systems
Wool proteins *	
Serum proteins	Immune-response genes
	Membrane receptors (hormone, cAMP)
Hemagglutins *	Membrane-transport systems
Serine esterases *	Embryonic antigens
Complement components	Blood-cell antigens
Hemocyanins *	
Nervous system	

Membrane molecules mediating specific cell–cell interactions
   Information storage

[a] Proteins indicated by * have been found to exist in multiple structural forms whose significance is generally unknown.
[From L. Hood *et al., Annu. Rev. Genet.* **9,** 305 (1975).]

3-13 Immunoglobulin genes evolved through the duplication and divergence of homology units

The existence of V- and C-region homology units (Figure 3–15) and the observation that the tertiary structures for the corresponding domains are very similar (Figure 3–16) suggest that the immunoglobulin genes probably evolved from a primordial gene for a polypeptide that corresponded to a single homology unit. A possible evolutionary scheme could be as follows (Figure 3–43). The hypothetical precursor gene could have duplicated very early to produce ancestral V and C genes. Subsequently, the V gene could have duplicated many times to generate a primordial multigene family that may have coded for primitive membrane receptor molecules (Essential Concept 3–14). This multigene family in turn could have been duplicated either by polyploidization or by duplication and translocation of a chromosomal segment to produce a primitive immunoglobulin gene family. Subsequent duplication could have produced the three families that evolved to become the contemporary λ, κ, and H families. Contiguous gene duplication could have led to C_H genes composed of three or four homology units in the heavy-chain family. If this scheme is correct, the evolution of antibody genes employed all of the major mechanisms of gene evolution—point mutation, discrete duplication, polyploidization, and translocation.

3-14 Immunoglobulin genes may have evolved from genes for other membrane receptor molecules

The evolution of the immune response has required development of at least four separate components: (1) a library of V and C genes, (2) a V–C translocation mechanism, (3) an amplification mechanism that initiates cell proliferation and protein synthesis when a membrane-bound receptor antibody molecule combines with antigen, and (4) the effector mechanisms of cellular and humoral immunity. Since immunoglobulins can function as membrane-associated receptors, it is tempting to speculate that V genes could have evolved from genes for other membrane receptor molecules (Figure 3–43). In ascending the evolutionary scale from single-celled organisms to complex metazoa, more and more cell-surface receptors are required for a variety of functions such as cell–cell recognition, scavenging of debris, and hormonal triggering. Families of related but variable proteins probably evolved to carry out these diverse receptor functions. A translocation mechanism may have evolved to unite the genes for variable receptor proteins to the gene for a common protein that served as an anchor whereby a variety of receptor molecules could be positioned appropriately in the membrane. Some classes of present-day antibodies are membrane proteins that function in precisely this fashion.

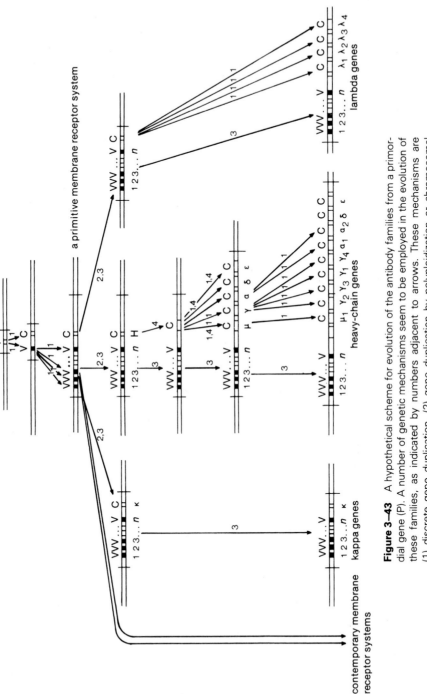

Figure 3–43 A hypothetical scheme for evolution of the antibody families from a primordial gene (P). A number of genetic mechanisms seem to be employed in the evolution of these families, as indicated by numbers adjacent to arrows. These mechanisms are (1) discrete gene duplication, (2) gene duplication by polyploidization or chromosomal translocation, (3) contiguous gene duplication, and (4) coincidental evolution of multiple genes. Mechanisms 1 and 4 may be identical (see text). [Adapted from G. Edelman and J. Gally, *Annu. Rev. Genet.* **6**, 1(1972).]

The property that distinguished early antibodies from other cell-surface receptors could have been the ability to initiate cell division upon combining with an antigen, thereby producing more cells with identical antibody receptors. Thus a primitive cellular immune system may have evolved first. In support of this possibility, preliminary studies suggest that certain invertebrates may exhibit primitive cellular transplant-rejection responses. Subsequently, lymphocytes could have evolved the sophisticated effector functions of humoral and cellular immunity seen in higher vertebrates.

The foregoing view suggests that V-gene families and translocation mechanisms antedated the emergence of the immune system, and that these phenomena may be common to other complex systems of cell-surface receptors in higher organisms. If so, other kinds of cell-surface receptor molecules are likely to yield additional examples of informational multigene systems. This possibility is discussed further in Chapter 4.

Selected Bibliography

Where to begin

Edelman, G. M., "Antibody structure and molecular immunology," *Science* **180**, 830 (1973). A Nobel Prize lecture on the structure of the antibody molecule.

General

"The origins of lymphocyte diversity," *Cold Spring Harbor Symp. Quant. Biol.* **41** (1976). The proceedings of an important meeting that includes references for all areas of immunology.

Cellular Selection and Regulation, in G. M. Edelman (Ed.), *The Immune Response,* Raven Press, New York, 1974. A collection of articles about different aspects of clonal selection.

Kabat, E. A., *Structural Concepts in Immunology and Immunochemistry,* Holt, Rinehart, and Winston, New York, 1976. An up-to-date text with a comprehensive discussion of antibody structure.

Sercarz, E., Herzenberg, L. A., and Fox, C. F. (Eds.), *The Immune System II: Regulatory Genetics,* Academic Press, New York, 1977. Proceedings of a recent meeting that covered many areas of immunology.

Smith, G., *The Variation and Adaptive Expression of Antibodies,* Harvard University Press, Cambridge, Mass. 1973. A detailed discussion of the genetic, structural, and serological arguments for various theories of antibody diversity.

Myeloma System

Potter, M., "Immunoglobulin-producing tumors and myeloma proteins of mice," *Physiol. Rev.* **52,** 631 (1972). A classic discussion of the biology and chemistry of the mouse myeloma system.

Homogeneous antibodies

Krause, R. M., "The search for antibodies with molecular uniformity," *Adv. Immunol.* **12,** 1 (1970). A detailed review article on how immunologists induce homogeneous antibodies.

Kohler, G., and Milstein, C. "Continuous cultures of fused cells secreting antibody of predefined specificity," *Nature* **256,** 495 (1975). A striking new technology for producing homogeneous antibodies that will revolutionize immunology and other disciplines employing antibody reagents.

Antibody specificity

Richards, F., Konigsberg, W., Rosenstein, R., and Varga, J., "On the specificity of antibodies," *Science* **189,** 130 (1975). A review of the case for the multispecificity of antibody molecules.

Three-dimensional structure of antibodies

Amzel, L. M., Poljak, R., Saul, F., Varga, J., and Richards, F., "The three-dimensional structure of a combining region–ligand complex of immunoglobulin NEW at 3.5 Å resolution," *Proc. Natl. Acad. Sci. USA* **71,** 1427 (1974). An x-ray analysis of an antibody molecule with its hapten in place.

Davies, D. R., Padlan, E. A., and Segal, D. M., "Three-dimensional structure of immunoglobulins," *Annu. Rev. Biochem.* **44,** 639 (1975). A review of research on the tertiary structure of antibody molecules.

Poljak, R., Amzel, L. M., Avey, H., Chen, B., Phizackerley, R., and Saul, F., "Three-dimensional structure of the Fab' fragment of a human immunoglobulin at 2.8 Å resolution," *Proc. Natl. Acad. Sci. USA* **70,** 3305 (1973). A classic paper on the three-dimensional structure of a human immunoglobulin.

Hypervariable regions

Capra, J. D., and Kehoe, J. M., "Variable-region sequences of five human immunoglobulin heavy chains of the V_{HIII} subgroup: definitive identification of four heavy-chain hypervariable regions," *Proc. Natl. Acad. Sci. USA* **71,** 845 (1974). A definition of the hypervariable regions of the heavy chain.

Wu, T. T., and Kabat, E. A., "An analysis of the sequences of the variable regions of Bence-Jones proteins and myeloma light chains and their implications for antibody complementarity," *J. Exp. Med.*

132, 211 (1970). The first clear discussion of hypervariable regions and their structural and genetic implications.

Antibody diversity

Cohn, M., Blomberg, B., Geckeler, W., Raschke, W., Riblet, R., and Weigert, M., "First-order considerations in analyzing the generator of diversity," in E. Sercarz, A. Williamson, C. F. Fox (Eds.), *The Immune System: Genes, Receptors, Signals,* Academic Press, New York, 1974, p. 89. A stimulating analysis of antibody structure and genetics, which concludes that somatic mutation is an important aspect of antibody diversity.

Edelman, G. M., and Gally, J., "The genetic control of immunoglobulin synthesis," *Annu. Rev. Genet.* **6,** 1 (1972). An excellent review on the genetics of antibody molecules.

Hood, L., Loh, E., Hubert, J., Barstad, P., Eaton, B., Early, P., Furhman, J., Johnson, W., Kronenberg, M., and Schilling, J., "The structure and genetics of mouse immunoglobulins," *Cold Spring Harbor Symp. Quant. Biol.* **41,** 817 (1976). A detailed review of immunoglobulin amino acid sequences and their implications, immunoglobulin diversity, and evolution of antibody genes.

Jerne, N. K., "The somatic generation of immune recognition," *Eur. J. Immunol.* **1,** 1 (1971). A classic paper on a somatic theory of antibody diversity.

Leder, P., Honjo, T., Seidman, J., and Swan, D., "Origin of immuno-globulin gene diversity: The evidence and a restriction-modification model," *Cold Spring Harbor Symp. Quant. Biol.* **41,** 855 (1976). An interesting model for antibody diversity based on an analysis of antibody genes at the nucleic acid level.

Two genes: one polypeptide chain

Hood, L., "Two genes: one polypeptide chain—fact or fiction?," *Fed. Proc.* **31,** 179 (1972). A review of the structural and genetic arguments that led to the "two gene–one polypeptide" hypothesis

Sledge, C., Fair, D. S., Black, B., Krueger, R. G., and Hood, L., "Antibody differentiation: apparent sequence identity between variable regions shared by IgA and IgG immunoglobulins," *Proc. Natl. Acad. Sci. USA* **73,** 923 (1976). A general analysis of the V–C translocation mechanism in heavy chains.

Tonegawa, S., Hozumi, N., Matthyssens, G., and Schuller, R., "Somatic changes in content and context of immunoglobulin genes," *Cold Spring Harbor Symp. Quant. Biol.* **41,** 877 (1976). Evidence at the DNA level that V and C genes are separate in the zygote and are rearranged during differentiation.

Tonegawa, S., Maxim, A. M., Tizard, R., Bernard, O., and Gilbert, W., "Sequence of a mouse germ-line gene for a variable region of an immunoglobulin light chain. *Proc. Natl. Acad. Sci. USA* **75**, 1485 (1978). A classic paper characterizing one of the first eucaryotic genes isolated from genomic DNA.

Antibody Evolution

Edelman, G. M., and Gally, J., "Arrangement and evolution of eucaryotic genes," in F. O. Schmitt (Ed.), *Neurosciences: Second Study Program*, Rockefeller University Press, New York, 1970, p. 962. A thoughtful review of multigene systems, which concludes that coincidental evolution may occur by gene conversion.

Hood, L., Campbell, J., and Elgin, S., "The organization, expression, and evolution of antibody genes and other multigene families," *Annu. Rev. Genet.* **9**, 305 (1975). A comparative review of the evolutionary, regulatory, and organizational features of most known multigene families.

Smith, G., "Unequal crossing-over and the evolution of multigene families," *Cold Spring Harbor Symp. Quant. Biol.* **38**, 507 (1973). An elegant computer simulation of crossing-over in multigene families.

Problems

3-1   Indicate whether each of the following statements is true or false. Explain the error in each statement you consider to be false.

(a)   The hinge region joins light and heavy chains in the immunoglobulin molecule.

(b)   One immunoglobulin molecule can have light chains with two different V-region sequences.

(c)   The V_H region is twice the length of the V_L region.

(d)   Homology units of immunoglobulin polypeptides are encoded by nucleotide sequences of about 330 nucleotide pairs in length.

(e)   The immunoglobulin active site is composed primarily of the light chain.

(f)   The V and C regions of the light chain have very similar tertiary structures.

(g) V_λ regions sometimes are associated with C_κ regions.

(h)   In the mammalian genome there are more genes for C regions than for V regions.

(i)   The immunoglobulin family to which a V region belongs can be determined from its amino acid sequence.

(j)   In the human genome, $C_{\lambda 1}$ and $C_{\lambda 2}$ are encoded by two distinct structural genes.

(k)   IgG1 and IgG2 molecules are distinguished by differences in their light-chain sequences.

(l)   A single antigen generally evokes the synthesis of a single molecular species of antibody.

(m)   Myeloma proteins from different humans always are identical in sequence.

(n)   The germ-line theory suggests that there are many V genes in the germ line.

(o)   V and C regions become joined at the protein level.

(p)   The presence of homology units in immunoglobulins suggests that genes for light and heavy chains evolved from a common precursor gene.

(q)   The clonal-selection theory states that a single antibody-producing cell generally synthesizes a single molecular species of antibody.

(r)   The observation that V regions generate a genealogic tree similar to those of other evolutionarily related proteins favors a germ-line theory of antibody diversity.

(s)   Genetic analyses of allotypes suggest that the three families of immunoglobulin genes are closely linked to one another.

(t)   The V regions that constitute a given subgroup are merely the terminal twigs on a common branch of the genealogic tree of variable regions.

(u)   Immunoglobulin genes are a multigene family, even from the viewpoint of most somatic theories.

(v)   Immunoglobulins constitute the only system in which two genes are known to encode a single polypeptide chain.

(w)   Species-associated V-region residues could indicate that V genes evolved prior to species divergence.

(x)   Antibody molecules are found on the cell surface of the B cell that synthesizes them.

(y)   A V–C translocation mechanism may have antedated the evolution of the immune system.

(z)   The phenomenon of allelic exclusion suggests that the immuno-globulin genes are located on the X chromosome.

3–2   Supply the missing word or words in each of the following statements.

(a)   The _____ theory of antibody formation suggests that the antigen plays a selective role in antibody synthesis.

(b)   The diversity of antigen-binding sites presumably is reflected in the amino-acid-sequence diversity of the subunit _____ regions.

(c)   _____ are serologic markers on immunoglobulins that segregate in a Mendelian fashion.

(d)   The _____ theory contends that the information content of the genome can be expanded during somatic differentiation.

(e)   _____ are homogeneous immunoglobulins derived from organisms with plasma-cell tumors.

(f)   The finding of _____ suggests that immunoglobulins evolved by a series of gene duplications.

(g)   The IgG antibody molecule folds into six discrete _____ .

(h)   The _____ regions fold to form the walls of the antigen-binding crevice.

(i)   The _____ functions of immunoglobulins from different classes are different, whereas the _____ function may be the same.

(j)   The two types of light chains are _____ and _____ .

(k)   The major branches on the genealogic tree of V regions for one antibody family represent _____ .

(l)   The set of antigenic determinants on the V domain of one antibody molecule is termed its _____ .

(m)   _____ refers to the observation that single antibody-producing cells in individuals heterozygous for an immunoglobulin allotype express only one allele or the other, but not both.

(n)   Immunoglobulin genes constitute an _____ multigene family.

(o)   Alanine is found at Position 1 in most rabbit κ chains. Aspartic or glutamic acids are found at this same position in most human κ chains. These amino acid alternatives are examples of _____ residues.

3-3   A myeloma patient excretes large quantities of a protein in his urine. The kidney generally permits only those molecules smaller than 45,000 daltons to pass from the blood to the urine. Assuming that no proteolysis occurs in the blood or kidney, what could this protein be?

3-4   Goat antibodies of the IgG class are induced with bovine serum albumin (BSA). These antibody molecules have a molecular weight of about 160,000, and can be fragmented into smaller pieces by chemical and enzymatic procedures. The patterns given in Figure 3-44 are obtained from gel filtration after the indicated chemical or enzymatic modification. Peak III can precipitate BSA from solution, whereas Peaks I, II, and IV do not combine with this antigen. Peak IV can fix complement under appropriate conditions, whereas none of the others can do so.

(a)   Sketch a model of the goat IgG molecule based on the information given, and indicate the cleavage sites that would give patterns (a) and (b).

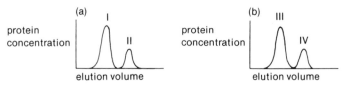

Figure 3-44   Gel filtration patterns of goat IgG after cleavage by (a) reduction and alkylation and (b) mild pepsin digestion (Problem 3-4). The fragments have the following molecular weights: I, 53,000; II, 23,000; III, ~100,000; and IV, ~50,000.

(b)   Suggest an explanation for the type of cleavage that occurs with mild pepsin digestion.

(c)   Where are the antigen-binding and effector functions located on this immunoglobulin molecule? Are both light and heavy chains necessary for each of these functions?

(d)   Papain digestion of the goat antibody gives two types of fragments that are about 50,000 daltons in molecular weight. Draw a model to explain this cleavage. The fragment with antigen-binding capacity no longer can precipitate BSA, although it does associate with BSA. Explain.

3-5   As a physician in a large medical center you have access to large numbers of myeloma patients. You decide to investigate their Bence–Jones proteins, which can be obtained easily in nearly pure form from their urine. You prepare antisera in rabbits against three of these light chains (A, B, C), and then analyze each of these antisera on Ouchterlony plates against a set of eight other Bence–Jones proteins, with the results shown in Figure 3–45.

(a)   Explain these results, based on your knowledge of human light chains. What experiments could you do to test your explanation?

(b)   Suggest an explanation for the spur formation seen opposite Well 2 in Figure 3–45C. What structural feature(s) of the light chain may correspond to this spur?

3-6   Myeloma tumors can be induced experimentally by injection of BALB/c mice with mineral oil. Various antigens have been added to the mineral oil in attempts to produce myeloma immunoglobulins with specific antibody activity, but all these attempts have failed. However, by screening large numbers of myeloma proteins against many different antigens, a few myeloma immunoglobulins have been found with apparently specific antibody activity. For example, one myeloma immunoglobulin has been found with an affinity constant of 10^7 moles/liter

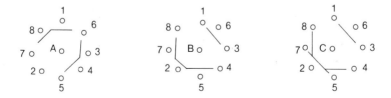

Figure 3–45 Analysis of three antisera to Bence–Jones proteins on Ouchterlony plates (Problem 3–5). One of the three antisera, A, B, or C, is placed in the central well of each plate, and the peripheral wells are filled with solutions of the eight Bence–Jones proteins. As the antigens and antibodies diffuse outward from their respective wells, precipitin lines appear as shown, thereby indicating formation of antigen–antibody complexes (Essential Concept A2–1B).

for the dinitrophenyl group (Dnp). This affinity is similar to that exhibited by biologically-induced antibody.

(a)   What functional and structural criteria must this myeloma protein fulfill to be considered a *bona fide* antibody?

(b)   Suppose that this immunoglobulin satisfies all of the criteria for antibody. Then it is discovered that, in addition, it has a high affinity constant (5×10^5 moles/liter) for menadione (vitamin K), a compound with little apparent steric similarity to Dnp. Offer three explanations for this paradoxical binding of apparently different antigenic determinants.

(c)   How could you test the possibilities that you suggest in Part (b)?

3-7   You are given two preparations of antibody against hen ovalbumen, each raised under similar immunization conditions in a different guinea pig. The specificities and binding constants of these preparations appear identical, yet one preparation fixes complement after combination with antigen and the second does not. Explain how antibodies with identical antigen-binding properties can have distinct effector functions.

3-8   The average mutation rate in human cells is about 10^{-9} substitutions per codon per DNA replication.

(a)   How many cell generations would be required for a lymphocyte clone to produce one mutation in a given V gene by ordinary somatic mutation?

(b)   How many generations would be required to obtain a second variation in this same V gene?

(c)   Assume that the average division time of a lymphocyte is 12 hours. How long does it take to produce one mutation in a given lymphocyte clone? Two mutations?

(d)   The mouse has a gestational period of 21 days. It is immunologically mature shortly after birth. Comment on the ability of ordinary somatic mutation to generate the antigen-independent diversification of the mouse immune system.

(e)   Some immunologists have suggested that during an immune response antigens selectively stimulate lymphocytes that produce V-region variants with higher antigen affinity, and that this antigen selection may drive the maturation of the immune process. The average immune response is over in 10–20 days. If V-region variation occurred by random somatic mutation, how many substitutions could be fixed in a given lymphocyte line during this time?

3-9   (a)   Classify the human myeloma V_κ sequences shown in Figure 3–46 into subgroups based on their relatedness.

(b)   Determine the nodal or prototype sequences for each of the subgroups.

sequence   position

	1								10												20			
1	D	I	Q	M	T	Q	S	P	S	S	L	S	A	S	V	G	D	R	V	T	I	T	C	
2	E	I	V	L	T	Q	S	P	G	T	L	S	L	S	P	G	E	R	A	T	L	S	C	
3	D	I	V	M	T	Q	S	P	L	S	L	P	V	T	P	G	E	P	A	S	I	S	C	
4	D	I	V	M	T	Q	S	P	L	S	L	P	V	T	P	G	E	P	A	S	I	S	C	
5	E	I	V	L	T	Q	S	P	G	T	L	S	L	S	P	G	Z	R	A	A	L	S	C	
6	D	I	Q	M	T	Q	S	P	S	S	L	S	A	S	V	G	D	R	V	T	I	T	C	
7	D	I	Q	M	T	Q	S	P	S	S	L	S	A	S	V	G	D	R	V	T	I	T	C	
8	D	I	V	M	T	Q	S	P	L	S	L	P	V	T	P	G	E	P	A	S	I	S	C	
9	E	I	V	L	T	Q	S	P	G	T	L	S	L	S	P	G	D	R	A	T	L	S	C	
10	E	I	V	L	T	Q	S	P	G	T	L	S	L	S	P	G	D	R	A	T	L	S	C	
11	D	I	Q	M	T	Q	S	P	S	T	L	S	A	S	V	G	D	R	V	T	I	T	C	
12	D	I	Q	M	T	Q	S	P	S	S	L	S	A	S	V	G	D	R	V	T	I	T	C	

Figure 3–46 N-terminal sequences of human V_κ regions (Problem 3–9).

(c) How many amino acid substitutions separate these prototype sequences?

(d) If the same extent of variation continued throughout the entire V region, how much would V regions from these subgroups differ on the average? Assume that the V region has 110 residues.

(e) Draw an approximate genealogic tree for the prototype sequences, using the differences obtained in Part (c). (See legend to Figure 3–31.)

(f) Assume that every individual can synthesize each V_κ region from each subgroup. Is it likely that these sets of proteins could be generated from a single V gene by somatic mutation? Consider ordinary somatic mutation and hypermutation in your explanation.

(g) Construct a difference matrix to show how many amino acid substitutions separate individual V regions from their respective prototype sequences. (Table 3–5 is an example of a difference matrix.)

(h) If the same extent of variation continues throughout the entire V region, by how many residues will the V regions within each subgroup differ from one of their respective prototypes?

(i) What is the most likely explanation for diversity within a subgroup?

(j) What reservations might you have about these human data?

3–10 Imagine that a detailed sequence analysis of myeloma κ-chain genes from the African elephant yielded the genealogic tree shown in Figure 3–31.

(a) Assume that these data come directly from analysis of the V genes themselves. If a random mutational mechanism were operating on the primordial V_κ gene (Level A), what would be the probability that two independent lymphocyte lines would incur identical nucleotide substitutions in their V_κ genes? (Such an identical substitution is termed parallel mutation.) Assume that the V region has 110 residues.

(b)   Would the probability of a parallel mutation in two lymphocyte lines be higher or lower at the protein level than at the nucleotide level? Why?

(c)   If two V_κ regions differed from the primordial V_κ gene by 20 substitutions, what would be the probability of Proteins 1 and 2 in Figure 3–31 arising in two independent lymphocyte lines? In view of your answer, what do you think would be the likelihood of observing parallel mutations in the V_κ regions of the African elephant?

(d)   Suggest two ways that the data given in Figure 3–31 could be reconciled with the reservations raised in Part (c) about parallel mutation.

(e)   How would you reconcile the data in Figure 3–31 with a theory that postulates ordinary somatic mutation as the mechanism for generating antibody diversity? What would be the level of germ-line genes? How would you explain two identical V_κ-region sequences arising from two independent tumors?

(f)   Answer Part (e) with regard to the theory of hypermutation. What types of selective pressures may account for some parallel mutation?

(g)   Answer Part (e) with regard to the theory of somatic recombination.

(h)   Answer Part (e) with regard to the germ-line theory.

3–11   The $C_{\lambda 1}$ and $C_{\lambda 3}$ regions of human λ chains are identical except for an arginine–lysine interchange at position 190 (Figure 3–25). Chemical analyses of the C_λ regions from ten normal individuals reveal that each individual has λ chains of both the λ1 and λ3 types.

(a)   Is it likely that this polymorphism is coded by alleles? Why? What is the probability of picking ten consecutive heterozygotes? (Assume that each variant represents 50% of the C_λ genes in the human population.)

(b)   Offer an alternative explanation for this C-region polymorphism.

3–12   The imaginary homologous C_H sequences shown in Figure 3–47 might have been obtained from gopher myeloma proteins. By inspection, group these C_H sequences into classes by relatedness of sequence.

3–13   Human heavy chains have C-region allotypes that can be recognized by serologic reagents or by sequence analysis. These allotypes represent variations within heavy chain subclasses that are designated as G1ᵃ or G1ᵇ, G2ᵃ or G2ᵇ, G3ᵃ or G3ᵇ, G4ᵃ or G4ᵇ, and A1ᵃ or A1ᵇ. Most Caucasians have the G1ᵃ, G2ᵃ, G3ᵃ, G4ᵃ, and A1ᵃ variants, whereas most Mongolians have the G1ᵇ, G2ᵇ, G3ᵇ, G4ᵇ, and A1ᵇ variants. Caucasian–Mongolian mixed marriages yield F1 offspring that produce both the a and b variants of each subclass. In a large-scale study, marriages between these F1 individuals and Caucasians (backcrosses) were found to yield offspring with the following phenotypes:

```
sequence                                position
                  1         5          10          15          20
      1       V K C A V V R S T A G M P S T A A A I L
      2       V K C A L V R S T A G M P S T A A A I L
      3       L R C A I V R T S A A F Y S A T S A V L
      4       A D C A M V R G N A G M P S G G G A L L
      5       V K C A V L R S T A G M P S T A A A I V
      6       V P P P V I K S T G A F P S G V G V L S
      7       V K C A L V R S T G G M P S T A A A I L
      8       L R C G I V R T S A A F Y S A T S A V L
      9       V K C A L L R S T A G M P S T A A A I L
     10       V P P P V I K S T G A F P S G V A V L S
```

Figure 3–47 Homologous C_H sequences from imaginary gopher myeloma proteins (Problem 3–12.)

$G1^a$ and $G1^b$, $G2^a$ and $G2^b$, $G3^a$ and $G3^b$, $G4^a$ and $G4^b$, $A1^a$ and $A1^b$; 337 offspring

$G1^a$, $G2^a$, $G3^a$, $G4^a$, $A1^a$; 321 offspring

$G1^a$ and $G2^b$, $G2^a$, $G3^a$ and $G3^b$, $G4^a$, $A1^a$ and $A1^b$; 1 offspring

(a)   What can you conclude about the genetic linkage of the heavy-chain genes that encode these allotypes?

(b)   How can the last phenotype be explained? Can you derive a gene order on the chromosome from this phenotype?

3–14   An experiment to show whether the joining of V and C regions occurs at the polypeptide level used cultured myeloma cells that produced a homogeneous κ chain of known sequence. In this experiment, a cell suspension was incubated for 15 minutes at 30° C in a medium that lacked leucine, in order to decrease the size of the internal leucine pool. ^{3}H-leucine then was added to the culture and the incubation temperature was raised to 43° C to inhibit further peptide-chain initiation. After 5 minutes, sufficient time to complete and release all previously initiated peptide chains, the cells were iced, washed, and lysed by homogenization. A ribosome-free supernatant fraction was obtained by high-speed centrifugation of the lysate. Carrier chains from the same myeloma, uniformly labeled with ^{14}C-leucine, were added to this fraction. The mixture of newly synthesized and carrier light chains then was isolated and digested with trypsin. The resulting peptides were separated by chromatography, and the ^{3}H$/^{14}$C ratio was measured for each peptide. Because the order of tryptic peptides in the protein was known, ^{3}H$/^{14}$C ratios could be plotted as a function of residue number along the polypeptide chain. The results obtained with myeloma cells from a hypothetical Martian gopher and from a BALB/c mouse are summarized in Figure 3–48. Interpret each of these results with regard to mechanisms for joining V and C genes or their products.

272

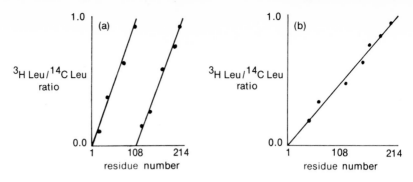

Figure 3–48 ^{3}H/^{14}C ratios in tryptic peptides of κ-light-chain myeloma proteins synthesized in cell-free systems from (a) Martian gopher and (b) BALB/c mouse (Problem 3–14).

set	sequence	position		
		1	10	20

(a)
1 D I Q M T Q S P S S L S A S V G D R V T I T C
2 D I K M T Q S P S S L S A S V G D R V T I T C
3 D I Q M T Q S P S S I S A S V G D R V T I T C
4 E I Q M T Q S P S S L S A S V G D R V T I T C
5 D I Q M T Q S P S S L S A S V G D K V T I T C
6 D I Q L T Q S P S S L S A S V G D R V T I T C
7 D I Q M T Q S P S T L S A S V G D R V T I T C
8 D I Q M T Q S P S S L S S S V G D R V T I T C
9 D I Q M T Q R P S S L S A S V G D R V T I T C
10 D I Q M T Q S P S S L S A S V G D R V S I T C

(b)
1 A V N L T Q S P S A L S A S L S D K V T I T C
2 D V Q L T Q S P S A L S G G L S D K V T I T C
3 D V Q L T Q S P S A L R A G L S D K V T I T C
4 E V H L S Q S P S A L S A S L G D R V T V T C
5 E V Q V S Q S P S G L S A S L G D R V T I T C
6 D I Q L T N P S [ ] A L S S S V G D R V T I T C
7 Q I Q L T Q T S [ ] A L S S S V G D R A T I T C
8 D M I L T Q T P S A L S S S V G D R A T I S C
9 E I Q L T Q T P S A L S S S I G D R A T I S C
10 D I Q L T Q T P S A L S S S I G E R A T I S C

(c)
1 D I Q M T Q S P S S L S A S V G D R V T I T C
2 E I V L T Q S P G T L S L S P G E R A T L S C
3 E I V L T Q S P S S L S A S V G D R V T I T C
4 D I Q M T Q S P S S L S A S V G E R A T L S C
5 D I Q L T Q S P G T L S L S P G E R A T L S C
6 D I Q M T Q S P S T L S L S P G E R A T L S C
7 D I Q M T Q S P S T L S L S C G D R V T I T C
8 E I V M T Q S P G T L S L S P G E R A T I T C
9 E I V L T Q S P G T L S L S P G E R A T I T C
10 D I Q L T Q S P S T L S A S V G D R V T I S C

Figure 3–49 Three sets of V-region sequences (Problem 3–17).

3-15   Assume that any light chain can combine with any heavy chain to generate antibody molecules with a spectrum of different combining sites. How many different antibody molecules could be assembled in an animal that could synthesize 10 different light and 10 different heavy chains? How many different antibodies could be assembled in an animal that could synthesize 100 of each chain? A thousand of each chain?

3-16   The mammalian haploid genome consists of about 3.2×10^9 nucleotide pairs of DNA.
(a)   How many V regions 107 residues in length could be encoded by this amount of DNA?
(b)   What percent of the mammalian genome would be required to encode 1000 V_L and 1000 V_H genes?

3-17   The sequence patterns obtained from V regions have placed important constraints on theories of antibody diversity. Analyze the sets of data in Figure 3-49. Indicate for each set (a, b, and c) whether the diversity could arise most simply by random mutation from one prototype sequence, recombination from two prototype sequences, or selection of a succession of random mutations from one prototype sequence. Justify each decision.

3-18   In the world of Pigmodia everything is small, creatures as well as molecules. Suppose, as a visiting expert biochemist, you are asked to examine and comment on the evolution of the representative Pigmodian antibody polypeptide chains given in Figure 3-50.
(a)   Can you distinguish V and C regions? How long are they?
(b)   Are internal homologies evident in the light or heavy chains?

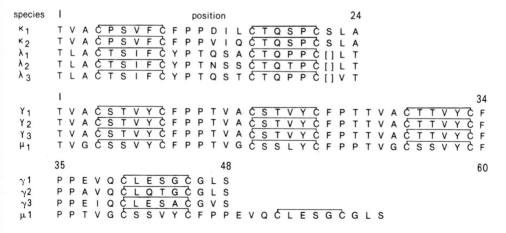

Figure 3-50 Amino acid sequences of Pigmodian immunoglobulin molecules. Bars indicate disulfide bridges (Problem 3-18).

If so, how long are they and how many homology units are present in each chain?

(c)   Do the V and C regions appear evolutionarily related? How?

3–19   You are given a protein sequenator by the National Science Foundation. As a young and enthusiastic protein chemist, you decide to learn how to use this instrument by determining the N-terminal sequences of rabbit and mouse κ chains. At the end of these experiments you are an expert on the sequenator. In addition, the data you have collected show that species-associated residues at Positions 11 and 17 distinguish rabbit chains from their mouse counterparts (Figure 3–51).

If one assumes that 50 or more V_κ genes were present in the common ancestor of both species, how can this observation be explained in evolutionary terms? Can you propose an evolutionary mechanism to account for your finding?

species							position									
	1							10								17
rabbit κ	A	I	V	M	T	Q	T	P	A	S	V	S	Z	P	V	G	G
	D	V	Q	V						S		T	A	A			
			L									Q	V				
mouse κ	D	I	V	M	T	Q	S	P	A	S	L	S	V	A	A	G	E
	E	V	Q	V			T	T	S	T		A	A	S	V	S	D
			L									P				L	
												M					

Figure 3–51   A comparison of the major residue alternatives at the N-termini of V regions from rabbit and mouse (Problem 3–19).

3–20   Heavy-chain disease (HCD) is a myeloma-like disorder in humans that is characterized by the presence in the serum and urine of an abnormally small protein of the gamma class of heavy chain. These γ-HCD proteins are not extracellular degradation products; rather, they are synthesized directly by neoplastic cells. They are characterized by sequence gaps, as indicated in Figure 3–52 for three γ-HCD proteins. In all such proteins

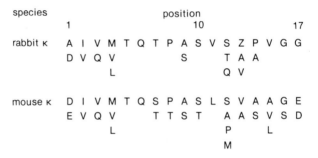

Figure 3–52   Sequence gaps in three γ-HCD proteins (Problem 3–20). The numbers on either side of the gap indicate the positions at which the normal sequence ends and begins again, respectively. The V_H region ends approximately at residue 119. [Data from B. Frangione, L. Lee, E. Haber, and K. Block, *Proc. Natl. Acad. Sci. USA* **70**, 1073 (1973).]

the normal sequences resume at position 216, a point that marks the beginning of the hinge region. The hinge region, a section of the heavy chain between the C_H1 and C_H2 domains (Figure 3–3), is unique in not being homologous to any other region in the heavy chain.

(a)   How are the deletions placed with respect to V and C regions?

(b)   Remember that V and C translocation occurs at the DNA level. Propose mechanisms by which the observed deletions could be produced.

3–21   Purified anti-*p*-azobenzoate antibodies (designated D) from donor rabbits will react with anti-idiotypic (anti-D) antisera. Suppose that you set out to determine which portion of the D antibody V regions combine with anti-D antisera. You purify D antibodies of the IgG class from a single donor rabbit. You prepare anti-D antiserum to these antibodies in allotypically matched recipient rabbits. You label $F(ab)_2$ fragments from these antibodies with ^{125}I and set up the following inhibition test. In a control experiment, you incubate ^{125}I-$F(ab)_2$ fragments from D with anti-D serum, and precipitate the resulting soluble complexes with goat anti-rabbit-Fc serum. You can determine the extent of the reaction by measuring the percent of the ^{125}I that is precipitated. This result establishes the fraction of the D antibodies that normally react with anti-D serum. You then repeat the experiment in the presence of various hapten inhibitors, with the results shown in Table 3–11. What are the implications of these data? Suggest two alternative interpretations.

Table 3–11

The effect of haptens and other small molecules on the reaction of ^{125}I-F (ab′)$_2$ derived from D antibodies of rabbit 114 with anti-D serum (Problem 3–21)

Competitor	Final molar concentration of competitor[a]		
	16×10^{-3}	5×10^{-4}	5×10^{-5}
	^{125}I-F (ab′)$_2$ precipitated as % of control[b]		
p-(p′-Hydroxy)-phenylazobenzoate	32	39	61
Benzoate	95	101	108
p-Nitrobenzoate	72	72	86
m-Nitrobenzoate	85	90	112
o-Nitrobenzoate	98	106	98

[a]Refers to concentration prior to the addition of goat anti-rabbit Fc antiserum.
[b]Expressed as percentage of the quantity precipitated in the absence of competitor.
[From B. Brient and A. Nisonoff, *J. Exp. Med.* **132**, 951 (1970). © 1970 by The Rockefeller University Press.]

3–22   Multiple myeloma occurs in about 1 out of 20,000 humans. About 1% of these patients express two different myeloma proteins. The first case of such a biclonal myeloma examined in detail produced an IgM and IgG myeloma protein with the N-terminal sequences shown in Figure 3–53.

(a)   If the two myeloma proteins were produced by independent neoplastic transformation events in two different lymphocyte clones,

class	chain												position																						
		1									10									20										30						

IgM:
κ: E I V L T Q S P G T L S L S P G E R A T L S C R A S Q S V S B S Y
μ: E V Q L L E S G G G V Q P G G S L R L S C A A S G P T P S T Y V M

IgG:
κ: E I V L T Q S P G T L S L S P G E R A T L S C R A S Q S V S B S Y
γ: E V Q L L E S G G G V Q P G G S L R L S C A A S G P T P S T Y V M

Figure 3–53 N-terminal sequences of light and heavy chains from myeloma immuno-globulins produced in a biclonal myeloma patient (Problem 3–22).

what would be the frequency of patients with two myeloma proteins? What does the observed frequency suggest?

(b)   The IgM and IgG myeloma proteins produced by this patient have identical idiotypic determinants. What do this finding and the sequence data in Figure 3–53 suggest about the independence of the two transformation events?

(c)   The IgM and IgG proteins appear to be produced by two distinct clones of myeloma cells. Explain how all these results may be reconciled with one neoplastic transformation in a single cell.

(d)   Suggest two possible genetic mechanisms that may explain your answer to Part (c).

3–23   In the mouse, homogeneous antibodies can be induced to the Group A streptococcal carbohydrate. An idiotype marker, designated A5A, has been defined for one clone of antibody-producing cells by preparing an anti-idiotype serum. This idiotype is expressed in more than 90% of all mice of the inbred strain A/J immunized with Group A streptococci, but the same idiotype is lacking in similarly immunized BALB/c mice. Interstrain matings were carried out with these two strains. Expression of the A5A marker in parental, F1, and backcross mice was as indicated in Figure 3–54. Ig-1e and Ig-1a are two alleles of a C_γ structural gene.

(a)   Comment on the segregation and expression of the A5A marker.

(b)   How is the segregation of the A5A marker related to that of the C_γ marker?

(c)   How would you explain the single variant animal with the Ig-1a/a allotype in the backcross of F1 × BALB/c? How would you test your explanation?

(d)   What do these results suggest about linkage between V_H and C_H genes?

(e)   What do these results imply about theories of antibody diversity?

3–24   The experiments of Tonegawa *et al.* described in Essential Concept 3–7B and Figure 3–19 place several constraints on the V–C translocation models diagramed in Figure 3–22.

(a)   Suppose that the data in Figure 3–19 are typical for kappa genes in a clone of normal antibody-producing cells. Why is the copy-insertion

relative level of
idiotypic antigen

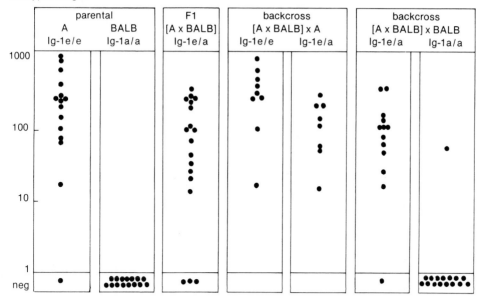

Figure 3–54 The expression of the A5A idiotype in the antibodies to group A streptococci from A/J (A) mice, BALB/c (BALB) mice, F1 hybrids, and backcross mice (Problem 3–23). Ig-1e and Ig-1a are two alleles of a C allotypic marker characteristic of the A/J and BALB/c strains, respectively. [Adapted from K. Eichmann and C. Berek, *Eur. J. Immunol.* **3,** 599 (1973).]

model (Figure 3–22) rendered unlikely by these observations? Can any of the other models be ruled out by these experiments?

(b)   What might the results of these experiments suggest about the role of V–C translocation in the mechanism of allelic exclusion?

(c)   Myeloma cells generally are subtetraploid, that is, they have somewhat fewer than double the diploid number of chromosomes. These cells also are aneuploid, which means that the number of copies of any given chromosome in the cell line may be one to three or more. In view of this information, how would you qualify your answer to Part (b)?

(d)   How would you use similar types of experiments to distinguish between the excision-insertion model and the looping-out model (Figure 3–22)?

3–25   An antigen Ms-1, discovered in a partially inbred rabbit colony, is inherited as an allotypic variant of IgM molecules, but not of other immunoglobulin classes. All the rabbits of this colony have heavy chains of allotype a1 and 12 light chains of allotype b4 (Table 3–6). In matings between outbred rabbits and one of the partially inbred rabbits, the pedigree in Figure 3–55 was observed.

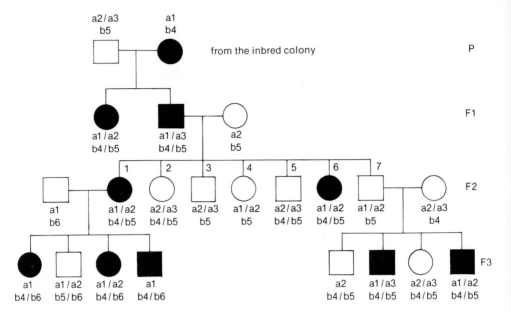

Figure 3–55 Family pedigree of a partially inbred rabbit and an outbred rabbit (Problem 3–25). Circles and squares represent females and males, respectively. Shaded symbols represent individuals that express the Ms-1 allotype. The markers a2, a3, and b5 are allotypes present in the outbred population. The designation a2/a3 indicates that an individual is heterozygous for allotypes a2 and a3; a2 indicates that the individual is homozygous for the a2 allotype.

(a)   Does the Ms-1 specificity appear to be determined by the genes that code for the a1 V regions? Why?

(b)   Propose a model for the pattern of inheritance observed in Figure 3–55. In particular, how can you account for the ability of two Ms-1-negative individuals (in the F2 generation) to produce Ms-1-positive progeny?

(c)   What regions in the IgM molecule might carry the Ms-1 specificity? How might you further localize the Ms-1 specificity?

3–26   Various inbred strains of rats have a serologically detectable polymorphism in their κ chains. The κ chains of the inbred DA strain react with antiserum A, whereas the κ chains of the inbred LEW strain react with antiserum B. Serological analysis of the two parental strains and the progeny of interstrain crosses gives the results shown in Table 3–12. The amino acid sequences of the C_κ regions from DA and LEW rats were determined, as shown in Figure 3–56.

(a)   What is the most likely explanation for the serological data in Table 3–12?

(b)   What is surprising about the data in Figure 3–56?

strain   position

	105												115										125										135
LEW	L	E	L	K	R	A	B	A	A	P	T	V	S	I	F	P	P	S	T	Z	Z	L	A	T	G	G	A	S	V	V	C	L
DA	L	E	L	K	R	A	B	A	A	P	T	V	S	I	F	P	P	S	M	Z	Z	L	T	S	G	G	A	T	V	V	C	F

				145										155									165
LEW	M	N	D	F	Y	P	R	B	I	S	V	K	W	K	I	D	G	T	E	[]	R	B	G	V	L	B	S	V	T	B
DA	V	N	D	F	Y	P	R	B	I	S	V	K	W	K	I	D	G	S	E	Z	R	B	S	V	L	B	S	V	T	B

				175									185									195
LEW	Z	B	S	L	D	S	T	Y	S	M	S	S	T	L	S	L	T	K	A	D	Y	Q	S	H	N	L	Y	T	C	Q
DA	Z	B	S	K	D	S	T	Y	S	M	S	S	T	L	S	L	T	K	V	Z	Y	Q	R	H	N	L	Y	T	C	Q

				205											
LEW	V	V	H	K	T	S	S	S	P	V	V	W	K	T	F	N	R	N	E	C
DA	V	V	H	K	T	S	S	S	P	V	V	W	K	T	F	N	R	N	E	C

Figure 3–56 C_K sequence of rat "alleles" (Problem 3–26). [ ] designates a residue deletion. [From V. Farnsworth *et al., Proc. Natl. Acad. Sci. USA* **73,** 1293 (1976).]

Table 3–12
Serological reactivity of rat κ chains (Problem 3–26)

	Reactivity with:	
Rats	Serum A	Serum B
20 DA rats	20	0
20 LEW rats	0	20
20 (DA × LEW) F1 rats	20	20
20 F2 rats	15	15

(c)   Offer three genetic models for the evolution of the two rat C_κ genes. Point out the limitations, if any, of the models you propose.

(d)   Suggest one experiment to distinguish the models offered in Part (c).

3–27   (a)   You have just trapped 766 Martian gophers, and you decide to characterize their immunoglobulins. You purify the immunoglobulin from Gopher 1 and inject it into 50 other gophers; then you inject purified immunoglobulin from gopher 2 into 50 different gophers; you continue until you have raised antibodies to the immunoglobulins purified from 15 individual gophers. You carry out quantitative antibody–antigen reactions and find that each of the 15 gophers used as a source of immunoglobulin can be placed into one of three groups, A, B, or C, each composed of animals that show no immunologic response to each other's immunoglobulins (Table 3–13). For example, Ig from an animal in Group A (Ig$_a$) injected into a second animal from Group A stimulates no antibody production. In contrast, Ig$_a$ injected into animals from Groups B and C elicits antibodies that can remove all of the immunizing antigen (Ig$_a$) from solution. What conclusions can you draw from these groupings?

Table 3–13

Immunologic reactions of Martian gopher immunoglobulins (Problem 3–27)

		Group of animals in which antiserum is raised:		
		A	B	C
	A (5)[a]	0[b]	100	100
Source of immunoglobulins:	B (5)	100	0	100
	C (5)	100	100	0

[a]Number of gophers falling into a given group.
[b]Percent of immunoglobulin precipitated by antiserum.

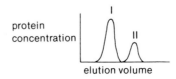

Figure 3–57 The gel-filtration pattern of Martian gopher immunoglobulins after reduction and alkylation (Problem 3–27).

Table 3–14

Immunologic reactions of Martian gopher immunoglobulin chains from Peaks I and II (Problem 3–27)

		Group of animals in which antiserum is raised:							
		A	B	C			A	B	C
Source of immunoglobulin for Peak I:	A	0[a]	100	100	Source of immunoglobulin for Peak II:	A	0[a]	100	40
	B	100	0	100		B	100	0	60
	C	100	100	0		C	40	60	0

[a]Percent of immunoglobulin precipitated by antiserum.

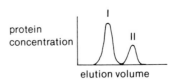

Figure 3–58 Gel-filtration pattern of Martian gopher immunoglobulins digested with pepsin (Problem 3–27).

Table 3–15

Immunologic reactions of Peaks I and II from pepsin-treated Martian gopher immunoglobulins (Problem 3–27)

		Group of animals in which antiserum is raised:							
		A	B	C			A	B	C
Source of immunoglobulin for Peak I:	A	0[a]	100	100	Source of immunoglobulin for Peak II:	A	0[a]	100	0
	B	100	0	60		B	100	0	100
	C	100	60	0		C	0	100	0

[a]Percent of immunoglobulin precipitated by antiserum.

(b)   Eager to move ahead, you submit one sample of immunoglobulin from each of the three groups to mild reduction, alkylation, and gel filtration on Sephadex G-100 (see Problem 3-4). For each group you obtain an identical pattern with two peaks (Figure 3-57), to give a total of six peaks.

You prepare antisera against each of the six peaks in animals from each of the three groups. Again you carry out a series of quantitative antibody–antigen reactions, with the results shown in Table 3-14. Assume that the individuals in each of the three groups are homozygous for their immunoglobulin genes. Also assume that antibody is not limiting in any of these reactions. What conclusions can you draw from these experiments? What is the significance of the 40% and 60% reactions in the table for Peak II?

(c)   You then carry out a pepsin digestion (see Problem 3-4) on the immunoglobulins from each of the groups, and once again you obtain identical patterns of two peaks (I and II) upon gel filtration on Sephadex G-200 (Figure 3-58). You prepare antisera to Peaks I and II as described above. Once again you carry out quantitative antibody–antigen reactions, with the results shown in Table 3-15. What final conclusions can you draw? How could you decide whether any of these markers are on the V_H regions?

(d)   How could you use these presumed genetic markers to ascertain something about the organization of genes for various immunoglobulin families in the Martian gopher genome?

Answers

3-1   (a)   False.   The hinge region joins the N- and C-terminal halves of the heavy chain.
(b)   False.   The light chains of a single antibody molecule always are identical, as are the heavy chains.
(c)   False.   The V_L and V_H regions are approximately the same size.
(d)   True
(e)   False.   Both chains contribute to the active site.
(f)   True
(g)   False.   The V regions of one immunoglobulin family never are associated with the C regions of another family.
(h)   False.   There are many more genes coding for V regions than for C regions.
(i)   True
(j)   True
(k)   False.   The C_H regions distinguish the classes and subclasses of antibodies.

(1)   False.   The immune response to a single antigen usually consists of a heterogeneous array of different antibody molecules.

(m)   False.   Identical myeloma proteins from different humans never have been observed.

(n)   True

(o)   False.   V and C regions become joined at the RNA level.

(p)   True

(q)   True

(r)   False.   The genealogic tree of V regions suggests that multiple germ-line V genes exist, but it does not prove that the diversity seen at the terminal twigs of the genealogic tree is coded in the germ line.

(s)   False.   The three families of immunoglobulin genes are genetically unlinked.

(t)   True

(u)   True

(v)   True

(w)   False.   The presence of species-specific V-region differences suggests that V genes evolved subsequent to species divergence.

(x)   True

(y)   True

(z)   False.   Immunoglobulin genes are autosomal. Allelic exclusion suggests that each antibody-producing cell can express only the maternal or the paternal allele for a particular immunoglobulin gene, but not both. The choice appears to be random, as for female X-chromosome inactivation in mammals, but may have an entirely different basis than X inactivation, as explained in Essential Concept 3–8G.

3–2   (a)   clonal-selection
      (b)   variable
      (c)   Allotypes
      (d)   somatic mutation
      (e)   Myeloma proteins
      (f)   homology units
      (g)   domains
      (h)   hypervariable
      (i)   effector, antigen-binding
      (j)   lambda and kappa
      (k)   subgroups
      (l)   idiotype
      (m)   Allelic exclusion
      (n)   informational
      (o)   species-associated

3–3   This protein probably is a light chain. Some myeloma patients synthesize an excess of light chain along with the myeloma immunoglobulin. Other myeloma patients synthesize just a light chain. The 23,000-dalton light chain can pass through the kidney and is excreted in the urine. Urinary light chains from myeloma patients are called *Bence–Jones proteins*, after their discoverer. Early structural studies were carried out on Bence–Jones proteins because they were easily obtained and readily purified of minor urinary protein contaminants.

3–4   (a)   Pattern (a), Figure 3–59; pattern (b), Figure 3–59.

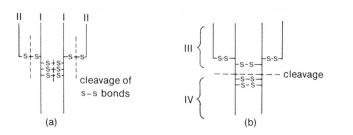

Figure 3–59 Cleavages of goat IgG (Answer 3–4a).

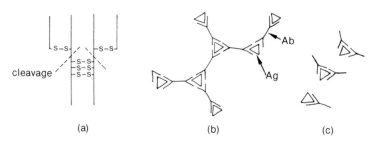

Figure 3–60 (Answer 3–4d.) (a) Sites of papain cleavage of goat IgG. (b) Lattice formed by association of bivalent antibodies (Ab) with antigen molecules (Ag). (c) Association of monovalent antibody fragments with antigen.

(b) Pepsin generally cannot cleave regions of polypeptide chains with a compact structure (the Fab and Fc fragments), but it can cleave unstructured or randomly oriented regions such as the hinge region.

(c) Fragment III (Fab) binds antigen. It is composed of the two light chains and the N-terminal halves of the heavy chains. Fragment IV (Fc) carries effector functions and is composed of the C-terminal halves of the heavy chains. Thus both light and heavy chains are required for antigen binding, but heavy chains alone can carry out some effector functions.

(d) The sites of papain cleavage are shown in Figure 3–60a. To precipitate an antigen, antibody must be bivalent so an antigen-antibody lattice can form (Figure 3–60b). Papain digestion produces univalent Fab fragments that can bind to antigen; however, they cannot form the lattice necessary for precipitation (Figure 3–60c).

3–5 (a) The results show two antigenically distinct types of light chains: Proteins 1, 3, 4, and 8 react with Antiserum A, and Proteins 2, 5, 6, and 7 react with Antisera B and C. These classes correspond to the λ and κ types of light chains. To confirm this explanation you could carry out amino-acid-sequence analysis on each of the eight proteins to determine their types. This kind of serologic analysis first suggested that there are two types of light chains in humans.

(b) Bence–Jones Protein 2 has antigenic determinants that are not present in Proteins 5 and 7, but that must have been present in the protein used to prepare antiserum C. There are two possible explanations for this observation. These determinants could be features of the V_L region of Protein 2 not present in Proteins 5 and 7 (i.e., idiotypic determinants). Alternatively, Antiserum C may be detecting a different type of C_L region in Protein 2. All humans have at least five different types of C_L regions: four C_λ subtypes and the C_κ type.

3–6   (a)   Fab fragments (which carry the antigen-binding sites on true antibodies), prepared from the immunoglobulin, must be shown to bind the Dnp group.

The Dnp group must be shown to bind in the active-site cleft. The hydrophobic Dnp group may associate nonspecifically with other hydrophobic clefts, which have nothing to do with the active site.

The stoichiometry of binding should be one mole of Dnp bound per mole of Fab, and the valence of the intact immunoglobulin should correspond to that of one of the known immunoglobulin classes. For example, IgG antibodies have a valence of two and IgM antibodies a valence of ten.

Upon binding to the antigen, the myeloma immunoglobulin should carry out the effector functions triggered by antigen binding to normal antibodies of the same immunoglobulin class. For example, complement fixation should occur with IgG1 molecules.

Normally the synthesis of antibodies is specifically induced by corresponding antigens. No one understands the nature of the induction process in myelomatosis. It would be interesting to make a specific antiserum (anti-idiotype) for the V regions of the myeloma protein and determine whether similar molecules are induced in a normal immune response to the Dnp group.

(b)   Dnp and menadione could share some unrecognized common structural features that permit binding to occur at the same antigen-binding site.

If menadione and Dnp have distinct antigenic determinants, there could be two distinct Fab binding sites, one for each antigen. Conversely, both antigens could bind to the same site in different orientations. The antigen-binding site could have two or more distinct subsites.

Menadione could bind nonspecifically to a region of the antibody molecule other than the active site.

(c)   You could locate the binding site for menadione.

You could carry out a competition experiment to determine whether Dnp can bind in the presence of excess menadione. If the sites are the same or if they hinder one another sterically, competition will occur. If the sites are independent, no competition will occur.

You could make a structural analysis of the two antigen–antibody complexes by x-ray crystallography.

3–7   Some immunoglobulin classes can fix complement, whereas others cannot. Therefore similar ovalbumen-specific V_H regions must be attached to different C_H regions in the two antibody preparations. This phenomenon, in general, allows the same antigen-binding site to be associated with many different types of effector functions. Thus antibody molecules allow a given antigen to trigger several different kinds of physiological responses.

3–8   (a)   In n cell generations, the clone will expand from 1 to 2^n cells, and $2^n - 1$ DNA replications will occur. There are about 110 codons in each V region gene, so the mutation rate is about 10^{-7} substitutions per V gene per DNA replication. Therefore, on the average, one mutation will occur in a given V gene when $2^n = 10^7$, or n $\cong$ 23 generations.
(b)   On the average, 23 more generations would be required to obtain a second mutation in the same V gene.
(c)   If the generation time is a half day, it will take, on the average, about 12 and 24 days to obtain one and two mutations, respectively.
(d)   Unless the rate of cell division is very rapid or the rate of mutation is much higher than the average in human cells, ordinary somatic mutation could account for no more than a small fraction of the observed V-gene diversity in this short time.
(e)   One to two substitutions would be fixed in 10–20 days. These types of calculation have led some immunologists to conclude that ordinary somatic mutation probably could not fix more than 1–4 substitutions in any given V gene for each lymphocyte line. Accordingly, theories of antibody diversity that invoke ordinary somatic mutation suggest that V regions differing by more than about eight residues (four mutations in each of two lymphocyte lines) probably are coded by separate germ-line V genes.

3–9   (a)   Three sets or subgroups of V_κ sequences are apparent:
I (1, 6, 7, 11, 12); II (2, 5, 9, 10); and III (3, 4, 8).
(b)   Prototype sequences are as follows:
I   D I Q M T Q S P S S L S A S V G D R V T I T C
II   E I V L T Q S P G T L S L S P G D R A T L S C
III D I V M T Q S P L S L P V T P G E P A S I S C
(c)   Prototype I differs from II by 10 residues; I differs from III by 11 residues; II differs from III by 11 residues.

(d)   I–II difference $= 110 \times \dfrac{10}{23} = 48$ residues

I–III difference $= 110 \times \dfrac{11}{23} = 53$ residues

II–III difference $= 110 \times \dfrac{11}{23} = 53$ residues

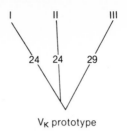

V_K prototype

Figure 3–61   A genealogic tree of V_K sequences (Answer 3–9e,f).

(e)   The genealogic tree is given in Figure 3–61.

(f)   To produce these V_K regions by somatic mutation from a single V gene, three unlikely constraints must be imposed on the mutational mechanism. First, 24 or more somatic mutations must occur in the V_K genes of three lymphocyte lines to generate the three V_K prototype sequences (Figure 3–61). Second, because each individual can synthesize every V_K sequence, precisely the same mutations must occur in each individual to generate the three V_K prototype genes. Third, the C_K gene must remain invariant in the face of numerous V_K gene mutations. Ordinary somatic mutation probably can produce only 1–4 mutations per lymphocyte line (see Problem 3–8); hypermutation can produce many more mutations. However, neither mechanism can account for the extensive parallel mutation that must occur in a single V_K gene to produce identical prototype V_K genes in every individual. Moreover, it seems unlikely that selective pressures could maintain the C_K gene invariant in the face of frequent V_K gene mutation, unless the somatic mutational mechanism were restricted to V genes. Thus it is likely that at least one germ-line V gene is present for each V-region subgroup.

(g)   The difference matrix for the prototype sequences and individual V_K regions is given in Figure 3–62.

(h)   For Protein 11 the difference is $110 \times \dfrac{1}{23} = 5$ residues.

For Protein 2 the difference is $110 \times \dfrac{1}{23} = 5$ residues.

For Protein 5 the difference is $110 \times \dfrac{2}{23} = 10$ residues.

(i)   Either somatic mutation or germ-line differences could account for the small differences between Proteins 11 and 2 and their respective prototypes. With ordinary somatic mutation, the two substitutions that differentiate Protein 5 and its prototype might be excessive (see Problem 3–8).

(j)   Since man is not inbred, some of these differences may reflect the polymorphisms of an outbred population.

prototypes	V regions				
	1	6	7	11	12
I	0	0	0	1	0
	2	5	9	10	
II	1	2	0	0	
	3	4	8		
III	0	0	0		

Figure 3–62 Difference matrices for intrasubgroup differences between V_K sequence and prototype I, II, and III (Answer 3–9g).

The remainder of the V region may not be comparable in variability to the N-terminal portion shown in Figure 46.

These selected myeloma proteins may fail to reflect the true diversity of the normal antibody population.

3-10 (a)   A sequence of 110 amino acid residues is coded by 330 nucleotide pairs. Each nucleotide may mutate to one of three other nucleotides. Hence the probability of two independent lymphocyte lines incurring precisely the same nucleotide substitutions in a given V-region gene is 1/990.

(b)   A parallel mutation at the protein level is more likely. Because a single amino acid generally can be specified by more than one codon, a given amino acid substitution could result from any one of two to six different nucleotide substitutions.

(c)   Proteins 1 and 2 require 19 parallel mutations from the primordial V_K gene. Assuming that all nucleotide substitutions are equally probable, the probability of getting 19 parallel mutations in two V genes (~321 nucleotides) can be calculated roughly in the following manner. Assume that one V gene has mutated at a single base. The probability of an identical mutation in the second V gene is $\left(\dfrac{1}{3} \times \dfrac{1}{321} \right)$, in which the second figure is the probability of mutation occurring in the same nucleotide base and the first figure is the probability that this base changes to the appropriate one of three other possibilities. Therefore the probability of 19 consecutive parallel mutations is $\left(\dfrac{1}{3} \times \dfrac{1}{321} \right)^{19}$ $= 2.05 \times 10^{-57}$. In view of this answer the likelihood of observing parallel mutations in the V_K regions of the African elephant would be extremely low.

(d)   The level of germ-line genes could be placed at about Level D in Figure 3–31. Moving the level of germ-line genes up the genealogic tree reduces the number of genetic events (and the number of parallel mutations) required to obtain the observed diversity.

Intense selective pressures could lead to a few parallel mutations.

(e)   One to four mutational events may occur in each lymphocyte line by ordinary somatic mutation (Problem 3–8). Thus the level of germ-line genes would be just above Level D. According to this theory, two identical V_κ regions of independent origin would be coded by a germ-line V_κ gene that had not undergone somatic mutation.

(f)   Hypermutation could generate large numbers of genetic events. It could not account, however, for extensive parallel mutation. Accordingly, to explain Proteins 1–6 in Figure 3–31, the level of germ-line V genes probably must be placed at D or higher. Among the selective pressures that could be invoked to account for the genealogic data by somatic mechanisms are antigen selection, requirements for light–heavy chain pairing, and mechanisms for eliminating antibodies to self.

(g)   Infrequent recombinational events among a large number of V genes is consistent with the genealogic tree of V-region sequences. Advocates of the recombinational theory argue that there are 10–100 germ-line V genes for each subgroup. Because mouse V_κ regions have more than 25 subgroups, there would be 250–2500 V genes, according to the somatic recombination theory. It is difficult, if not impossible, to distinguish between this alternative and the germ-line theory by any of the techniques currently available to immunologists.

(h)   The germ-line theory would suggest that all V-region genes are present in the germ line, and would predict that V-region sequences should be related by genealogic trees similar to those observed for other evolutionarily related proteins. Such relationships have been observed among the sequences analyzed so far.

3–11   (a)   It is unlikely that these variants are allelic forms of the same structural gene. If each variant represents 50% of the C_λ genes in the human population, then the probability of picking ten consecutive heterozygotes is $(1/2)^{10}$ or $1/1024$. If the variants were present in unequal frequencies in the population, then the probability of selecting 10 consecutive heterozygotes would be even lower.

(b)   This polymorphism may be coded by duplicate germ-line genes that have diverged by one base substitution.

3–12   There are four distinct classes. They are I: 1, 2, 5, 7, 9; II: 3, 8; III: 4; IV: 6, 10.

3–13   (a)   These genes must be closely linked because each group of polymorphisms segregates as a unit.

(b)   The last individual must carry one Caucasian chromosome and a recombinant chromosome that arose in the F1 parent, as shown in Figure 3–63. The phenotype of this individual suggests that the genes in parentheses are grouped together, although a precise order cannot be determined.

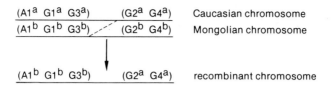

Figure 3–63 Recombination between genes for human C_H allotypes (Answer 3–13).

3-14 The labeling regimen should produce a low $^3H/^{14}C$ ratio near the N-terminus of each polypeptide, increasing to a high ratio at the C-terminus. Light chains from the Martian gopher show two gradients of $^3H/^{14}C$ ratios: one extends from residue 1 to 107 (V region) and the other from 108 to 214 (C region). This observation suggests that the V and C regions are translated as two separate polypeptides. Accordingly, the joining of V and C regions must occur at the polypeptide level. Light chains from the BALB/c mouse show a single gradient, indicating that they are synthesized as one continuous polypeptide chain. Therefore, in this system, V–C joining occurs at the nucleic acid level. These experiments actually have been carried out for mouse light chains, with results similar to those shown in Figure 3–48b.

3-15 With random association, the number of different antibodies that could be assembled is $p \times q$, in which p = number of light chains and q = number of heavy chains. Therefore, with 10 light and 10 heavy chains, $10^2 = 100$ antibodies could be formed; with 100 of each chain, $100^2 = 10^4$; and with 1000 of each chain, $1000^2 = 10^6$.

3-16 (a) Specification of a V region 107 residues in length requires a gene of at least 321 nucleotide pairs. The maximum number of such genes that could be encoded by the mammalian haploid genome is $\dfrac{3.2 \times 10^9}{3.2 \times 10^2}$ $= 10^7$ V genes.

(b) If the entire haploid genome represents 10^7 V-gene equivalents, then the percent of haploid DNA required for 1000 V_L and 1000 V_H genes is $\dfrac{2 \times 10^3}{10^7} \times 100\% = 0.02\%$. For random association of V_L and V_H regions, this percentage of the genome could provide the information for 10^6 different antibody molecules.

3-17 (a) In this set the diversity can arise most simply by random mutation without selection. Each sequence can be generated by a single base substitution from the prototype sequence (Sequence 1). The substitutions seem to be randomly distributed throughout the 23 residues. Therefore the diversity in Sequences 2–10 is generated by single, random substitutions from the prototype sequence (Figure 3–64).

(b)   In this set the diversity can arise most simply by mutation plus selection. In several cases two or more of the sequences shown have some of the same substitutions (e.g., the deletion at Position 9 in Proteins 6 and 7). Because of the enormous number of possible substitutions that could occur it is unlikely that two of ten sequences would have the same random substitutions unless selective forces were operating

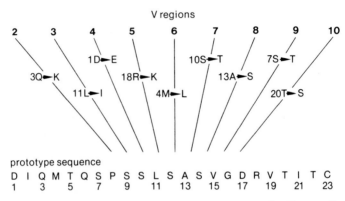

Figure 3–64   Diversification of V regions by random mutation (Answer 3–17a).

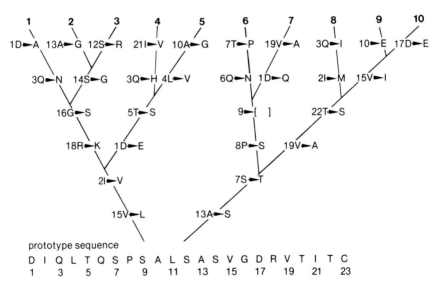

Figure 3–65   Diversification of V regions by mutation and selection (Answer 3–17b).

(see Problem 3–10). In support of this conclusion, the variants can be arranged into a genealogic tree in which each sequence differs from an ancestral sequence by six single base substitutions (Figure 3–65).

Remember that each sequence is generated in a different lymphocyte clone. If random somatic mutation from a single V gene were postulated, the two clones that are to produce Sequences 2 and 3 would have to undergo five parallel mutations to generate Genes 2 and 3 from the ancestral gene. Intense selective pressures would be required to explain this number of parallel mutations. One of the controversial questions in contemporary immunology is whether such selective pressures can operate effectively during the short time span of somatic differentiation.

(c)   In this set the diversity can arise most simply by recombination. The critical observation here is that each residue position shows no more than two amino acid alternatives, apart from one mutation at Position 15. Sequences 1 and 2 are the parental sequences. All the remaining sequences are linear combinations of the two parental sequences. Sequences 3, 4, 5, 6, and 9 show one recombinational event. Sequence 7 shows two, 8 shows three, and 10 shows four recombinational events. No genealogic tree can be constructed from these sequences.

3–18   (a)   The V regions for each family are the C-terminal 12 residues. The C regions for light chains are 12 residues, whereas those for heavy chains are 36 (γ) and 48 (μ) residues.

(b)   The light chains are composed of two homology units, each 12 residues in length, with symmetrically placed disulfide bridges. The heavy chains have 4 (γ) or 5 (μ) similar homology units. The μ chain in man also appears to have five homology units.

(c)   The V regions and the C regions share at least two features: (1) they can be broken down into homology units 12 residues in length, and (2) these homology units have symmetrically disposed disulfide bridges that span four residues. The V regions are related to one another by sequence homology, as are the C-region homology units.

3–19   Species-associated residues indicate that most rabbit V_κ genes have diverged from their mouse counterparts in parallel at these positions. The following two mechanisms can be postulated:

1.   Mutation and selection: with intense enough selective pressures, multiple genes could evolve in parallel.

2.   Homologous but unequal crossing-over: this hypothesis suggests that multigene families are continually being expanded and contracted by gene duplication and deletion, respectively, and by unequal crossing-over during recombination. If different genes are duplicated (or deleted) in different evolutionary lines, species-associated residues will result (Figure 3–41).

3-20   (a)   The deletions include portions of both the C and V regions in all three proteins.

(b)   The V_H and C_H genes could have been translocated prior to the deletion event.

A deletion event unrelated to normal translocation could join the V and C genes by removing all of the chromosomal region between these nucleotide sequences. It is extremely unlikely that the V and C genes would incur independent deletions and subsequently become joined.

A deletion could result from malfunction of the translocation mechanism itself. If this explanation is correct, then study of γ-HCD polypeptides and the genes that encode them could help to elucidate the translocation mechanism.

3-21   Haptens related structurally to the immunizing antigen compete with the anti-D antibody for binding to the D antibodies. This result might be explained in either of the following two ways:

1.   The region of the combining site of the D antibody may include a major fraction of its idiotypic antigenic determinants. If so, the presence of hapten could sterically inhibit the reaction with anti-D antibody.

2.   Combination of the hapten with the active site of the D antibody may cause a conformational change that alters idiotypic determinants, which need not be confined to the region of the active site.

X-ray structural studies indicate no variable-domain conformational changes upon reaction of an antibody with a hapten. Accordingly, most immunologists favor the first explanation.

3-22   (a)   If 1 in 20,000 individuals undergoes a neoplastic transformation that leads to multiple myeloma, then the probability of two independent transformations in the same individual would be $1/20,000 \times 1/20,000$ or 1 in 4×10^8. Patients with two myeloma proteins occur with a far higher frequency (1 in 2×10^6). Therefore, individuals with one multiple myeloma protein appear predisposed to express a second myeloma protein, that is, the events that produce a biclonal myeloma are not independent.

(b)   The V_L sequences are identical, even throughout most of the first hypervariable region. The same is true of the V_H sequences. Moreover, the indistinguishable idiotypes suggest that these identities extend throughout the variable regions. Randomly chosen V_L and V_H sequences are very different from one another. Therefore it seems almost certain that the two transformation events are related, which supports the conclusion that they do not occur independently.

(c)   Perhaps the neoplastic transformation occurs in a single precursor lymphocyte that is committed to expression of a particular IgM protein. A cell from the resulting clone subsequently may differentiate, thereby undergoing a heavy-chain class switch that leads to production of an

IgG protein with the same V_L and V_H regions as before. This same differentiation is believed to occur in the course of a normal immune response.

(d)   Mechanism 1: During the differentiation of a lymphocyte, a single V_H gene first may be associated with a C_μ gene and later be translocated to a C_γ gene.

Mechanism 2: A single V_H gene may be replicated and then inserted near every C_H gene. Then lymphocyte differentiation would reflect simply the sequential expression of complete $V_H C_H$ genes, analogous to the expression of ε, γ, and then β chains of hemoglobin at successive stages of human development. Currently these two mechanisms cannot be distinguished (see Figure 3–21).

3–23   (a)   The A5A marker exhibits Mendelian segregation, and its expression is dominant or codominant because it is present at similar levels in A/J mice and Fl hybrids.

(b)   With only one exception the A5A marker segregates with the Ig-1e allele; therefore, these two markers are closely linked.

(c)   This animal probably is a recombinant in which the A5A marker is now associated with the Ig-1a allele. You could test this hypothesis by determining whether the linkage of A5A to Ig-1a persists in subsequent crosses.

(d)   The A5A marker represents a specific V_H gene, which encodes a variable region that reacts with the Group A streptococcal antigen, whereas the C_γ allotypic marker represents a C_H gene. Therefore the results suggest that V_H and C_H genes may be linked as a general rule. This suggestion can be tested by investigating the linkage of other idiotypic markers.

(e)   The absence of the A5A marker from the BALB/c strain, and its Mendelian segregation in interstrain crosses, suggest strongly that a V_H gene that codes for A5A is present in the germ line of A/J mice. Additional results of this kind would provide further support for the theory that V_H sequences are encoded in the germ line.

3–24   (a)   The copy-insertion model proposes that a copy of the V gene is inserted nearer a C gene (V_2 in Figure 3–22). The original V gene remains in its site on the chromosome. If this model were correct, the restriction-enzyme experiments would have revealed two DNA fragments that contain V-gene sequences in the differentiated myeloma DNA, one peak representing the original V gene, and a second peak representing the V-gene copy translocated to the C gene. None of the other models can be ruled out by these experiments.

(b)   Mammalian cells contain two copies of each chromosome. The experimental results in Figure 3–19 suggest that V–C joining must have occurred in both of the chromosomal homologues that carry the κ gene family, because in the myeloma DNA all the V gene copies appear to be in the same DNA fragment as the C gene copies. If V–C joining had occurred on only one of the two homologues, then 50% of the myeloma DNA should have shown the embryonic pattern of fragmentation. Furthermore, the translocated V genes on both chromosomes must be very similar, if not identical, because both hybridize with the same mRNA. If this result is representative of normal antibody-producing cells as well as myeloma cells [see Part (c) of this problem], then the V–C joining mechanism does not play a role in allelic exclusion.

(c)   Since the myeloma tumor used in these experiments was aneuploid, it may have carried just a single copy of the chromosome on which the κ gene family is located. To test this possibility, similar experiments should be carried out in a normal diploid cell line.

(d)   The looping-out model postulates that in the process of V–C joining, all the intervening V genes between the joined V gene and the C genes are lost from the chromosome. The excision-insertion model predicts that no V genes will be lost. To distinguish between these models a population of mRNA's that code for many κ chains could be hybridized with embryonic and myeloma DNA to determine whether any of the corresponding genes are lost in the process of differentiation.

3–25   (a)   The Ms-1 allotype does not appear to be coded by a1 V genes because several a1 individuals in the pedigree are Ms-1-negative; for example, Individuals 4 and 7 in the F2 generation.

(b)   Ms-1 must be a variant of the μ constant region because the Ms-1 allotype is observed only on IgM molecules. However, expression of the Ms-1 allotype occurs only in individuals that produce the b4 light-chain allotype as well. Individuals that carry only the Ms-1 C_μ gene or the b4 C_κ gene alone do not exhibit the Ms-1 allotype. The two mated Ms-1-negative individuals in the F2 generation each contribute one of the genes necessary to produce Ms-1-positive progeny. Close linkage between the V_H and C_H (including C_μ) genes accounts for the observation that a1 and Ms-1 always segregate together in these experiments.

(c)   The $C_\mu 1$ and C_κ regions are the only constant-region homology units that interact with one another in the IgM molecule. Therefore the Ms-1 specificity probably is produced by the interaction of these two homology units. This supposition could be verified by testing Fab and Fc fragments of the IgM molecule for the Ms-1 specificity, and if possible, by isolating and testing the $C_\mu 1$ domain alone.

3–26   (a)   The most likely explanation for the serologically detectable polymorphism is that the two rat strains have different κ-chain allotypes. If the DA rats are (A/A) and the LEW rats are (B/B), the F1 rats will be (A/B). If A and B are codominant alleles, all of the F1 rats will react with both serum A and serum B. The ratios of F2 rats will be (for 20 total progeny) 5(A/A):10(A/B):5(B/B). Because the 10(A/B) rats react positively with both sera, there are 15 out of 20 positive reactions for each serum.

(b)   It is surprising that there are so many sequence differences between the two κ "allotypes." Usually allotypes differ by only one or a few residues. These κ-chain variants are examples of complex allotypes.

(c)   Three possible evolutionary models for complex allotypes are given in Figure 3–29.

Model 1: The allotypes may have arisen as classical alleles (Figure 3–29a). This model would require that a surprisingly high number of mutations must occur and be fixed in each allele during the evolution of rats as a species.

Model 2: The allotypes may have evolved by gene duplication and deletion (Figure 3–29b). There is a precedent for this model in the β hemoglobin genes of the mouse and the C_λ genes of the rabbit. Accordingly, this model seems most plausible.

Model 3: The allotypes may be duplicated genes whose expression is regulated by a polymorphic control mechanism (Figure 3–29c). It is unclear why such a complex mechanism would evolve to regulate the expression of two genes.

(d)   Model 3 could be verified by demonstrating that all rats have both C_κ genes or that they can synthesize both C_κ regions. Model 2 would be supported if some rats have and express both C_κ genes, whereas others have only one gene or the other. The observation that some rats have C_κ genes intermediate in sequence between the LEW and DA allotypes would be consistent with the idea of successive single base substitutions in a single gene, as suggested by Model 1.

3–27   This pattern of precipitation is similar to that which occurs with rabbit immunoglobulins and antisera directed against their various allotypes. The simplest explanation assumes that gopher immunoglobulins are similar to other mammalian immunoglobulins in their chain structure.

(a)   The gophers in each group exhibit serologic (genetic) markers on their immunoglobulins that differ from those of the other groups.

(b)   The gopher immunoglobulins separate into subunits resembling the familiar mammalian light and heavy chains. There are serologic differences in both chains from all three groups.

Because a fraction of Peak II (light) chains precipitates and a fraction does not when reacted with antisera from other strains, Peak II must include at least two types of chains that carry distinct serologic markers. We may call these two types κ and λ by analogy with humans. An explanation of the results could be that the kappa to lambda ratio of gopher is 60:40 (as in man) and that Groups A and C have identical κ chain markers; B and C have identical λ chain markers; whereas A and B have different markers on both the κ and λ chains.

(c)   Pepsin digestion produces an $F(ab)_2$ fragment, which consists of two Fab fragments joined by a disulfide bridge (Figure 3–59b). Remember that these fragments contain the N-terminal halves of the heavy chains.

Because the $F(ab)_2$ fragments from animals of groups A and C differ completely (100%), as opposed to a 40% difference for the light chains, there must be an antigenic difference in the N-terminal half of the heavy chain. $F(ab)_2$ fragments from animals of Groups B and C do not differ in the N-terminal half. No clear conclusion can be drawn about the extent of differences on the N-terminal half of the heavy chains of strains A and B because of the difference in light chain markers; however, since A differs from C and B does not, A must differ from B.

The experiments with Peak II show that there also are serologic differences in the Fc fragment, that is, the C-terminal half of the heavy chain. Groups A and B differ in the C-terminal half. Perhaps surprisingly, Groups A and C differ in the N-terminal half (Peak I results) but not in the C-terminal half, whereas Groups B and C differ in the C-terminal half but not in the N-terminal half (Peak I results). If alternative N-terminal markers are designated n_1 and n_2 and alternative C-terminal markers are designated c_1 and c_2, then the pattern of markers on heavy chains of the three groups could be represented as A: n_1, c_1; B: n_2, c_2; and C: n_2, c_1.

Whether the heavy-chain N-terminal serologic marker is on the N-terminal portion of the C_H region or on the V_H region can be established by determining whether this marker is shared by all classes of heavy chains. If so, it must be a V_H-region marker. If the marker is found only on a single class of H chain, it must be in the N-terminal half of the C_H region.

(d)   One interesting experiment would be to carry out appropriate crosses to investigate the linkage of the various genetic markers, especially those on the two halves of the heavy chain. If the two markers on the heavy chain are unlinked, it would indicate that the heavy chain is the product of more than one gene. In the rabbit the genes for λ, κ, and heavy chains are unlinked.

4 MOLECULAR RECOGNITION AT CELL SURFACES

In the vertebrate immune system, diverse immunologic functions are initiated by events at the lymphocyte cell surface. These functions include transmission of positional information by cell-cell recognition, as in the homing of B cells and T cells to specific areas of lymphoid tissue, and they include the triggering of differentiation and proliferation by specific macromolecules, as in the response of B-cell and T-cell precursors to a circulating cognate antigen. Since new genes evolve from previously existing genes, the vertebrate immune system must have had its origins in more primitive recognition systems. From a variety of evidence such recognition systems appear to operate in the development and physiological functioning of all metazoan organisms, and they appear to be mediated by recognition elements in the surface plasma membranes of cells. This chapter considers the general structure and function of the plasma membrane, the characteristics of some simple metazoan cellular-recognition systems, and the properties of the membrane-associated molecules that participate in various aspects of vertebrate immunity.

Essential Concepts

4-1 Membranes are fundamental components of biological organization

A. Membranes perform a variety of general functions in all cells and tissues.

1. Membranes are barriers to macromolecules and most polar molecules, but they are relatively permeable to water and small hydrophobic molecules. Membranes separate cells from their environment and from one another, and permit the specialization

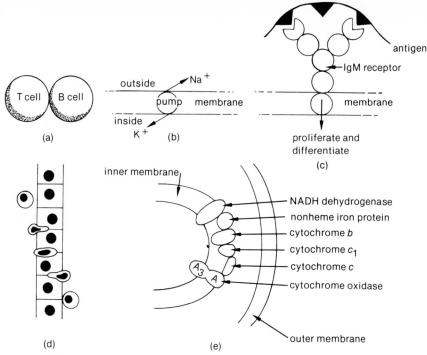

Figure 4–1 General functions of membranes. (a) Compartmentalization of cells to permit functional specialization. (b) Transfer of materials into and out of cells. (c) Transfer of signals from the environment into cells. (d) Mediation of cell movement, for example, movement of a lymphocyte through a postcapillary venule. (e) Organization of proteins, for example, of the electron transport enzymes in the inner mitochondrial membrane.

of cellular function that is characteristic of metazoa (Figure 4–1). In addition, membranes compartmentalize the interior of cells into areas of distinct specialization, such as the nucleus, the mitochondria, the endoplasmic reticulum, and the Golgi apparatus.

2. Membranes mediate the transport of ions, metabolites, and macromolecules into and out of cells. Membrane pumps and gates allow active or passive transport, respectively, of certain ions and metabolites (Figure 4–1b). In nerve and muscle-cell membranes the cooperative action of pumps and gates leads to propagation of action potentials along cells. Endocytosis and exocytosis are employed to move macromolecules into or out of cellular compartments, respectively.

3. The plasma membrane and associated cytoskeletal elements mediate cell movement. In the many types of eucaryotic cells that are capable of amoeboid movement, the plasma membrane is a dynamic structure that appears to be sending out pseudopodia in all directions, as if to explore its environment (Figure 4–2).

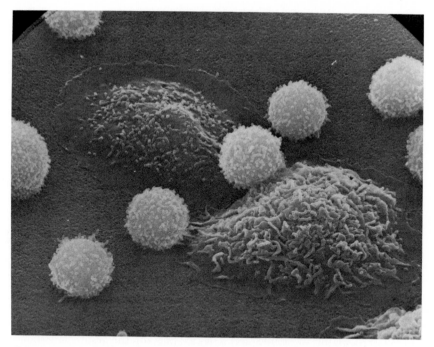

Figure 4–2 A scanning electron micrograph of several lymphocytes (round cells) and macrophages. [Courtesy of J. Orenstein and E. Shelton.]

4.   The plasma membrane mediates transfer of information from the exterior to the interior of cells. Most eucaryotic cells carry a variety of membrane-associated receptor molecules that are capable of transducing external stimuli into appropriate cellular responses. Cells within a tissue recognize and specifically adhere to one another via cell surface structures. Certain cells such as T cells, B cells, and macrophages recognize one another and communicate differentiation signals at the cell surface (Figure 4–1a). In addition, small molecules or macromolecules can interact with cell-surface receptors to produce an appropriate cellular response, as in the stimulation of target cells by hormones, the triggering of lymphocyte differentiation by antigen (Figure 4–1c), and the initiation of action potentials at nerve synapses.

B.   The general structure of the plasma membrane is a mosaic of proteins in a lipid bilayer.

1.   By weight, 50–60% of the plasma membrane is protein and 30–40% is lipid. These categories include some glycoproteins and glycolipids, which carry covalently-linked carbohydrate side chains. The lipids are responsible for the sheetlike structure of

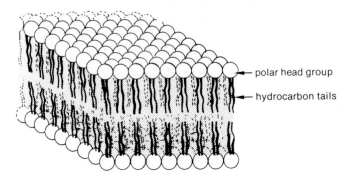

Figure 4-3 Diagram of a section of a bilayer membrane formed from phospholipid or glycolipid.

membranes and for their general properties as hydrophobic barriers, whereas the proteins mediate specific membrane functions.

2. The lipid and protein molecules of membranes have polar and nonpolar regions, that is, they are *amphipathic*. The lipids often are symbolized by a circle for the hydrophilic polar "head" of the molecule and a wavy line for the hydrophobic nonpolar hydrocarbon "tail." Such lipids can aggregate spontaneously in aqueous solution to form a bilayer, with the hydrophobic tails in the interior and the hydrophilic heads at the surface (Figure 4-3). Hydrophobic interactions of the tails are primarily responsible for the strong tendency toward bilayer formation. Because edges with exposed hydrocarbon chains are energetically unfavorable, bilayers tend to close upon themselves to form spherical vesicles. The proteins of membranes "float" in the lipid bilayer with their hydrophobic regions in the nonpolar interior and their hydrophilic regions exposed to the solvent (Figure 4-4).

3. The three major membrane lipids are phospholipids, glycolipids, and cholesterol. Phospholipids are derived from either of the two alcohols, glycerol or sphingosine, one or two fatty acids, and a phosphorylated alcohol (Figure 4-5). Phospholipids derived from glycerol are called phosphoglycerides. The hydroxyl groups at C1 and C2 of glycerol are esterified to the carboxyl groups of two fatty acids. The C3 hydroxyl group of the glycerol backbone is esterified to any one of several phosphorylated alcohols (Figure 4-6). For example, the phosphoglyceride with choline as the alcohol is *phosphatidyl choline*, a common membrane phospholipid. The only phospholipid not derived from glycerol is *sphingomyelin*, in which a hydroxyl group of sphingosine is esterified to choline (Figure 4-5). The fatty acid chains in

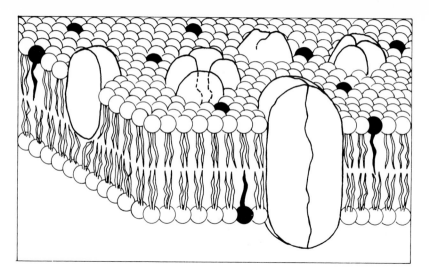

Figure 4–4 The fluid-mosaic model of membrane structure. Black lipid molecules represent glycolipids; large white inclusions are protein molecules "floating in the bilayer, with their hydrophobic regions in contacting lipid side chains and their hydrophilic regions exposed to the external medium." [Adapted from J. S. Singer in *Cell Membranes: Biochemistry, Cell Biology and Pathology*, G. Weissmann and R. Claiborne (Eds.), H. P. Publishing Co., Inc., New York, 1975, p. 35.]

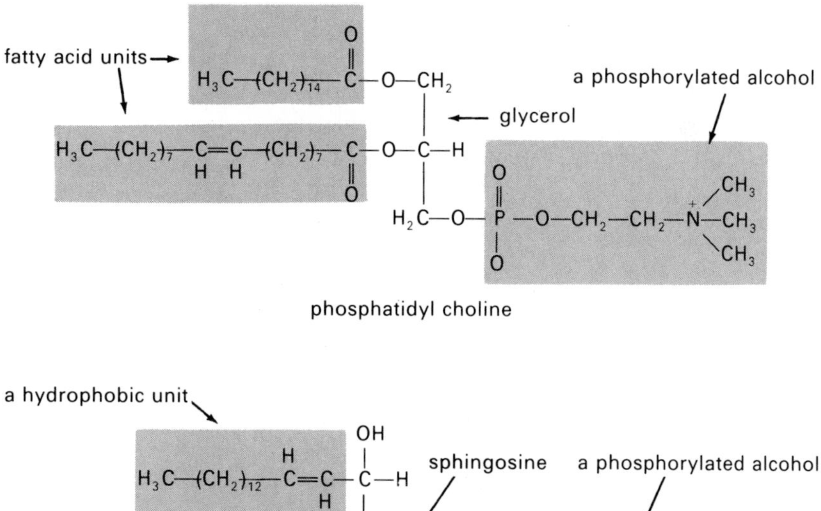

fatty acid units →

a phosphorylated alcohol

← glycerol

$$H_3C-(CH_2)_{14}-\overset{\overset{O}{\|}}{C}-O-CH_2$$

$$H_3C-(CH_2)_7-\underset{H}{C}=\underset{H}{C}-(CH_2)_7-\overset{\overset{}{}}{C}-O-\overset{}{C}-H$$

$$H_2C-O-\overset{\overset{O}{\|}}{\underset{O}{\underset{|}{P}}}-O-CH_2-CH_2-\overset{+}{N}{\overset{CH_3}{\underset{CH_3}{-}}}CH_3$$

phosphatidyl choline

a hydrophobic unit

sphingosine   a phosphorylated alcohol

$$H_3C-(CH_2)_{12}-\underset{H}{\overset{H}{C}}=C-\overset{\overset{OH}{|}}{C}-H$$

fatty acid unit →

$$R-\overset{\overset{}{}}{\underset{\overset{\|}{O}}{C}}-\underset{H}{N}-\overset{}{C}-H$$

$$H_2C-O-\overset{\overset{O}{\|}}{\underset{O^-}{\underset{|}{P}}}-O-CH_2-CH_2-\overset{+}{N}{\overset{CH_3}{\underset{CH_3}{-}}}CH_3$$

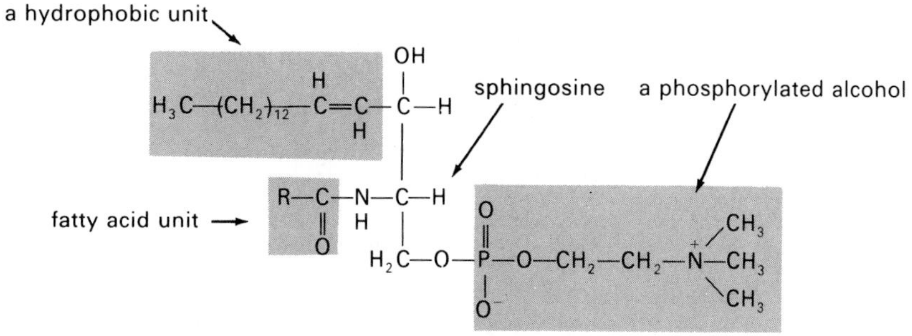

sphingomyelin

Figure 4–5 Two types of phospholipids (see text).

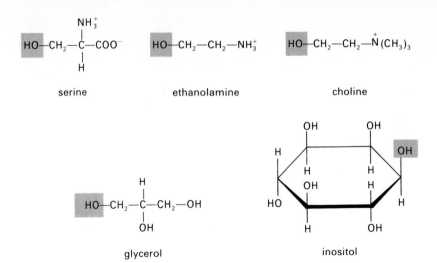

serine

ethanolamine

choline

glycerol

inositol

Figure 4–6 Alcohols commonly attached to phospholipids. The shaded hydroxyl group indicates the point of attachment.

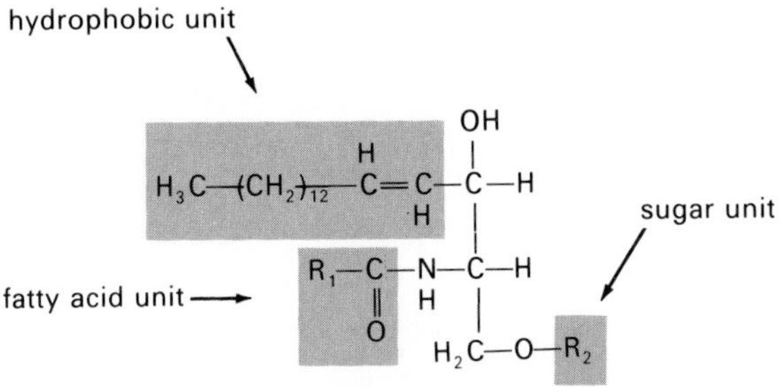

hydrophobic unit

sugar unit

fatty acid unit

Figure 4–7 The general structure of a glycolipid.

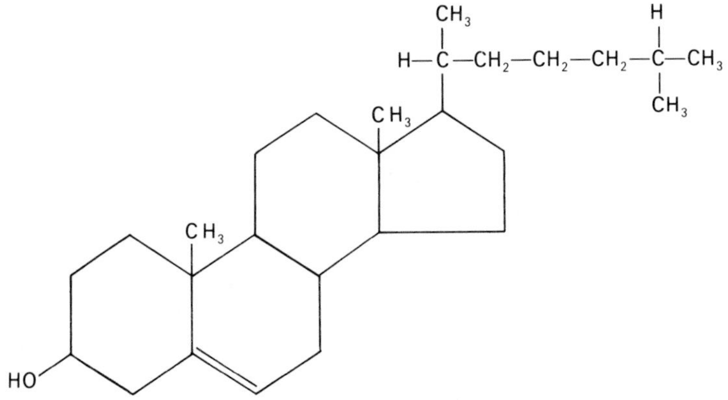

Figure 4–8 The structural formula of cholesterol.

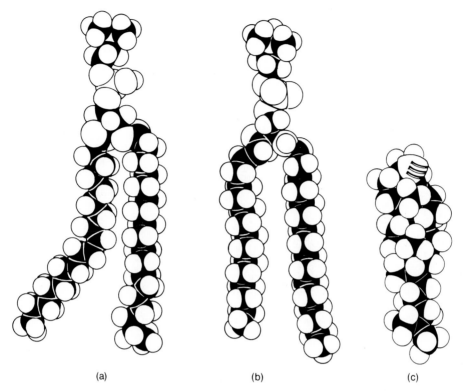

(a)   (b)   (c)

Figure 4–9 Space-filling models of (a) phosphatidyl choline, (b) sphingomyelin, and (c) cholesterol.

phospholipids usually contain between 14 and 24 carbon atoms and may be saturated or unsaturated. Double bonds are nearly always in the cis configuration, which produces a kink in the fatty acid chain.

Glycolipids are derived from sphingosine, a fatty acid unit, and a sugar unit (Figure 4–7). In glycolipids one or more sugars may be attached to the lipid moiety. Cholesterol, a steroid, is the biosynthetic precursor of bile acids and steroid hormones, as well as an important component of cells. The plasma membranes of certain cells are rich in cholesterol and its esters (Figure 4–8).

Membrane lipids are similar in three-dimensional configuration (Figure 4–9). The phosphatidyl choline molecule resembles a tuning fork with the fatty acid "prongs" pointing in one direction and the choline "handle" in the opposite direction. Its three dimensional shape is roughly that of a cylinder. Sphingomyelin, glycolipids, and cholesterol have similar cylindrical structures, with polar heads and nonpolar tails (Table 4–1).

Table 4–1
Hydrophobic and hydrophilic regions of membrane lipids

Membrane lipid	Hydrophobic region	Hydrophilic region
Phosphoglycerides	Fatty acid chains	Phosphorylated alcohol
Sphingomyelin	Fatty acid chain	Phosphoryl choline
	Hydrocarbon chain of sphingosine	
Glycolipid	Fatty acid chain	One or more sugar residues
	Hydrocarbon chain of sphingosine	
Cholesterol	Entire molecule except for OH group	OH group

4. Membrane fluidity is determined by several factors. The fatty acid chains of the lipid molecules in a bilayer can exist in an ordered crystalline state or in a relatively disordered fluid state. A transition from the frozen to the fluid state for a given membrane occurs at a characteristic temperature called the melting temperature. The melting temperature is determined by the degree of saturation and length of the fatty acid side chains, and by the amount of cholesterol in the membrane.

The crystalline state is favored by the presence of saturated fatty acid chains because their straight hydrocarbon tails can participate in van der Waals interactions with one another along the full length of contiguous chains (Figure 4–10a). As a corollary, longer hydrocarbon chains favor the crystalline state because they interact more strongly than shorter ones; each additional methylene group adds about 0.5 kcal/mole to the energy of interaction of adjacent chains (Figure 4–10c). Conversely, cis double bonds may lower the melting temperature, favoring the fluid state, because they cause kinks in the hydrocarbon chains which interfere with the packing of adjacent fatty acids (Figure 4–10b).

The presence of cholesterol in the bilayer has two effects on the fluidity. Cholesterol breaks up the orderly packing of fatty acid side chains and therefore lowers the melting temperature. Above the melting temperature, however, its rigidity decreases membrane fluidity.

Animals have the ability to adjust the melting temperature of their membrane lipids to the surrounding environmental temperatures. For example, Lapland reindeer have significantly more unsaturated fatty acids in the membranes of cells in their extremities than in those of their other body cells. Likewise, poikilothermic (cold blooded) animals increase the fraction of unsaturated

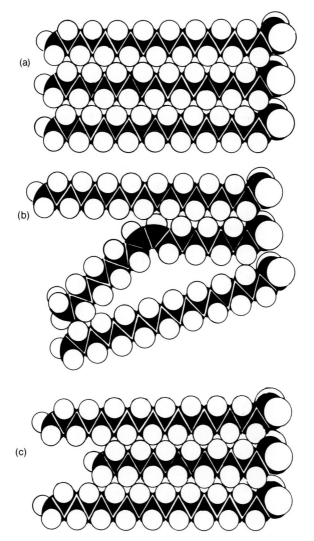

Figure 4–10 Space-filling models illustrating the packing of various fatty-acid chains. (a) Three molecules of a saturated C_{18} fatty acid. (b) An unsaturated C_{18} fatty acid with a single double bond between two saturated C_{18} fatty acids. (c) Two molecules of a saturated C_{18} fatty acid separated by a saturated C_{14} fatty acid.

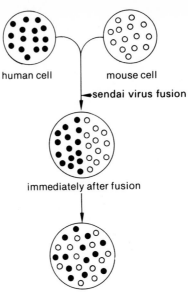

human cell   mouse cell

←sendai virus fusion

immediately after fusion

after 40 minutes at 37°C

Figure 4–11 A diagram showing the fusion of a mouse cell and a human cell followed by diffusion of membrane proteins in the plane of the plasma membrane. The human (●) and mouse (o) proteins are completely intermingled after forty minutes. [Adapted from L. Frye and M. Edidin, *J. Cell Sci.* **7**, 319 (1970).]

fatty acids in their membranes at colder temperatures. Such adjustments maintain the plasma membranes of cells in the fluid state.

5. In a fluid membrane both the lipid and protein components are capable of rapid rotational and translational diffusion in the plane of the membrane. Such diffusion is illustrated by interspecific cell-fusion experiments, in which the protein antigens of two cells can be shown to intermingle with one another rapidly following membrane fusion (Figure 4–11). Lipid components occasionally can undergo transverse (flip-flop) diffusion from one side of the membrane to the other, but the rate of flip-flop is 10^9 times slower than the rate of translational diffusion. Transverse diffusion of proteins presumably is even less frequent because of the high free energy required to transport a hydrophilic domain through the hydrophobic lipid bilayer.

6. Different plasma membranes differ in the types and the amounts of proteins present, corresponding presumably to the distinct functions that various plasma membranes perform. For example, the red blood cell, the lymphocyte, and the kidney tubule cell plasma membranes have quite distinct membrane-protein compositions. The molecular weights of membrane proteins vary from approximately 10,000 to several hundred thousand. A few membrane proteins are present in high concentrations

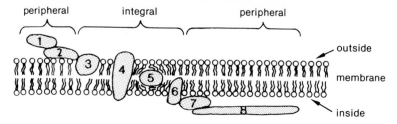

Figure 4–12 Possible locations of peripheral and integral membrane proteins.

of 10–50% of total membrane protein, but most are present at concentrations of only a fraction of a percent.

7.   Membrane proteins can be classed in two distinct groups, designated *integral* and *peripheral,* which are distinguished by the nature of their association with the lipid bilayer. Integral proteins are characterized by resistance to isolation from the membrane; hydrophobic bond-breaking agents such as detergents and organic solvents are required to dissociate them from the bilayer. By contrast, peripheral proteins can be dissociated from the bilayer by mild techniques such as changing the ionic concentration of the medium or adding a chelating agent such as ethylenediaminetetracetate (EDTA). Thus integral proteins probably interact directly with the membrane lipids, whereas peripheral proteins appear to be attached primarily to the polar surfaces of the bilayer (Figure 4–12). It is difficult to define the set of peripheral proteins precisely, because many of them may be attached so loosely that they are lost during membrane isolation.

8.   Integral membrane proteins, like membrane lipids, have an amphipathic structure that permits them to associate simultaneously with hydrophobic membrane lipids and the hydrophilic external environment (Figure 4–13). In theory, an integral protein

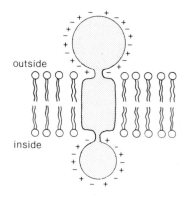

Figure 4–13   A model of an ampnipathic membrane protein. [Adapted from J. S. Singer in *Structure and Function of Biological Membranes,* L. I. Rothfield (Ed.), Academic Press, New York, 1971, p. 145.]

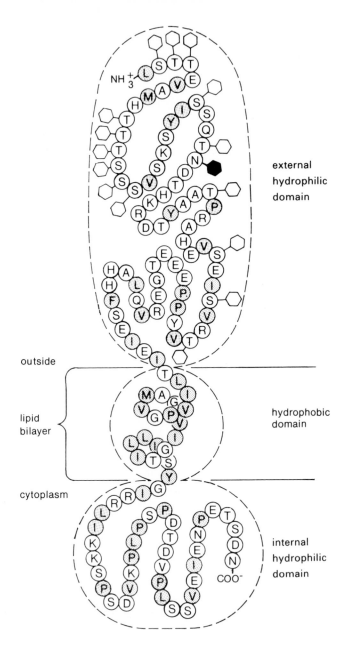

Figure 4–14 A diagrammatic representation of the three domains of glycophorin, an integral amphipathic membrane protein of the red blood cell. The single-letter designations for amino acid residues are as listed in Table 3–1. Hydrophobic residues are stippled to show their distribution more clearly. Hexagons attached to certain amino acids indicate attached carbohydrate groups.

309

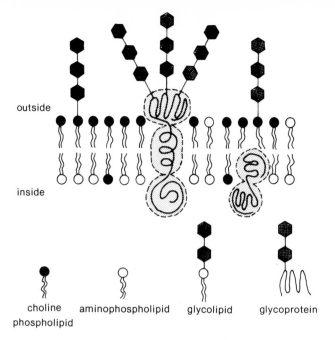

Figure 4–15 Three types of asymmetries found in the red blood cell membrane. (1) Glycolipids and glycoproteins are found only on the outer surface. (2) Choline phospholipids (phosphatidylcholine and sphingomyelin) predominate in the outer monolayer, whereas amino phospholipids (phosphatidylethanolamine and phosphatidylserine) predominate in the inner monolayer. (3) The integral membrane proteins are themselves asymmetrically distributed.

may be positioned in several different ways relative to the lipid bilayer (Figure 4–12, types 3–6). In the red blood cell membrane, which is the best studied plasma membrane of eucaryotic cells, the majority of the seven or eight major integral proteins are of Type 6, whereas two are of Type 4. No integral proteins of Type 3 or 5 have been identified yet in red blood cells. The best studied integral membrane protein is glycophorin, a red blood cell protein of Type 4. Its polypeptide chain of 131 amino acid residues is divided into three distinct domains. External and internal hydrophilic domains are separated by a membrane-associated hydrophobic domain (Figure 4–14). The N-terminal portion of the molecule forms the external domain, the middle forms the hydrophobic membrane domain, and the C-terminal portion forms the internal domain. Thus the glycophorin molecule is linearly amphipathic. It will be interesting to determine whether this arrangement is general for integral membrane proteins.

9. All plasma membranes probably are asymmetric in the sense that their inner and outer surfaces are different. The red blood cell membrane exhibits asymmetry in all of its major components: phospholipids, proteins, and carbohydrates (Figure 4–15). Choline phospholipids predominate in the outer half of the lipid bilayer, whereas amino phospholipids predominate in the inner half. The integral membrane proteins are asymmetrically inserted; for example, all of the glycophorin molecules are oriented with their N-terminal polar domains to the outside. Glycolipids and gly-coproteins are found only on the external membrane surface. Presumably, similar asymmetries will be found in other plasma membranes in keeping with the different functions of the inner and outer surfaces.

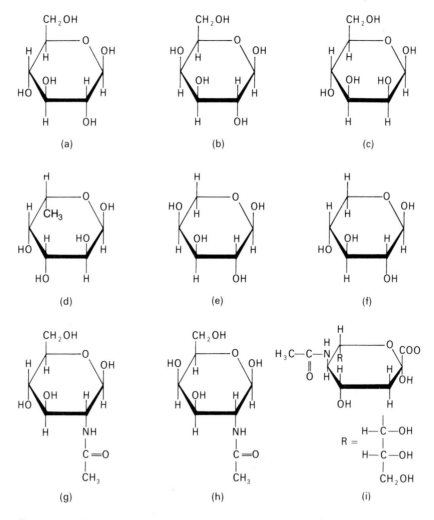

Figure 4–16 The nine sugars from which membrane oligosaccharides are constructed. (a) D-glucose (Glc); (b) D-galactose (Gal); (c) D-mannose (Man); (d) L-fucose (Fuc); (e) L-arabinose (Ara); (f) D-xylose (Xyl); (g) N-acetyl-D-glucosamine (GlcNAc); (h) N-acetyl-D-galactosamine (GalNAc); and (i) N-acetylneuraminic acid, or sialic acid (NANA).

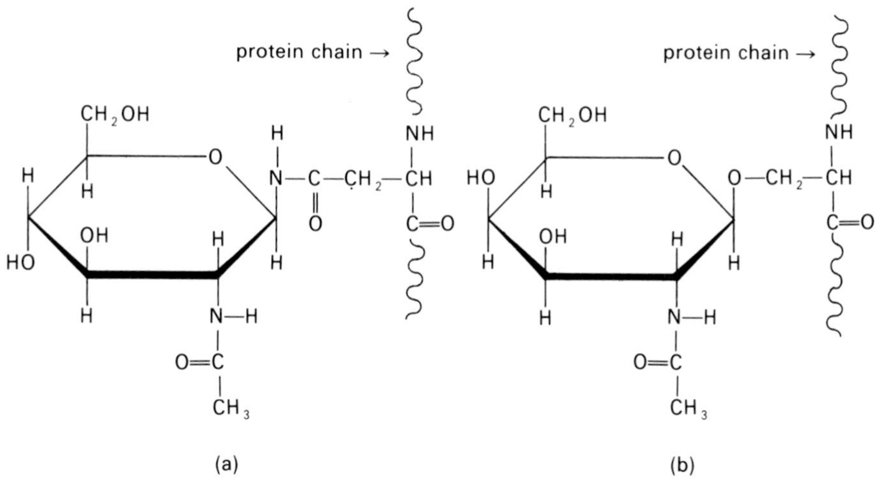

Figure 4–17 Two types of carbohydrate linkages to glycoproteins. (a) N-glycosidic linkage of N-acetylglucosamine to asparagine. (b) O-glycosidic linkage of N-acetylgalactosamine to serine.

4-2   Oligosaccharides are attached to glycoproteins and glycolipids on the external side of the plasma membrane

A.   Glycophorin, a typical membrane glycoprotein, is 60% carbohydrate by weight (Figure 4–14). The carbohydrates of membrane glycoproteins and glycolipids are oligosaccharides composed of two to fifteen monosaccharides each.

1.   Membrane oligosaccharides are constructed from only nine different components (Figure 4–16). Six of these components are simple sugars: four six-carbon sugars, fucose, glucose, galactose, and mannose, and two five-carbon sugars, arabinose and xylose. Two of the components are amino sugars, glucosamine and galactosamine, which carry an acetyl amino group. The remaining component is N-acetyl-neuraminic acid, also called sialic acid. This component is the most complex of the membrane sugars and provides most membranes with the bulk of their negative charge.

2.   Five sugars are involved in attaching oligosaccharides to glycoproteins through five different amino acids and two different types of bonds (Figure 4–17 and Table 4–2). Apart from N-acetylgalactosamine, each sugar can join with just a single amino acid. A glycoprotein can have many points of oligosaccharide attachment, and generally the carbohydrate groups attached to the same amino acid residue are identical. For example, glycophorin has 15 oligosaccharides attached through O-glycosidic

Table 4–2
Types of glycoprotein and oligosaccharide linkages

Sugar	Amino acid	Type of linkage
N-Acetylglucosamine	Asparagine	N-Glycosidic
Xylose	Serine	O-Glycosidic
N-Acetylgalactosamine	Threonine or serine	O-Glycosidic
Galactose	Hydroxylysine	O-Glycosidic
Arabinose	Hydroxyproline	O-Glycosidic

bonds to serine or threonine, and a sixteenth oligosaccharide attached to asparagine (Figure 4–14). Glycolipids have a single oligosaccharide moiety linked to a sphingosine backbone (Figure 4–7).

B. The biosynthesis of oligosaccharide units in glycoproteins and glycolipids probably occurs in the Golgi apparatus and requires three steps (Figure 4–18). These are the synthesis of monosaccharides from glucose, their activation by conversion to nucleotide derivatives, and their linkage onto the oligosaccharide chain.

1. Three features are of particular interest in the biosynthesis of glycoproteins. First, oligosaccharides are not synthesized by a template mechanism as are proteins and nucleic acids. Instead, oligosaccharides are built up by a series of enzymatic reactions in which individual glycosyltransferases add carbohydrate monomers to specific substrates (Figure 4–19). Second, oligosaccharide chains generally are synthesized by adding monosaccharides to the nonreducing ends or branch points of growing oligosaccharide chains. Third, multiglycosyltransferase systems govern the synthesis of individual oligosaccharide chains, as illustrated in Figure 4–19.

2. In a multiglycosyltransferase system, each transferase is specific for the sugar to be added and for one particular amino acid or oligosaccharide acceptor sequence. Thus oligosaccharide assembly proceeds in a stepwise fashion, beginning with the attachment of the first sugar to the protein. A different transferase catalyzes each step of chain elongation, and each transferase is able to catalyze its reaction only when the preceding steps of synthesis have occurred. For example, when a galactose unit appears more than once in the final product, as in Steps 2 and 3 in Figure 4–19, distinct transferases are required for each step.

3. The genetic information for the synthesis of a particular oligosaccharide chain is expressed as a multiglycosyltransferase system. Consequently, if a particular transferase gene is not

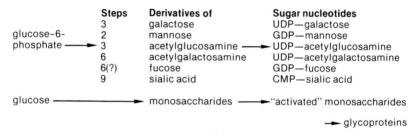

glucose-6-phosphate →	Steps	Derivatives of	Sugar nucleotides
	3	galactose	UDP—galactose
	2	mannose	GDP—mannose
	3	acetylglucosamine →	UDP—acetylglucosamine
	6	acetylgalactosamine	UDP—acetylgalactosamine
	6(?)	fucose	GDP—fucose
	9	sialic acid	CMP—sialic acid

glucose ————————→ monosaccharides ———→ "activated" monosaccharides

———→ glycoproteins

Figure 4–18 Biosynthesis of oligosaccharide units in glycoproteins and glycolipids. The overall process consists of three stages: (a) the synthesis of monosaccharides from glucose, where the number of enzymatic reactions is indicated under "steps"; (b) activation of the monosaccharides by conversion to the corresponding nucleotide derivatives (some of the monosaccharides are formed as sugar-nucleotides); (c) polymerization of monosaccharides, or incorporation into complex carbohydrates. [Adapted from S. Roseman, *Chem. Phys. Lipids* **5,** 270 (1970).]

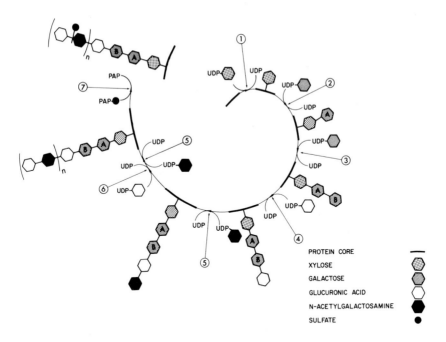

Figure 4–19 Biosynthesis of the glycoprotein chondroitin-4-sulfate. Numbers 1 through 7 refer to the enzymes that catalyze the various steps: (1) xylose transferase; (2) galactose transferase 1; (3) galactose transferase 2; (4) glucuronic acid transferase 1; (5) *N*-acetyl-D-galactosamine transferase; (6) glucuronic acid transferase 2; (7) sulfotransferase. UDP is uridine diphosphate. PAP designates the sulfate donor 3-phosphoadenosine 5'-phosphosulfate. [Courtesy of A. Dorfman.]

expressed (such as the galactose transferase 2 in Figure 4–19), the oligosaccharide chain will terminate at that point.

The sequence of saccharides on a particular protein in a cell is determined by the set of glycosyltransferases that is expressed by that cell. If compartmentalization of glycosylation does not occur within that cell, the same sequence of saccharides will be attached to each protein that has the appropriate recognition site for the first glycosyltransferase.

4. The optimal pH, sugar–nucleotide concentrations, and other cofactor requirements vary markedly for different transferases. Consequently, under physiological conditions, there is variable completion and therefore considerable heterogeneity among oligosaccharide chains.

C. Oligosaccharides are capable of greater sequence diversity than proteins. Multiglycosyltransferases of different specificities can join

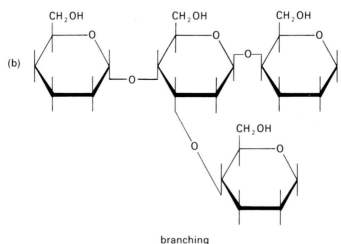

Figure 4–20 Two ways of generating oligosaccharide diversity not available to proteins and nucleic acids: (a) α or β linkages; (b) branching.

the nine basic subunits together in many different combinations. Moreover, sugars can form α or β linkages through any of their hydroxyl groups, so that an enormous number of continuous-chain and branched oligosaccharide structures is possible (Figure 4–20). To illustrate the combinatorial effects of these properties on oligosaccharide diversity, there are about 10^{24} possible structures for a 12-residue oligosaccharide of three mannose, three N-acetylglucosamine, three galactose, and three sialic acid residues. Even if one particular sequence of these residues is specified, the number of possible isomers still is approximately 6 × 10^6.

D.   Lectins are plant proteins or glycoproteins that bind to various sugars and sugar residues in oligosaccharides. The remarkable specificity of lectins has made them useful in studying the architecture of the cell surface. Moreover, recent studies with cellular slime molds (Essential Concept 4–8) suggest that lectinlike molecules may play a fundamental role in cell–cell recognition. Table 4–3 gives the specificities, sources, and molecular weights of some commonly used lectins.

Table 4–3
Properties of some commonly used lectins

Lectin	Source	Approximate molecular weight	Saccharide specificity[a]
Abrin	*Abrus precatorius*	134,000	D-Gal
Concanavalin A (Con A)	*Canavalia einsformis* (Jack bean)	55,000	α-D-Man, α-D-Glc
DBA	*Dolichos biflorus*	135,000	α-D-GalNAc
Soy bean agglutinin (SBA)	*Glycine max* (soybean)	110,000	D-GalNAc, D-Gal
Lentil lectins (LCA)	*Lens culinaris* (lentil)	42,000–60,000	α-D-Man, α-D-Glc
LP	*Limulus polyphemus*	400,000	sialic acid
Lima bean agglutinins	*Phaseolus limensis*	270,000	D-GlcNAc, D-Man
Phytohemagglutinin (PHA)	*Phaseolus vulgaris* (red kidney bean)	140,000	D-GalNAc
Pokeweed mitogen (PWM)	*Phytolacca americana*	32,000	
RCA$_I$	*Ricinus communis* (castor bean)	60,000–120,000	β-D-Gal
RCA$_{II}$ ricin			D-Gal, D-GalNAc
Wheat germ agglutinin (WGA)	*Triticum vulgaris* (wheat germ)	23,000	(D-GlcNAc)$_2$, sialic acid

[a]See legend to Figure 4–16 for saccharide names.
[Condensed from G. L. Nicolson, *Int. Rev. Cytol.* **39**, 89, 1974.]

E.   The human blood-group substances, also called the ABO and Lewis antigens, are cell-surface oligosaccharides whose genetics and chemistry are better understood than those of any other cell-surface carbohydrate system. These blood-group oligosaccharides are attached to glycolipids in the plasma membranes of red blood cells and other human cells. In addition, they may be attached to soluble glycoproteins that are found in secretions such as saliva, tears, and gastric juice. Large quantities of soluble glycoproteins that exhibit blood-group specificities can be obtained from certain individuals with ovarian cysts or tumors. These glycoproteins contain 85% by weight of carbohydrate in the form of multiple short oligosaccharides attached to a polypeptide backbone (e.g., see Figure 4–14).

1.   Five distinct blood-group specificities related to the ABO and Lewis systems can be detected by "natural" antibodies present in humans who lack the corresponding cell-surface antigens. These specificities are designated A, B, H(O), Le^a (Lewis a), and Le^b (Lewis b). Antibodies that react with four of these specificities can be inhibited by prior reaction with the corresponding monosaccharide (Table 4–4).

All natural antibodies to these blood-group antigens are IgM immunoglobulins. Because they are specific for relatively common saccharides, it is believed that these antibodies are induced by environmental polysaccharide antigens, which would explain both their ubiquitous presence and their IgM (thymus-independent) nature. These natural antibodies are absent only from individuals with congenital or acquired agammaglobulinemia (Essential Concept 2–5), and are therefore useful in the diagnosis of these disorders. The relationships among ABO phenotypes, genotypes, and natural serum antibodies are given in Table 4–5.

2.   Three genetically unlinked but functionally related gene systems, designated ABO, Hh, and Lewis, code for glycosyltransferases that determine the structure of blood-group oligosaccharides for the ABO and Lewis systems (Table 4–6). Each of these glycosyltransferases operates on two closely related oligosaccharides, which are the precursors to the blood-group substances (Figure 4–21). The synthetic pathways of the various blood-group oligosaccharides are given in Figure 4–22.

3.   The multiple precursor oligosaccharides on a single polypeptide backbone are modified to differing extents by the transferase genes. For example, in an individual with A, B, H and Le genes, the A, B, H, Le^b and even Le^a specificities can be detected on the same glycoprotein molecule. Because the glycosyltransferase systems are not very efficient, carbohydrate chains are completed to varying extents on the same glycoprotein backbone. Accordingly, some oligosaccharide chains are finished to the

Table 4–4

Monosaccharides that inhibit antibodies to specific blood-group substances[a]

	Blood-group specificity	Inhibiting monosaccharide
	A	N-Acetyl-D-galactosamine
	B	D-Galactose
	H	L-Fucose
	Le[a]	N-Acetyl-D-glucosamine

[a]See Figure 4–16.

Table 4–5

Relation between genotype, red blood cell antigens, and serum antibodies in the ABO blood-group system

Group (phenotype)	Genotype	Antigen on red cell	Antibodies in serum
A	AA AO	A	anti-B
B	BB BO	B	anti-A
AB	AB	AB	neither anti-A nor anti-B
O	OO	—	anti-A and anti-B

Table 4–6

Gene systems, alleles, and gene products responsible for the ABH and Lewis specificities

Gene system	Alleles	Gene product
ABO	A B O	N-Acetyl-D-galactosamine transferase D-galactosyl transferase No functional gene product
Hh	H h	L-fucosyl transferase No functional gene product
Lewis	Le le	L-fucosyl transferase No functional gene product

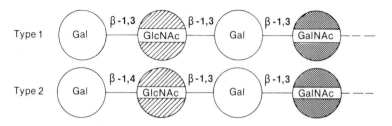

Figure 4–21 Two types of precursor oligosaccharides for the ABO and Lewis blood-group substances. Gal, D-galactose; GlcNAc, N-acetyl-D-glucosamine; GalNAc, N-acetyl-D-galactosamine.

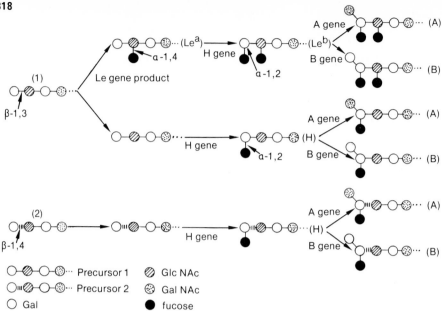

Figure 4–22 Pathways for the synthesis of the ABO-Lewis blood-group substances. (1) and (2) indicate the precursor oligosaccharides (see Figure 4–21). The blood-group specificities detectable at each step are indicated in parentheses. UDP is uridinediphosphate; GDP is guanosinediphosphate; β-1,3, β-1,4, α-1,4, and α1,2 indicate linkages between adjacent sugar residues. Gal, galactose; GlcNAc, N-acetyl-D-glucosamine; GalNAc, N-acetyl-D-galactosamine.

extent of expressing the Le^a specificity, others to the extent of expressing the H specificity, and so on (Figure 4–22). Thus the normal process of synthesis generates a family of closely related glycoproteins (or glycolipids). As indicated in Table 4–6, the transferase alleles O, h, and le represent lack of the corresponding enzyme functions. Consequently, when these alleles are present in the homozygous state, oligosaccharide synthesis is blocked at specific sites of monosaccharide addition.

4. An additional gene, secretor (Se), plays a different role in determining the expression of blood-group specificities. The effects of this gene indicate that there are two distinct systems for the synthesis of blood-group substances. The soluble blood-group substances attached to glycoproteins and found in various body secretions are produced by the *secretory blood-group system.* The insoluble blood-group substances, attached to glycolipids and found on certain plasma membranes such as those of the red blood cells, are produced by the *membrane blood-group system.* The secretor gene, in its homozygous (Se/Se) or heterozygous (Se/se) state, allows blood-group substances to be secreted in the soluble system. An individual homozygous for the recessive form of this gene (se/se) is termed a nonsecretor, and has no A, B, or H specificities in his secretions, although these specificities are expressed on his red blood cells. It appears that the se/se genotype leads to lack of H gene activity in the secretory system.

The Le glycosyltransferase acts only in the secretory system. The resulting glycoproteins are adsorbed from the serum onto the red blood cell membrane to confer the Le specificity on these cells. Most of the structural studies just described have been carried out on glycoproteins obtained from various secretions. More recent studies on glycolipids from the red blood cell membrane suggest that the oligosaccharides responsible for the membrane ABO specificities are identical to those found in secretions.

5. The ABO–Lewis blood-group systems demonstrate that a relatively limited number of glycosyltransferases can generate a variety of different genetically controlled oligosaccharides. The function of the blood-group antigens still is unknown; individuals who are homozygous for the alleles O, h, le, and se do not appear to suffer ill effects from their lack of the corresponding enzymes. However, these antigens do exhibit the diversity and genetic regulation that are fundamental requirements for any cell-surface recognition system.

4-3   Membrane biosynthesis, budding, and fusion are still poorly understood

A.   Membrane components are in a constant state of turnover. The half-life of lipids in the membrane may be on the order of minutes, whereas the proteins have half-lives ranging from hours to days.

Membrane biosynthesis is still poorly understood. It is likely, however, that most membrane components are synthesized and inserted into a lipid bilayer in the endoplasmic reticulum. This system gives rise to the membranous vesicles of the Golgi apparatus, where oligosaccharides become attached to sites on inner vesicle surfaces to form glycoproteins and glycolipids. Vesicles from the Golgi then are transported to the cell boundary, where they fuse with the plasma membrane in such a way that their inner glycosylated surface becomes continuous with the outer surface of the cell. The means by which the asymmetric arrangements of lipids are generated and the mechanism by which integral proteins are inserted in the correct orientation into the bilayer are unclear. Factors that control the rates of turnover of the various membrane components also are poorly understood.

B.   Membrane budding and fusion are fundamental aspects of plasma membrane physiology (Figure 4–23). Besides playing a role in membrane

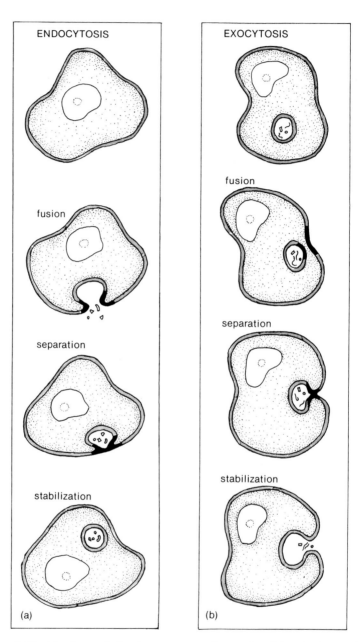

Figure 4–23 Membrane fusion in processes of normal cellular physiology. Shaded portions of membranes denote sites of membrane fusion. [Adapted from J. A. Lucy in

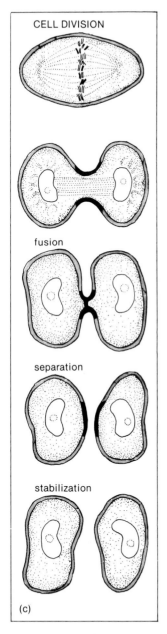

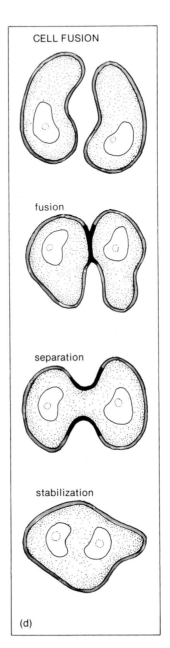

Cell Membranes: Biochemistry, Cell Biology and Pathology, G. Weissmann and R. Claiborne (Eds.), H. P. Publishing Co., Inc., New York, 1975, p. 75.]

turnover, budding and fusion also are important in many normal processes that increase or decrease the number of membrane-bounded compartments in a cell or tissue. Exocytosis and endocytosis involve vesicle fusion with and budding off from the plasma membrane, respectively (Figure 4–23a and b). Cell division requires one plasma membrane-bounded compartment to bud into two (Figure 4–23c). Reproduction requires the fusion of sperm and egg membrane (Figure 4–23d). During embryonic development, somatic cells can fuse to form syncytial tissues, as in the fusion of myoblasts to form myotubules in muscle development, and the fusion of osteoblasts in vertebrate bone development.

C.   Membrane fusion is involved in the phagocytic response of macrophages to foreign antigens. In addition, experimentally-induced cell fusion has become an important technique for research in cell physiology and somatic-cell genetics.

1.   In two steps the macrophages of the immune system phagocytose antigens that have been coated with antibodies. First, Fc or C3b receptors on a small area of the macrophage cell surface interact with their corresponding ligands, the Fc region of antibody or the C3b component of complement on the antigen surface. Then the remaining Fc or C3b receptors on the macrophage interact with their corresponding ligands by extension of membrane leaflets over the antigen surface to initiate a zippering process that results in membrane fusion on the opposite side, forming a phagosome (Figure 4–24). Receptor–ligand binding in this system leads to a highly local phagocytic response; antigens that have been bound experimentally by lectins to other regions of the macrophage membrane at the same time are not phagocytosed (Figure 4–25).

2.   Certain viruses such as *Sendai* can promote cell fusion by binding to the plasma membrane (see Figure 4–11). This process has been a useful tool for somatic-cell genetics. In the presence of Ca^{2+}, agents that increase membrane fluidity, such as unsaturated or short-chain fatty acids and increased temperature, also promote cell fusion. However, the molecular mechanisms of cell fusion are not yet understood.

4-4   Membranes appear to be associated with a filamentous cellular cytoskeleton

A.   Beneath the plasma membrane, eucaryotic cells have a cytoskeleton that consists of three types of filamentous structures: microtubules, microfilaments and 10-nm filaments (Figure 4–26). These filaments are responsible for a variety of cellular functions. To carry out these

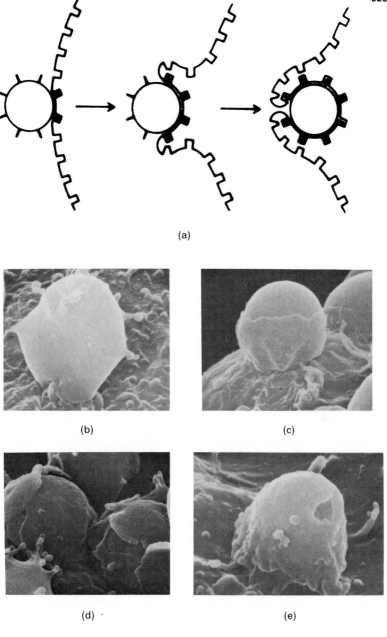

(a)

(b)

(c)

(d)

(e)

Figure 4–24 The formation of a phagosome in a macrophage interacting with IgG-coated red blood cells via the Fc receptor on the macrophage plasma membrane. (a) Attachment, engulfment, and membrane zippering, leading to formation of the phagosome. Symbols: O, red blood cell; –, IgG, ⊔, Fc receptor. [Adapted from F. M. Griffin, Jr., J. A. Griffin, J. E. Leider, and S. C. Silverstein, *J. Exp. Med.* **142,** 1263 (1975).] (b)–(e) Sequential scanning electron micrographs of the zippering of macrophage membrane leaflets around IgG-coated red blood cells. [Electron micrographs courtesy of J. Orenstein and E. Shelton.]

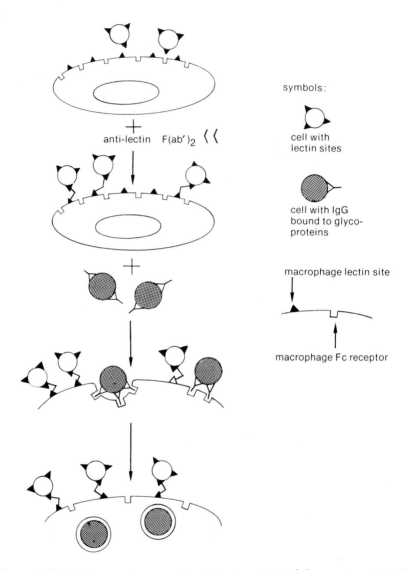

symbols:

cell with
lectin sites

cell with IgG
bound to glyco-
proteins

macrophage lectin site

macrophage Fc receptor

Figure 4–25 A diagram of an experiment to show that IgG-Fc receptor-mediated phagocytosis is a local, segmental response on the macrophage membrane. Macrophages bearing lectin-binding sites and Fc receptors are bound to target red blood cells either via Fc receptors or via lectin cross-linking. Only Fc-receptor binding triggers phagocytosis, and only membrane areas with IgG-coated red blood cells participate in the formation of a phagosome. Red blood cells bound by lectin cross-links stay on the macrophage surface.

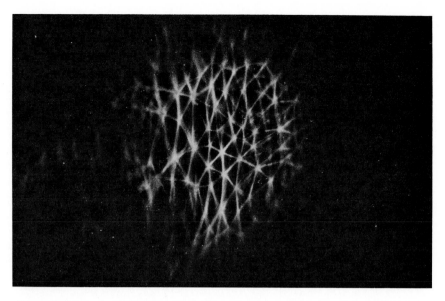

Figure 4–26 Actin filaments in rat embryo cells visualized by the fluorescent antibody technique. The embryo cells are separated from one another by treatment with the proteolytic enzyme trypsin. The cells are then fixed and stained after attachment to glass slides. [Courtesy of E. Lazarides.]

functions, elements of the cytoskeleton presumably must interact directly or indirectly with the cell membrane (Figure 4–26).

1. Microfilaments are found as networks or bundles in an ill-defined region called the cell cortex, just beneath the plasma membrane. These bundles appear to be aggregates of filamentous actin, myosin, and tropomyosin (Figure 4–27). They are connected through foci that contain actin and another muscle protein, α-actinin, to form a polygonal lattice around the cell interior. Microfilaments have been implicated in a variety of cellular functions including motility, exocytosis, membrane ruffling, formation of the mitotic contractile ring that separates two anaphase cells during division, and the maintenance of cell shape.

2. Microtubules effect shape changes in some cells by poly-merization and depolymerization, and they may serve as static tracks along which other elements move through the cytoplasm. However, tubulin, the subunit of microtubules, does not appear to be associated directly with membranes.

3. The 10-nm filaments are composed of a protein called desmin. This protein also is found as a structural component of muscle, where it may serve to link myofilaments at their Z lines to the

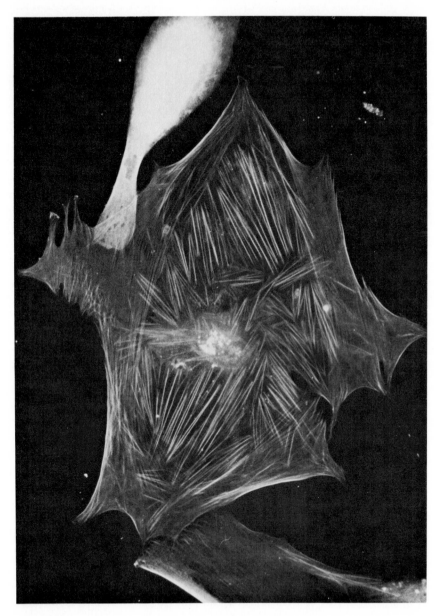

Figure 4–27 Actin filaments of a mouse fibroblast visualized by the fluorescent antibody technique. [Courtesy of E. Lazarides.]

plasma membranes of muscle cells. Little is known about the functions of 10-nm filaments, but it appears likely that they do interact directly with components of the plasma membrane.

B.   The cytoskeleton may interact with integral membrane proteins to alter their mobility.

    1.   Spectrin is a protein of approximately 200,000 molecular weight that is found associated with the inner surface of the plasma membrane in red blood cells. According to the scheme in Figure 4–12, spectrin is a Type 8 protein. It is rodlike and tends to aggregate in solution, but appears to be distinct from myosin. A similar protein, designated filamin, has been found in smooth muscle and in association with the plasma membranes of other nonmuscle cells. Spectrin appears to interact with various integral membrane proteins to reduce their mobility. Thus spectrin filaments may provide mechanical support for the red blood cell membrane by linking together integral membrane proteins (Figure 4–28).

    2.   The plant lectin, concanavalin A, does not bind directly to receptor immunoglobulins. However, binding of concanavalin A to the cell surface inhibits the capping and endocytosis of receptor immunoglobulins. This inhibition can be reversed by the addition of colchicine, a drug that depolymerizes microtubules. The

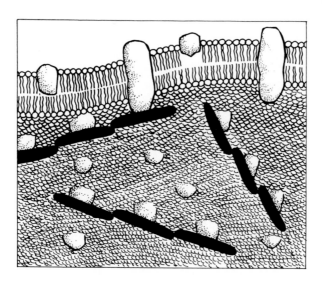

Figure 4–28   A possible mode of interaction of spectrin (dark rods) with integral membrane proteins of the human red blood cell. [Adapted from J. S. Singer in *Cell Membranes: Biochemistry, Cell Biology and Pathology*, G. Weissmann and R. Clairborne [Eds.], H. P. Publishing Co., Inc., New York, 1975, p. 35.]

inhibition of capping also is achieved if concanavalin A is applied to only a small portion of the cell surface. While the molecular mechanisms involved in these effects are not known, it is apparent that concanavalin A attaching to a small fraction of its binding sites on a B cell somehow restricts the mobility of the receptor immunoglobulins and perhaps of other integral membrane proteins in the membrane. The finding that colchicine reverses this effect suggests that microtubules may be involved, although the drug effects of colchicine are complex.

4-5   Cell-surface receptor molecules share a number of general properties

A.   Responses to the many extracellular signals that coordinate metazoan growth and development begin at the cell surface. Hormones, drugs, neurotransmitters, and antigens are some examples of such extracellular signals. The cell-surface receptor molecules that recognize these signals must be highly specific, because a given stimulus usually triggers only a highly selective cellular response. In addition, these molecules must be as diverse as the population of external signals to be received. This dual requirement for specificity and diversity argues strongly that cell-surface receptor molecules must be proteins.

B.   Receptor proteins must transduce information from the external environment into meaningful intracellular signals. To do so, these molecules must carry out three distinct functions: recognition of a specific external stimulus, transduction of a signal across the plasma membrane, and initiation of a response inside the cell (Figure 4–29). Although few receptor proteins have been characterized at the molecular level, we can make several reasonable assumptions about their common properties. It is likely that these proteins span the membrane, and thus belong to the class of integral membrane proteins. In addition, by analogy with immunoglobulins, it is likely that receptor proteins have discrete domains which perform the three receptor functions, according to the following model (Figure 4–29).

   1.   Specific interaction of the recognition domain with external stimuli in the form of molecular ligands involves the usual molecular complementarity typical of enzyme–substrate and antigen–antibody reactions.

   2.   Transduction of the external binding signal across the membrane probably involves conformational changes in the transducer domain, which could occur by one of two general mechanisms (Figure 4–30). Ligand binding could cause either changes in individual receptor molecules, or aggregation of identical membrane receptors, whose interaction with each other could induce conformational changes.

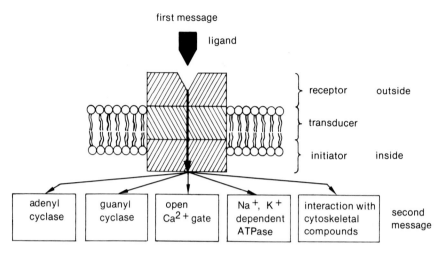

Figure 4–29 A model of cell-surface receptor and its three primary functions— specific reception of a first (external) message, transduction of this signal, and initiation of a second (internal) message. The second message acts through one of a relatively limited number of effector mechanisms to initate the appropriate cellular response. [Adapted from M. F. Greaves in *Cellular Recognition,* Chapman and Hall, Ltd., London, 1975, p. 11.]

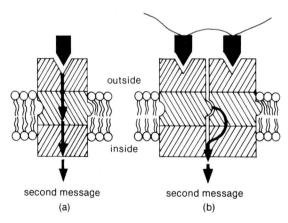

Figure 4–30. Two models for the transduction of external signals through membrane receptors. (a) Direct conformational alteration of a monomer by ligand binding. (b) Conformational change in transducer regions initiated by aggregation of identical membrane receptors.

3. The initiator functions of receptor proteins can act on any of a number of intracellular effector pathways. The possibilities include direct interaction with the cytoskeletal system to initiate or terminate movement, opening or closing of specific ion gates, activation or deactivation of specific ion pumps, and activation of nucleotide cyclases to produce the "second messengers," cyclic AMP or cyclic GMP, which in turn modulate the activities of soluble enzymatic or regulatory proteins.

4-6   Immunoglobulins are the most thoroughly characterized cell-surface receptors

A.   The receptor immunoglobulin molecules associated with the plasma membrane of a given lymphocyte appear to be very similar, if not identical, to the specific antibodies secreted by the same cell or its clonal descendants. The number of receptor immunoglobulins on a lymphocyte has been estimated to be between 5×10^4 and 2×10^5 molecules.

1.   Immunoglobulins M, D, G, and A have been identified by immunofluorescence as cell-surface receptors on lymphocyte membranes. Most lymphocytes appear to have receptor IgM and/or IgD immunoglobulins. These molecules appear to be integral membrane proteins, in that they can be isolated from lymphocyte membranes only by strong detergents. The C-terminal domain of the heavy chain appears to be anchored to the membrane, because antibodies specific to the C_H2 domain of the IgG molecule react with membrane bound IgG, whereas antibodies specific for the C_H3 domain do not (see Figure 3–13).

2.   Antisera directed against the idiotype, allotype, and isotype of the secreted immunoglobulin from individual clones of lymphocytes also react with the corresponding membrane-bound immunoglobulins. These observations suggest that the V domains as well as the C domains of secreted and membrane-bound immunoglobulins from a given lymphocyte are very similar, if not identical.

3.   Using detergents, monomeric IgM, IgD, and IgG have been isolated from lymphocyte membranes. The sizes of the light and heavy chains appear to be very similar in the membrane-bound and secreted molecules. So far there is insufficient evidence to distinguish among the following four possibilities regarding the relationship between the C_H regions of membrane-bound and soluble antibody: the C_H regions could be identical; they could differ only in their attached carbohydrate groups; they could be different in amino acid sequence, although related; or they could be identical except for a hydrophobic polypeptide belt attached to the terminal C_H homology unit.

4. Proof that membrane-bound immunoglobulins are the receptors for antigen is still somewhat indirect. Anti-immunoglobulins block antigen binding to lymphocytes. Antigen receptors and cell-surface immunoglobulin molecules can be induced to cap together (cocap) by the addition of antigen (Essential Concept 1–6C). This observation implies that cell-surface immunoglobulins and antigen receptors are identical or associated with one another. Finally, when radiolabeled Dnp–hemocyanin is bound to specific lymphocytes and incubated *in vitro,* the labeled complexes that are shed into the tissue culture medium can be precipitated equally well by antibodies to Dnp or immunoglobulin. Each of these observations implies, but does not prove, that the antigen receptors and the specific membrane-associated immunoglobulins are the same molecules.

5. The role that immunoglobulins play in B-cell triggering is still controversial. Several models are discussed in Essential Concept 1–6 and are illustrated in Figure 1–28.

B. There are preliminary indications that immunoglobulin molecules undergo conformational changes upon binding antigen.

1. Intramolecular interactions in the immunoglobulin molecule may occur between neighboring domains on the same chain (cis interactions) as well as between paired homology units on separate chains (trans interactions). Strong trans interactions occur between V_L and V_H, C_L and $C_H 1$ and the paired $C_H 3$ homology units (Figure 3–13). X-ray studies indicate that there is little or no interaction between the paired $C_H 2$ homology units.

2. Spectroscopic studies of soluble antibody in the presence or absence of antigen suggest that the environments of tryptophan and tyrosine residues in the Fc as well as the Fab regions change when antigen is bound. This apparent conformational change requires that the antigen fill most of the antigen-binding site and that the inter-heavy-chain disulfide bridge be intact. Monomeric antigens of appropriate size can induce this change, implying that it is intramolecular rather than intermolecular. It is an attractive hypothesis that this conformational change could serve the transducing function of receptor immunoglobulins. However, spectroscopic studies are difficult to interpret unambiguously, so that these conclusions are tentative.

C. In summary, the evidence so far available indicates that receptor immunoglobulins exhibit properties expected of cell-surface receptors in general. Given that immunoglobulins probably evolved from more general recognition systems, it is fruitful to explore simpler organisms than vertebrates for immunoglobulinlike receptor molecules and for recognition events analogous to antigen–antibody interactions.

4-7   Cell-cell recognition occurs through complementary molecular interactions

A.   In all organisms that are multicellular or that go through a multicellular stage in their life cycle, positional information appears to be transmitted through cell-cell recognition via cell-surface receptors. The molecular basis for this recognition must be complementary interaction between cell-surface components. The possible recognition mechanisms can be classified conveniently into three types (Figure 4–31).

1.   *Self-self interaction* may occur between identical receptor molecules on two different cells to form an intermolecular complex with two-fold rotational symmetry (Figure 4–31a). A familiar example of such an interaction is the association of two $\alpha\beta$ dimeric subunits of hemoglobin to form the $\alpha_2\beta_2$ tetramer. Cell-cell recognition via self-self interaction requires only one gene product, which is expressed on the surface of all associating cells.

2.   *Complementary interaction* may occur between a receptor protein on one cell and a different macromolecule on another (Figure 4–31b). Familiar examples of such complementary interactions include the association of the hemoglobin α chain with the β chain and the recognition of a macromolecular carbohydrate by an enzyme or a specific antibody molecule. Cell-cell recognition via complementary interaction requires a minimum of two different gene products. Both may be expressed on all cells, or each may be expressed on only one of two populations of cells that interact.

3.   A special case of complementary interaction may involve identical surface-receptor molecules on all cells that recognize a multifunctional heterologous linker molecule (Figure 4–31c). Such recognition also requires a minimum of two gene products: one for the receptor and another for the linker.

B.   Complex metazoa, which require many distinct sets of cell-cell recognition elements, must have multiple genes to code for these molecules. Conceivably, the genes for cell-surface receptors have evolved as multigene families like those of the immunoglobulins, so that new recognition specificities or families of specificities can be generated readily. Whether such multigene families exist, all three of the mechanisms outlined in the preceding section require that genes or portions of genes that code for complementary recognition elements must *coevolve*, so that complementarity is maintained in the course

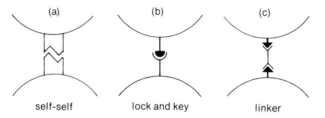

Figure 4–31   Three types of specific interactions between cell-surface receptors.

of inevitable evolutionary changes. In view of this requirement for coevolution, recognition systems would be expected to evolve relatively slowly. Evidence in support of a slow evolutionary rate is the lack of species specificity among cells of a given tissue in vertebrate embryos. For example, if cells of embryonic liver and kidney tissue from two unrelated species are dissociated, mixed, and allowed to re-sort, then the two species of kidney cells will recognize each other as "self" and cohere, as will the two species of liver cells. By contrast, liver and kidney cells from the same embryo will separate by virtue of their differing tissue specificity.

The following sections review evidence for specific cell-cell interactions in the development of slime molds, simple metazoa, and finally, the vertebrate immune system.

4-8   Slime molds exhibit specific cellular interactions that are mediated by lectinlike molecules and their receptors

The life cycle of the cellular slime mold *Dictystelium discoideum* begins with a vegetative or nonsocial phase in which unicellular amoebae consume bacteria and divide about every three hours. When the food supply is exhausted, the amoebae aggregate over the next 9–12 hours into a multicellular slug that contains up to 10^5 cells, which form stable intercellular contacts. Cells of the slug, which is motile and phototactic, differentiate into two types, prespore and prestalk cells. During the next 12 hours the slug becomes sessile and the cells rearrange to form a stalk topped by a sporangium, which contains stable spores (Figure 4–32). Because cells can be isolated in the vegetative state and at various stages during the development of the cohesive multicelled organism, slime molds are an ideal model system for studying the development of cellular cohesiveness. Cohesiveness is due to developmentally controlled lectinlike cell surface molecules.

1. Fab fragments from antibodies raised against cells from the cohesive state, after absorption with the vegetative state, block the aggregation of amoebae.

334

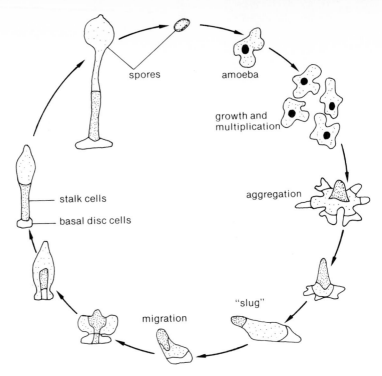

Figure 4–32 The life cycle of the cellular slime mold *Dictystelium discoideum.* [Adapted from James D. Watson, *Molecular Biology of the Gene,* 3rd ed., © 1976 by J. D. Watson: W. A. Benjamin, Inc., Menlo Park, Calif., p. 508.]

2. Several experiments suggest that a lectinlike cell-surface carbohydrate-binding protein mediates these cell-cell interactions. *D. discoideum* produces two proteins of approximately 100,000 molecular weight termed discoidin I and II. These proteins, which can be purified from the cohesive form of the slime mold, specifically bind to *N*-acetyl-D-galactosamine. Antibodies directed against the discoidins bind to the cell surface of cohesive but not vegetative cells, demonstrating that the discoidins are present on the cell surface. The appearance of the discoidins parallels the development of cohesiveness as the cells aggregate.

There is also evidence for developmentally regulated high-affinity cell-surface receptors for the discoidins. Vegetative cells are not significantly agglutinated by added discoidins, but as the cells differentiate they become increasingly agglutinable. Thus, both the lectins and their receptors appear to be developmentally controlled.

N-Acetyl-D-glucosamine can specifically block the aggregation of developing cells. This finding suggests that interactions between the discoidins and their receptors are responsible for the cohesiveness of the multicellular form of the slime mold.

3. A lectinlike molecule apparently responsible for the cohesion of a second cellular slime mold, *Polysphondylium pallidum,* has been isolated and shown to have a different molecular weight (250,000) and sugar affinity (glucuronic acid) from the discoidins. Thus the cell-aggregation factors for slime molds appear to be species-specific.

4. A mutation that prevents cohesion in *D. discoideum* at high temperature has been described recently. Hence, genetic as well as biochemical approaches can be employed in the analysis of the function and regulation of this system. It will be interesting to determine whether the two different cell types of the slime mold (prestalk and prespore) employ different lectinlike molecules and receptors.

4-9   Metazoan development depends upon specific cell-cell interactions

A.   Metazoa are made up of many cells that specifically rearrange themselves and differentiate into distinct cell types during development. These differentiation events appear, at least in part, to be mediated by specific cell-surface molecules. In a few systems the most general features of cell-cell interactions are becoming apparent.

The construction of tissues and organs in vertebrate embryos involves extensive cell migrations and rearrangements. Many organs, including the heart, gonad, adrenal medulla, and various components of the skeleton and the nervous system arise in the embryo from cells that are distant from their final location (Figure 4–33). These cells migrate to predetermined sites and selectively aggregate with other cells to form tissue primordia.

One explanation for specific embryonic cell recognition is that each tissue may have characteristic cell-surface *recognition molecules* that allow appropriate cells to aggregate into tissues and organs (Figure 4–34). The discriminating properties of these recognition molecules may increase as development progresses. For example, initially cells of the three embryonic layers, the ectoderm, mesoderm, and endoderm, may specifically recognize cells of their own type. Then these embryonic layers further differentiate into the major tissue classes, and finally the cell types within tissues sort out.

B.   Tissue-specific cell surface antigens, termed *differentiation antigens* have been demonstrated in several systems. Rabbit antisera raised against mouse embryonic neural retina tissue, after absorption with heterologous tissues, react with the surfaces of neural retinal cells but not with other cell types. Similar antisera have been prepared for myocardium, liver and skeletal muscle. Obviously, these antisera may

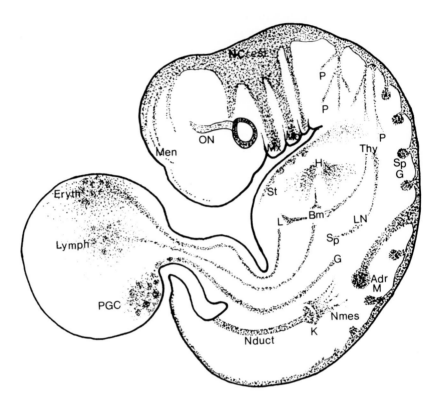

Figure 4–33 The migration pathways of various cells in the vertebrate embryo. [Courtesy of A. A. Moscona.]

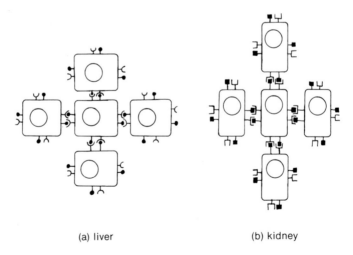

(a) liver   (b) kidney

Figure 4–34 A diagram of tissue-specific cell-surface recognition systems utilizing lock-and-key interactions.

be directed against differentiation antigens with a variety of different functions; however, their existence is consistent with the hypothesis of cell-surface recognition systems.

C.   An *in vitro* system has been developed to study the specific aggregation of embryonic cells (Figure 4–35). For example, the embryonic neural retina is composed of three layers of discrete cell types. When the embryonic retina is treated with trypsin, it disassociates into a single-cell suspension. When this suspension is agitated to promote cell collisions, the cells go through two stages of reaggregation. Initially, cells send out microvilli that contact other cells of the various cell types (Figure 4–36). Over the next 24 hours the cell types in these mixed aggregates sort out to reconstitute the initial neural retinal tissue pattern with similar cells associated in discrete layers. Almost all mammalian and avian embryonic tissues sort out in a similar manner. Several interesting observations have come from *in vitro* studies of this type.

> 1.   When single-cell suspensions of two different tissues such as embryonic liver and neural retina are mixed, they sort out in a tissue specific fashion. Hence there must be *tissue-specific* cell-surface recognition molecules.

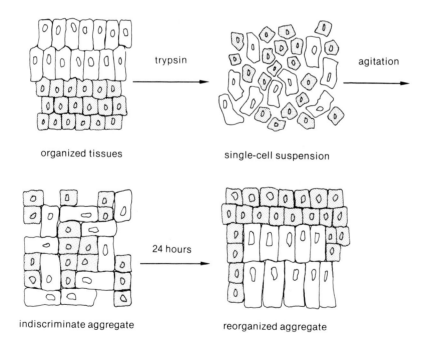

Figure 4–35 A diagram of *in vitro* dissociation and reaggregation of an embryonic tissue with two layers of different cell types.

2. Distinct cell types within a single tissue can specifically reaggregate. Thus there must be *cell type-specific* cell-surface recognition molecules within a tissue.

3. When single-cell suspensions of neural retina from chick and mouse are mixed, the ordinary neural retinal tissue pattern is reconstituted with the avian and mammalian cells intermingled. This observation suggests that both the *cell type*-specificity and *tissue*-specificity recognition molecules have been *highly conserved* during vertebrate evolution.

4. Seven-, 10- and 14-day embryonic neural retinal cells show a progressive decline in their ability to reassociate specifically. There is a corresponding loss in the fluidity of the cell membrane as embryonic cells mature. These two changes may be related, because cell-cell recognition appears to require clustering of receptors, which in turn requires mobility of receptors in the membrane. Thus cellular association may be regulated either by the expression of specific cell-interaction molecules or by altering the fluidity, and thus the potential distribution, of receptors in the cell membrane.

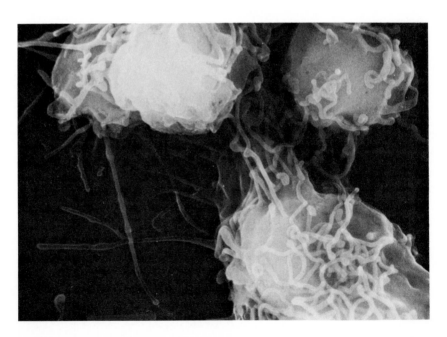

Figure 4–36 A small aggregate of retinal cells formed after 30 minutes of reaggregation. Note the microvilli interconnecting these cells. [From Y. Ben-Shaul and A. A. Moscona, *Exp. Cell Res.* **95,** 191, 1975.]

5. A glycoprotein that specifically promotes the reaggregation of neural retinal cells, but not other embryonic cells, has been isolated from the medium over monolayers of these cells grown in tissue culture. This glycoprotein, 50,000 in molecular weight, can be isolated from neural retinal membranes and binds to the cell surface of neural retinal but not of other embryonic cells. Antibodies to this factor bind only to neural retinal cells. A second glycoprotein of 50,000 molecular weight that promotes the specific reaggregation of cerebral cells also has been isolated. It is interesting that two glycoproteins of similar size possess similar specific functions. This finding raises the possibility that there may be a related family of specific cell-recognition molecules.

D. The specific glycoproteins just discussed promote the specific aggregation of cells over a 24-hour period, a time span sufficient for many complex changes to occur in the cell membranes. A more rapid recognition assay can be carried out by measuring the binding of radiolabeled plasma membrane vesicles (microspheres) prepared from one type of embryonic cells to cells of homologous and heterologous embryonic tissues. Several interesting observations have been made using this assay.

1. Membrane vesicles from chick neural retina and cerebellum bind to homologous but not to heterologous cells. In addition, specific aggregation of homologous cells can be blocked by the addition of these membranes. These observations suggest that the molecules responsible for specific recognition are present on the plasma membrane vesicles.

2. Chick plasma membrane vesicles from 7-, 8-, and 9-day-old optic tectum and neural retina show specificity for homologous cells of the same age. Seven-day membrane vesicles do not interact with 8- or 9-day-old cells, whereas 8- and 9-day membrane vesicles react only weakly with cells of the earlier developmental stage. Thus the cell-surface recognition molecules appear to change rapidly over short time spans in development.

3. Glycoproteins with similar physical properties have been partially purified from the plasma membranes of embryonic optic tectal and neural retinal tissues. These glycoproteins inhibit the aggregation of homologous but not heterologous cells, and show the same temporal ontogenic specificity as the plasma membrane vesicles.

4. Monolayers of embryonic cells on an appropriately modified glass surface can be used as an assay to measure the rate of binding of single radiolabeled cells. This assay system reveals a dorsoventral gradient of adhesive specificity in neural retina cells. That is, the highest cellular affinities are exhibited between cells derived from the extremes of the gradient. The simplest interpretation of these results is that there is a dorsoventral gradient of cell-surface specificities within the neural retina.

E.   In summary, the recognition molecules of vertebrate embryos appear to be located on the cell surface, highly specific, and possibly homologous in their physical properties. These findings suggest that related families of membrane recognition molecules have evolved to facilitate cell sorting and organization in vertebrate embryos.

4-10   Cell-cell recognition events in some simple metazoa are coupled with effector functions

A.   In addition to cell sorting, some lower metazoa exhibit phenomena that appear more directly related to vertebrate cell-mediated immunity. The colonial ascidian (sea squirt) *Botryllus* produces star-shaped colonies by the fusion of several individuals (zooids). Each zooid (ray) has individual functions but shares a common vascular system with other zooids. The colony is initiated by a larva that develops from a fertilized ovum and forms the star-shaped colony by cell proliferation. Thus each colony is a clone of cells that comprises partially differentiated individual rays. *Botryllus* colonies show the following recognition phenomena.

1.   If a colony (A) is divided in two, the parts grow separately as independent colonies. If these colonies are brought together again, they fuse and regenerate a single colony.

2.   If an unrelated colony (B) of the same species is brought into contact with Colony A, rejection and cell death occur, and a barrier of dead or necrotic material develops between the two colonies.

3.   If a colonial ascidian of another species, *Botrylloides,* comes into contact with either *Botryllus* Colony A or B, the ascidians grow over one another as if each were an inert surface for the other.

4.   *Botryllus* is a hermaphroditic organism, that is, it contains both male and female gonads. This organism has a self-sterility barrier which prevents self-fertilization. Thus genetically identical eggs and sperm do not give rise to viable progeny, whereas genetically nonidentical eggs and sperm do.

B.   These recognition phenomena can be explained by the hypothesis that *Botryllus* has a species-specific self-recognition system and in addition a recognition locus that can differ genetically among different

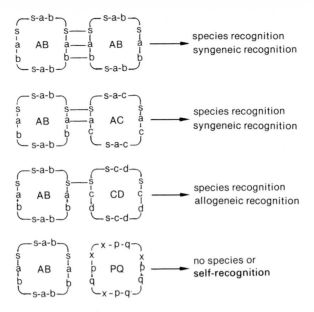

Figure 4–37 A model of two types of possible cell-surface recognition elements in colonial tunicates. Species markers (s and x) and syngeneic recognition units (a, b, c, d, p, and q) represent cell-surface molecules that may interact with their identical counterparts on other cells (a straight line indicates this interaction). These recognition units may be of the complementary type or the syngeneic interaction types (see Figure 4–31). Capital letters indicate the genotypes of each cell for the genes that control the syngeneic recognition elements.

clones within the species. The recognition locus in *Botryllus* is extremely polymorphic with many allelic alternatives. These alleles may code for cell-surface recognition units (Figure 4–37). If two cells of the same species are similar in their recognition units, then *syngeneic* recognition occurs. If two cells of the same species are dissimilar in their recognition units, then *allogeneic* recognition occurs (Figure 4–37). The cells of two different species ignore one another because the species-specific self-recognition systems are unrelated. The two types of recognition, syngeneic and allogeneic, each trigger distinct effector reactions.

1. Syngeneic recognition between somatic cells leads to cooperation between cells to form a multicellular heterotypic colony.

2. Allogeneic recognition between somatic cells leads to a necrotic reaction.

Thus colonial tunicates, in recognizing self and nonself, exhibit several features characteristic of vertebrate immunity. In particular, allogeneic or nonself-recognition is an important aspect of the mammalian T-cell response. In addition, tunicates have coupled various types of effector mechanisms to these recognition events.

C.   Angiosperm trees also have an incompatibility system that prevents self-fertilization in a manner similar to that of tunicates. Allogeneic recognition may have been fundamental in the evolution of metazoan sexual systems that promote genetic diversity among the organisms of a given species.

4-11 Earthworms may exhibit a primitive form of cellular immunity

A.   Earthworms may represent a link between primitive cell-recognition systems involved in development and the immune cell-recognition characteristic of vertebrates. Skin allografts between earthworms from the same geographical area often remain intact, presumably because of genetic similarity. Allografts between earthworms from different areas generally are rejected. Xenografts (between different species) almost always are rejected. The rejection of both allografts and xenografts is of the chronic type, that is, some grafts survive more than 250 days. The graft-rejection process occurs in two phases.

> **1.**   About two days after transplantation, varying proportions of donor cells die, presumably due to inadequate vascularization and nutrition. This phase is nonspecific and nonimmunologic in nature.

> **2.**   About 12 days after transplantation, the degenerated musculature of the graft is infiltrated by coelomocytes (macrophage-like cells present in the coelomic fluid), which surround and eliminate the grafted tissues by engulfing dead cells.

B.   When a second graft is placed on a recipient that has previously rejected a first graft, an accelerated or second-set graft rejection generally occurs, particularly in the case of xenografts. Just five days after the second graft is transplanted, the coelomocytes begin destroying the graft. This second-set rejection process is specific. Furthermore, if coelomocytes are harvested after the rejection of the first graft and injected into an untreated recipient, this worm will show accelerated rejection of a graft from the same donor. Thus effector specificity and perhaps immunologic memory appear to reside in the macrophagelike coelomocytes.

C.   In attempting to trace the evolutionary precursors of the immune system, it is useful to review the major features of vertebrate immunity (Table 4–7). The essence of vertebrate immunity is the free wandering lymphocyte that expresses a single type of receptor from a large library and can be stimulated by appropriate antigens to undergo proliferation and differentiation to effector functions, which include reactions of tolerance and allogeneic recognition.

To summarize the preceding sections, several of these features are present in invertebrates and vertebrate tissues other than those of the immune system. Slime molds and vertebrate embryonic cells have cell-surface receptors capable of self-recognition. In vertebrates

Table 4-7
Fundamental features of the vertebrate immune system

1. Wide diversity of molecular specificities for lymphocyte receptors and antibodies
2. Phenotypic restriction of lymphocyte clones to expression of only one specificity for both surface receptors and any secreted antibody
3. Elimination of lymphocyte clones specific for antigenic determinants present and accessible in the body, thus allowing the system subsequently to distinguish self from nonself
4. Antigenic stimulation of specific lymphocytes to proliferate, producing descendant lymphocytes of the same specificity
5. Differentiation of lymphocytes into those that can synthesize and secrete specific receptors and those that remain as effector cells and memory cells
6. Ability to eliminate most foreign cells and microorganisms through the actions of antibodies and effector cells

these recognition molecules are clonally expressed (e.g., kidney cells have kidney-specific recognition molecules and liver cells have liver-specific recognition molecules). Moreover, there appears to be a large library of specific recognition molecules for the many tissues of the vertebrate organism. Presumably the same will be true of other metazoa with tissue differentiation. Accordingly, the library of receptors for lymphocytes may have evolved from a more primitive multigene family of recognition molecules.

Colonial ascidians have developed a dual recognition system for self and for unrelated members of the same species. *Botryllus* has effector mechanisms that are triggered by the allogeneic recognition system, including somatic-cell killing and germ-cell fusion. Earthworms exhibit several features of vertebrate immunity, including chronic graft rejection and mobile immunospecific coelomocytes, which are the effector cells and perhaps memory cells for graft rejection. Thus various features of vertebrate immunity are seen in diverse representatives of the invertebrate branch of the animal kingdom.

These subvertebrate recognition systems may be evolutionarily related to the major histocompatibility complex of vertebrates—an important multigenic cell-cell recognition system that appears to be involved in developmental interactions, immunologic recognition of foreign antigens, and internal immunological surveillance throughout chordate species.

4-12 The major histocompatibility complex of mammals controls a variety of phenomena related to immune recognition

A. The major histocompatibility complex (MHC) is a cluster of loci occupying a single chromosomal region in all mammals so far examined for it. The gene products of this region are involved in a variety of immune phenomena, some of which have been discussed in other chapters.

1. The MHC was first recognized by its ability to control allograft rejection (Essential Concept 2–11). The ability to identify and destroy foreign cells may be important in protecting the developing fetus against invading maternal cells (or vice versa) and in immune surveillance for cancer cells (Essential Concept 5–7).

2. Ia, D, and K gene products of the MHC are recognition elements in the cellular interactions among T cells, B cells, and macrophages. These elements may be either cell-surface or soluble factors and may either facilitate or inhibit immune responses (Essential Concept 1–13).

3. Ir genes of the MHC regulate the magnitude of thymus-dependent immune responses to a variety of antigens. This regulation extends to cellular as well as humoral responses (Essential Concept 1–11).

4. Ir genes play a fundamental role in the phenomena of associative recognition (Essential Concept 1–13).

5. Genes in the MHC control the synthesis of certain complement components. These genes may be either structural or regulatory in nature (Essential Concept 1–9c).

The presence of the MHC in all mammals and its many effects on immune responses indicate that its functions must be important. However, the nature of many of these functions, and the mechanisms by which most genes of the complex act, are not understood. In attempts to understand the MHC, immunologists are actively exploring its genetics, its distribution among vertebrates, its possible evolutionary antecedents in invertebrates, and the molecular properties of the proteins coded by MHC genes. The current status of these investigations is reviewed in the following sections.

B.   In different species the major histocompatibility complexes have different designations (Table 4–8). *Classes* refer to loci or regions within the MHC that appear to be functionally related. Class I loci control the major transplantation antigens; Class II loci control immune responsiveness; and Class III loci control elements of the complement system.

The two best studied MHC's are those of the mouse, designated the H-2 complex, and the human, designated the HLA complex. The human complex appears to play an important role in the susceptibility to certain diseases (Essential Concept 2–15). The mouse has served as a useful model system for understanding the MHC of mammals because of its ready manipulation as an experimental system.

Table 4–8

Nomenclature and class identifications of the major histocompatibility complexes of various animals

Species	Designation of MHC	Class I	MHC regions of: Class II				Class III
			Ia	Ir	LD	H	
Mouse	H-2	2[a]	+	+	+	+	+
Human	HLA	3	+	+	+		+
Rhesus monkey	RhL-A	2	+	+	+		+
Chimpanzee	ChL-A	1					
Rat	AgB (H1)	2	+	+	+		
Rabbit	RL-A	1			+		
Dog	DL-A	2			+		
Pig	SL-A	1					
Guinea pig	GPL-A	2	+	+	+	+	+
Chicken	B	1		+	+		
Syrian hamster	none				+		
Clawed toad	none				+		

[a]Numbers indicate how many Class I regions have been identified.

[Adapted from J. Klein in *Major Histocompatibility Complex,* D. Gotze (Ed.), Springer-Verlag, Berlin, 1977, p. 339.]

1. The H-2 locus of the mouse is genetically complex. It has been possible to characterize it extensively because of the availability of *inbred* and *congenic* strains. Individuals from an inbred strain of mice, produced by repeated brother–sister matings, have very similar if not identical genetic constitutions. More than 100 different inbred strains now have been constructed. Congenic strains of mice are genetically identical except for a single genetic region or locus. A method for construction of congenic strains is illustrated in Figure 4–38. By this method, for example, the H-2 complex of a B-strain mouse may be placed in the background of an A-strain genome. The resulting congenic strain is designated A.B. Experiments with inbred and congenic strains of mice have led to construction of a detailed genetic map of the H-2 region (Figure 4–39).

2. The H-2 complex of the mouse is located on Chromosome 17. It can be divided into five major *regions* designated K, I, S, G, and D marked by the H-2K, Ir-1, Ss-Slp, H-2G, and H-2D genes, respectively (Figure 4–39). The boundaries of each region are determined by intra H-2 recombinations between these traits. Whenever two traits are clearly separated by a crossover and are unaltered by the recombinational event, the traits are assumed to be controlled by two separate genes. In a similar manner

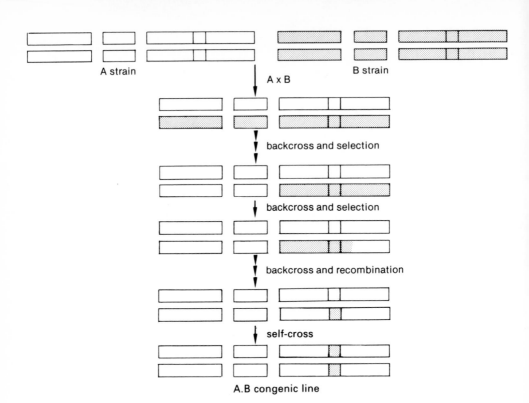

Figure 4–38 Diagram of the steps required to produce a congenic A.B strain of mice. Pairs of chromosomes for the inbred A and B strains of mice are designated by open and dark rectangles, respectively. The MHC is designated by boundary lines on one chromosome. With an appropriate assay system (e.g., allograft rejection), the B-strain MHC from F₁ progeny can be followed through repeated backcrosses to the A strain. This backcrossing process leads to (1) the loss of all B-strain chromosomes other than the one that carries the H-2 locus and (2) the loss of B genes from the B chromosome that carries the H-2 locus by crossing over with the homologous A chromosome. These two processes are depicted as occurring successively, although they actually occur simultaneously. After a large number of backcrosses, the B chromosome that carries the H-2 locus will have primarily A genes except in the H-2 complex of one chromosome. Two such F₁ animals can be crossed to produce a homozygous congenic strain.

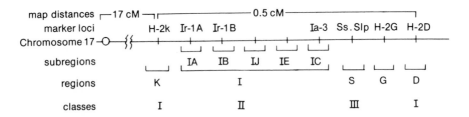

Figure 4–39 A genetic map of the mouse H-2 complex on Chromosome 17. Map distances (centimorgans), marker loci, regions, and subregions are indicated. ⭕ represents the centromere.

the I region has been subdivided into at least five distinct, but functionally related, *subregions* designated I-A, I-B, I-J, I-E, and I-C. A unique combination of alleles at loci within the H-2 complex is termed a *haplotype.* Different inbred strains of mice generally have different H-2 haplotypes, which are denoted H-2^a, H-2^b, and so on.

The number of genes in the H-2 complex is not known. The recombination frequency between the H-2K and H-2D loci is 0.5 centimorgans, which corresponds to enough DNA to code for up to 2,000 polypeptides, 200 amino acids in length. Nevertheless, some immunologists believe the MHC may include just 7 or 8 genes, whereas others feel it may encode hundreds. If the MHC does include hundreds of structural genes, then one or more libraries of cell-surface receptors could be included. However, if the MHC includes only 7 to 8 genes, they must carry out more general types of functions.

3. The HLA complex of man is located on the sixth chromosome. It also can be divided into five regions (Figure 4–40), which are homologous to their mouse counterparts. The map distance across the human HLA complex is 1.6 centimorgans, more than three times the extent of the H-2 complex.

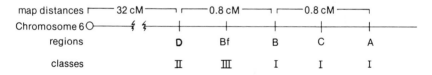

Figure 4–40, A genetic map of the human HLA complex on human Chromosome 6. Map distances (centimorgans) and regions are indicated. The circle represents the centromere.

C. The Class I regions, which encode the classical transplantation antigens, are K and D in the mouse and A, B, and C in the human. The known numbers of Class I regions in other mammals are indicated in Table 4–8.

1. The Class I-region gene products identified so far are integral membrane glycoproteins about 45,000 in molecular weight (Figure 4–41). They are noncovalently associated with β_2-microglobulin, a molecule of about 100 amino acid residues that exhibits significant homology to the C_H homology units of the IgG molecule. The transplantation antigen appears to be divided into four units each about 100 amino residues in length. The two central units have centrally-placed disulfide bridges that span about 60 amino acid residues. This structure demonstrates some

Table 4–9
K and D antigenic determinants of the mouse[a]

H-2 haplotype	K determinants Public																				K determinants Private	D determinants Public															D determinants Private
	1	3	5	7	8	11	25	27	28	29	34	35	36	37	38	39	42	45	46	47		1	3	5	6	13	27	28	29	35	36	41	42	43	44	49	
b	−	−	+	−	−	−	−	+	+	+	−	+	+	−	−	+	−	−	+	−	33	−	−	−	+	+	+	+	+	−	−	−	−	−	−	−	2?
d	−	+	−	−	+	−	−	+	+	+	+	−	−	−	−	−	−	−	+	+	31	−	+	−	+	+	+	+	+	+	+	+	+	+	+	+	4
f	−	−	+	+	+	−	−	+?	+?	+?	−	−	−	+	−	+	−	+	+	−	?	−	−	−	+	+	+	−?	−?	−	−	−	−	−	−	+	9
j	+?	−	c	+	−	−	−	·	·	·	−	−	−	−	+	−	−	+	+?	+?	15	+	+	·	+	−	−	+	+	−	−	−	−	−	−	−	2
k	+	+	+	−	+	+	+	−	−	−	+	−	−	+	+	−	−	+	+	+	23	+	+	+	−	−	−	−	−	+	−	+	−	−	−	+	32
p	+	−	+	+	−	−	−	−′	−	−	+	−	−	+	+	−	−	+	−	·	16	−	+	−	+	+	+	+	+	c	c	−	−	−	−	+	?
q	+	+	+	+	+	+	+	−	−	−	+	−	−	−	−	−	−	+	−	+	17	+	+	+	+	+	+	+	+	−	−	+	−	−	−	−	30
r	+	+	−	−	+	+	+	−	−	−	−	−	−	−	−	−	+	+	−	−	·	−	−	−	−	−	−	−	−	c	c	−	+	−	−	+	18?
a	+	−	+	+	−	−	−	−	−	−	−	−	−	−	−	−	+	+	·	−	19	−	+	−	+	+	−	+	−	c	+	+	−	−	−	+	12
u	c	−	+	−	+?	−	−	−	−	−	−	+	+	−	−	−	−	+	·	·	20	−	+	−	·	+? +?	+?	+	−	c	+	+	42	+	+	+	4
v	+	+	+	−	−	−	−	+	·	+	−	−	−	−	−	−	−	+?	−	·	21	−	−	−	+	−? +?	−? +?	+	−	−	−	−	−	+	−	+	4
z	−	·	+	−	−	−	−	+	+	+	−	−	−	−	−	−	−	−	+	+	·	−	−	−	+	−	·	·	+	−	−	−	−	−	−	·	30

[a] (−) = absence of an antigen; (·) = unknown; (?) = presence or absence of antigen is uncertain; (c) = some antisera cross-react with the indicated H-2 haplotype.

[From J. Klein, *Biology of the Mouse Histocompatibility-2 Complex*, Springer-Verlag, New York, 1975, p. 126.]

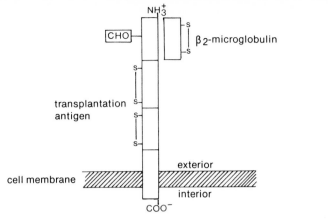

Figure 4–41 The general structure of a Class I-region gene product (transplantation antigen), showing its association with the cell membrane and with β_2-microglobulin. The transplantation antigen appears to be divided into four homology units of approximately 100 amino acid residues each, and the β_2-microglobulin may be associated with either of the two homology units closest to the N-terminus. The positions of cysteine residues that participate in disulfide bridges and of an attached carbohydrate group are indicated by S and CHO, respectively.

gross homologies to immunoglobulins (see Figure 3–13), and raises the possibility that these two genetically complex membrane systems may share a common evolutionary origin.

2. The Class I molecules are expressed on all mammalian cells except some in the terminal stages of differentiation and those in the early stages of embryonic development. The transplantation antigens are found in the highest density on nucleated blood cells, including B cells, mature T cells, and macrophages.

3. The class I molecules induce strong humoral responses following allogeneic immunization. For these reasons they also have been designated *s*erologically *d*etermined (SD) molecules. Each Class I molecule carries a number of determinants antigenic to most allogeneic hosts. These determinants, which can be defined by the *alloantisera* they elicit, fall into two categories (Table 4–9): determinants that are unique to the immunizing haplotype (*private specificities*), and determinants that are shared by other haplotypes (*public specificities*).

4. The Class I molecules of mouse and man exhibit striking genetic polymorphism. For example, at the K and D loci the domestic inbred strains of mice have 11 and 10 alleles, respectively, that are are expressed in more than 25 different chromosomal combinations or haplotypes (Table 4–9). Moreover, when wild mice from different areas are examined, each small breeding unit (deme) generally has new private K and D specificities distinct from all known private specificities and from those of mice in nearby breeding units. Given the worldwide distribution of mice, the potential polymorphism of Class I gene products may be larger than that of any other known genetic system.

5.   The Class I molecules evoke strong cell-mediated lymphocytotoxic and allograft rejection responses, but poor mixed lymphocyte and graft-versus-host responses. These responses can be used to distinguish tentatively between MHC gene products of Class I and Class II.

D.   The Class II regions, which control immune responsiveness, are designated I in the mouse and D in the human (Table 4–8). Class II regions also may be called the *lymphocyte-defined* (LD) regions. Several assay systems have defined four distinct phenotypic expressions of the Class II regions: *Ia, Ir, Ld,* and *H.* The corresponding genetic determinants are distributed among the I subregions I-A, I-B, I-C, I-E, and I-J, as shown in Figure 4–39.

1.   The *I* region-*a*ssociated or Ia loci code for integral cell-surface glycoproteins that generally have two subunits, one approximately 35,000 in molecular weight and the other approximately 28,000. The Ia molecule is not associated with β_2-microglobulin. Ia molecules are expressed predominantly on B cells, and in lower concentrations on T cells, epidermal cells, and macrophages. The Ia molecules also are serologically complex and highly polymorphic, exhibiting public and private specificities.

2.   The immune response or Ir loci control the level of the immunoglobulin response to thymus-dependent antigens. The responses to a wide variety of antigens are under control of the immune response genes (Table 4–10). This diversity of antigens implies either that the Ir region must contain a large number of different genes that encode receptors with diverse binding sites, or that a few Ir gene products somehow modify either the specificity of T-cell receptors or cell-cell interactions between T cells and other cells (Figure 1–45). The latter model could apply to helper or suppressor T cells. Indeed, one Ir subregion of the mouse, I-J, appears to encode an antigen-specific T-cell suppressor factor.

Three additional Ir loci have been described: Ir-1A in the I-A subregion, Ir-1B in the I-B subregion and Ir-1C in the I-C subregion. Complementation for T-cell suppression is known to occur between genes located in different I subregions. Gene complementation means that appropriate gene products from at least two separate loci must be present to have a particular phenotype expressed (e.g., T-cell suppression). One simple interpretation of this complementation is that the corresponding pairs

Table 4–10

A partial list of antigens under the control of immune response genes in the mouse

poly-L(Tyr,Glu)-poly-D,L-Ala-poly-L-Lys[a]
poly-L(His,Glu)-poly-D,L-Ala-poly-L-Lys[a]
poly-L(Phe,Glu)-poly-D,L-Ala-poly-L-Lys[a]
ovalbumin
benzylpenicilloyl$_6$ conjugate of ovalbumin
benzylpenicilloyl$_{25}$ conjugate of bovine gammaglobulin
benzylpenicilloyl$_4$ conjugate of ovomucoid
benzylpenicilloyl$_4$ conjugate of bovine pancreatic ribonuclease
dinitrophenyl$_{42}$ conjugate of bovine gammaglobulin
ovomucoid
2,4,6-trinitrophenyl conjugate of mouse serum albumin
$(\text{L-Glu}^{60}\ \text{L-Ala}^{30}\ \text{L-Tyr}^{40})n$[b]
$(\text{L-Glu}^{58}\ \text{L-Ala}^{38}\ \text{L-Tyr}^4)n$[b]
$(\text{L-Glu}^{58}\ \text{L-Lys}^{38}\ \text{L-Phe}^4)n$
thyroglobulin
IgA
IgG$_{2a}$
IgG$_{2b}$
Thy-1
male histocompatibility antigen (H-Y)
antigen 2 controlled by the H-2 complex (H-2.2)
erythrocyte alloantigen 1 (Ea-1)
sex limited protein (Slp)
nuclease from staphylococcus aureus

[a]Synthetic branched multichain polypeptide.
[b]Random linear copolymer with the superscript indicating the molar ratio of amino acids in the polymer
[From J. Klein, *Biology of the Mouse Histocompatibility-2 Complex,* Springer-Verlag, New York, 1975, p. 126.]

of genes code for two cell-surface receptors that are complementary and possibly present on different cell types (e.g., B cells and T cells).

3. The LD loci, which code for *lymphocyte-activating determinants,* are defined by their ability to stimulate mixed lymphocyte or graft-versus-host reactions. These cell-surface determinants are certainly present on B cells and probably on T cells and macrophages. It is not known whether they are present on other cell types. MHC-associated LD loci have been identified in a variety of mammals (Table 4–8). In the mouse, two such loci have been identified: LD-1 in the I-A subregion and LD-2 in the I-C subregion.

4. Class II *histocompatibility* or H loci are assayed by the graft-rejection response. H loci have been identified in the mouse and guinea pig. In the mouse, two H loci have been described. One in the I-A subregion controls acute or rapid graft rejection,

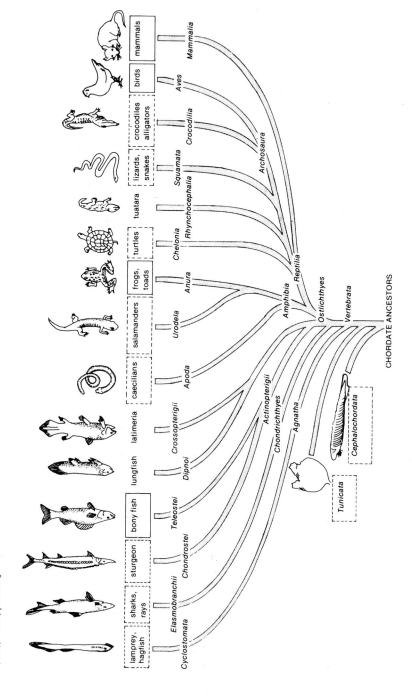

Figure 4–42 Occurrence of the MHC among *Chordata*. A solid box indicates presence of an MHC in at least some species of a class; a dashed box indicates absence of an MHC in all species, and no box indicates that no MHC data are available for that class. [Adapted from J. Klein in *Major Histocompatibility System in Man and Animals*, D. Gotze (Ed.), 1977, p. 353.]

and the other in the I-C subregion controls a more chronic rejection.

The number of loci in the Class II region and the interrelationships of the Class II loci are not understood. It is possible that most of the diverse traits associated with Class II loci may be controlled by just a few genes.

5. Although close linkage of the Class I and Class II genes has been found in all mammals studied (Table 4–8), the order of these regions can vary. For example, in the mouse the Class II region is between the two Class I regions, whereas in the human the Class II region is outside the two Class I regions (see Figures 4–39 and 4–40).

E. Class III regions control the expression of complement components or receptors. Several MHC loci that code for complement components have been reported in four different mammals (Table 4–8). In the mouse, the Ss protein is probably a C4 complement component. The H-2 complex has also been reported to influence the time of appearance of the C3 receptor on B cells and the level of the C3 complement component.

F. The G region of the H-2 complex codes for a polymorphic system of cell-surface antigens found on red blood cells. Little is known about the structure or functions of these molecules.

G. The evolution of the major histocompatibility complex may provide some clues as to its function. Nothing in evolution is created *de novo;* each new gene must arise from an already existing gene. Thus the evolution of a gene or gene system may be analyzed by comparing the genes, gene products, or gene phenotypes for a particular system from more and more distantly related animals. It is difficult to make such a comparison with a system as poorly defined as the MHC. Nonetheless, certain limited generalizations can be drawn from the analysis of MHC-like traits in vertebrates and invertebrates.

1. An evolutionary tree of *Chordata,* showing the presence or absence of the MHC, where known, is given in Figure 4–42. All vertebrates exhibit allograft rejection. These rejections fall into one of two categories. *Chronic* rejections exhibit a delayed onset of months and a prolonged rejection process often of several weeks. *Rapid* rejections have a rapid onset of one to three weeks and a short rejection process, often of a few days. The rapid rejections are found in some fish, some amphibia, birds, and mammals (Figure 4–43). Rapid graft rejection probably indicates the presence of mammalianlike Class I molecules. These same animals give strong mixed lymphocyte reactions that probably indicate the presence of Class II molecules (Figure 4–43). Thus the mammalianlike Class I and II molecules appear to evolve

354

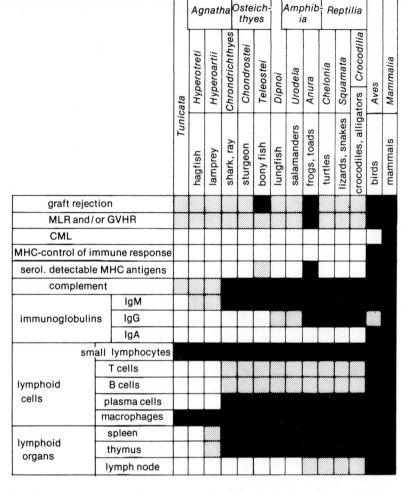

Figure 4–43 The evolution of immunological traits among *Chordata*. Dark boxes indicate presence of mammalianlike traits; stippled boxes indicate presence of atypical or incompletely developed traits; empty boxes indicate either the absence of traits or absence of knowledge about these traits in the indicated species. [Adapted from J. Klein in *Major Histocompatibility System in Man and Animals,* D. Gotze (Ed.), 1977, p. 358.]

together. Moreover, these traits appear to have evolved independently in a number of vertebrate evolutionary lines (Figure 4–42). Finally, the complement system is present in all vertebrates studied to date, indicating the presence of Class III molecules.

2. Invertebrate histocompatibility-like systems may have given rise to the vertebrate MHC locus. The evolutionary drive for genetic diversification possibly could have generated an allogeneic recognition system in invertebrate germ cells that could prevent self-fertilization and allow only dissimilar eggs and sperm to unite. However, it is difficult to imagine a selective advantage for recognition and destruction of allogeneic somatic cells, unless such cells could arise spontaneously and threaten the animal. Given that systems of recognition exist at both the germ cell and somatic cell level, one could postulate that perhaps both self and nonself-recognition capacities in invertebrates evolved into more complex vertebrate systems responsible for generation of developmental patterns and surveillance over neoplastic or infected cells. Class I molecules may interact with viral or neoplastic cell-surface molecules to trigger cytotoxic killing (Essential Concept 1–13). Class II molecules may have evolved to promote B cell–T cell interactions and, accordingly, more sophisticated effector functions. Class III molecules are an effector system in themselves, triggered by immune reactions that can lead in various ways to the elimination of foreign cells and invaders.

4–13 Partial amino-acid-sequence data pose intriguing questions about the organization and evolution of MHC genes

A. The partial amino acid sequence of mouse, human, and guinea pig transplantation antigens (Class I molecules) are presented in Figure 4–44. Several conclusions are indicated about the homology relationships of the transplantation antigens with one another and with the immunoglobulin gene families.

1. The K and D gene products are homologous to one another and probably descended from a common ancestral gene (Figure 4–44). Moreover, the Class I products of mouse, man, and guinea pig are homologous to one another. Thus all the Class I molecules in these species are descended from a common ancestral gene.

2. The K and D gene products both associate with β_2-microglobulin, a free immunoglobulin domain (Figure 4–41). In addition, immunoglobulins and transplantation antigens share several general features: extreme polymorphism, location in the cell membrane, and involvement in the immune response. Therefore, it has been suggested that the K and D gene products may be homologous to immunoglobulins. Although the N-termini of K and D gene products demonstrate marginal amino-acid-sequence homology to immunoglobulins, an internal fragment of a human transplantation antigen shows striking homology to a portion of the V region of immunoglobulins (Figure 4–45). This homologous relationship suggests either that the transplantation antigens and immunoglobulins share a common ancestor and arose by divergent evolution, or that these particular regions in the two molecules

Figure 4-44 Partial amino acid sequences of Class I molecules from mouse, human, and guinea pig.

position

MHC		1	2	3	4	5	6	7	8	9	10	11	12	13	14	15	16	17	18	19	20	21	22	23	24	25	26	27
mouse H-2	K^d	Met		His			Arg	Tyr	Phe		(Thr)				Arg	(Pro)						Arg	Phe					Tyr
	K^b	Met	Pro	His		Leu	Arg	Tyr	Phe	Val	(Thr)	Ala	Val		Arg	(Pro)		Leu		—	(Pro)	Arg	Tyr	Met			(Leu)	Tyr
	K^k	Met	Pro	His		Leu	Arg	Tyr	Phe	His		Ala	Val		Ile	Pro		Leu		Lys	Pro	Phe	Ala					Tyr
	D^d	Met		His		Leu	Arg	Tyr	Phe	Val	(Thr)	Ala	Val	(Thr)	Arg	Pro		Phe		—	Pro	Arg	Tyr					Tyr
	D^b	Met	Pro	His		—	Arg	Tyr	Phe	—	(Thr)	Ala	Val		Arg	Pro		Leu		—	Pro	Arg	Tyr					Tyr
human HLA	A2	Gly	Ser	Ser	Ser	Met	Arg	Tyr	Phe	Phe	Thr	Ser	Val	Ser	Arg	Pro	Gly		Gly	Gly	(Ser)	Asx	Phe	Ile	Ala	Val		
	B7	Gly	Ser	Ser	Ser	Met	Arg	Tyr	Phe	Tyr	Thr	Ser	Val	Ser	Arg	Pro	Gly		Gly	Glu			Phe	Ile		Val		
	B7,12	Gly	Ser	Ser	Ser	Met	Arg	Tyr	Phe	Tyr	Thr	Ala	Val	Ser	Arg	Pro	Gly		Gly	Glu			Phe	Ile	Ala	Val		
							Val																					
	B7,14	Gly	Ser	Ser	Ser	Met	Arg	Tyr	Phe	Tyr	Thr	Ser	Val	Ser	Arg	Pro	Gly		Gly	Glu	(Ser)	Asx	Phe					
	A1,2								Phe	Phe	Thr	Ser		Ser														
	B8,13		Ser					Tyr	Tyr	Ser	Ser	Ala	Val	Ala	Ala	Pro	Gly											
guinea pig GPLA	B.1			His		Leu	Arg	Tyr	Phe	Tyr		Ala	Val			Pro							Phe	Val				Tyr

Figure 4-44 Partial amino acid sequences of Class I molecules from mouse, human, and guinea pig. Boxes indicate positions at which one or more sequences show identity between species. ( ) indicates probable but not certain residue assignment. — indicates that the residue found at that same position in other K or D sequences is *not* present in the indicated sequence. A blank indicates an unidentified residue. These data were obtained by newly developed microsequencing techniques which yield, for technical reasons, only partial amino-acid-sequence data. [A compilation of data presented by B. Cunningham et al., S. Nathenson et al., B. Schwartz et al., J Silver et al., and J. Uhr et al. in *Cold Spring Harbor Symp. Quant. Biol.* **41**, 1976.]

	1			5					10				15				
HLA fragment	Lys	Arg	Thr	Val	Thr	Arg	Pro	Leu	Asp	Glu	Ala	Ile	Tyr	[ ]	Cys	Ala	Leu
human V_H	Thr	Met	Thr	Asp	Val	Asp	Pro	Val	Asp	Thr	Ala	Thr	Tyr	Tyr	Cys	Ala	Arg
human V_λ	Thr	Ile	Thr	Gly	Thr	Arg	Thr	Glu	Asp	Glu	Ala	Asp	Tyr	Phe	Cys	Ala	Thr
mouse V_λ	Thr	Ile	Thr	Gly	Ala	Glu	Thr	Glu	Asp	Glu	Ala	Ile	Tyr	Phe	Cys	Ala	Leu

Figure 4–45 Sequence comparison of a fragment of a human transplantation antigen with portions of three immunoglobulin V regions. Boxes indicate identical residues. [ ] indicates a deletion assumed in order to maximize homology relationships. [From C. Terhorst et al., *Proc. Natl. Acad. Sci. USA* **74**, 4002, 1977.]

must fold in a similar manner and therefore attained similar structures by convergent evolution. More amino-acid-sequence data on transplantation antigens will be required to resolve this issue unambiguously.

3. At certain positions in their sequences, both the K and D molecules exhibit common amino acid residues that distinguish these polypeptides from the human A and B transplantation antigens (Figure 4–44). One explanation for such *species-associated residues* could be that the gene duplication event that presumably created the K and D genes occurred after the divergence of the mouse and human evolutionary lines (Figure 4–46a). An alternative explanation is that the ancestral D and K genes duplicated before mammals diverged and that parallel evolution occurred within each species by some process of gene conversion or correction (Figure 4–46b). Thus either repeated gene duplication has occurred among Class I genes during the mammalian divergences or some type of "communication" (gene conversion or correction) between genes separated by 0.5 map units is required to explain species-associated residues. A similar phenomenon is observed among immunoglobulin sequences (Essential Concept 3–12).

4. The K^k and K^b gene products differ by 5 out of 17 residues, or $\sim 30\%$, and the D gene products differ by 4 out of 14 residues, or $\sim 29\%$ (Figure 4–47). Furthermore, three out of the four K^k amino acid substitutions correspond to two base substitutions in the genetic code dictionary, further emphasizing the evolutionary separation of these "alleles." These differences are consistent with the finding that these transplantation antigens differ in several serological specificities (Table 4–9). These sequence differences constitute some of the largest ever reported for "alleles." Thus the K and D gene products are *complex allotypes*, that is, apparent alleles that differ by multiple amino acid residues

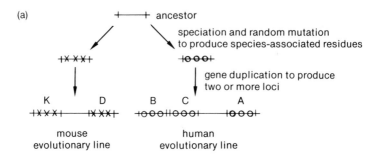

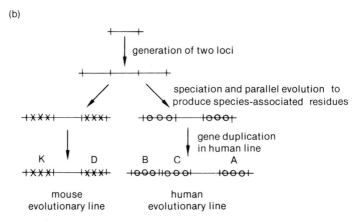

Figure 4–46 A schematic diagram of two hypotheses for the evolution of genes with species associated residues for mammalian transplantation antigens (see text). (a) Duplication *after* speciation. (b) Duplication *before* speciation. The X's and O's designate species-associated residues in the mouse and human evolutionary lines, respectively.

(Essential Concept 3–9c). These transplantation "alleles" may represent closely linked duplicated genes with a control mechanism that permits only one of the genes to be expressed (Figure 3–30c). In support of this model are recent preliminary reports that mouse lymphocytes infected with certain viruses may express Class I genes supposedly not present in the strain supplying the lymphocytes.

5.   A partial amino acid sequence of the α polypeptide (35,000 molecular weight) of an Ia molecule derived from subregion I-E or I-C is shown in Figure 4–48. The α polypeptide shows striking homology to its human counterpart. Thus homology relationships now have been demonstrated between two categories of genes in the major histocompatibility complex of man and mouse—Ia molecules and transplantation antigens. Moreover, the genes that

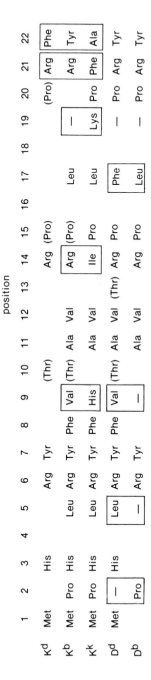

Figure 4–47 Partial amino acid sequences of Class I gene products from the mouse. Boxes indicate positions at which alleles of the K locus or alleles at the D locus differ from one another. For additional details see legend to Figure 4–49. [A compilation of data presented by B. Cunningham et al., S. Nathenson et al., J. Silver et al., and J. Uhr et al. in *Cold Spring Harbor Symp. Quant. Biol.* **41**, 1976.]

position

	1	2	3	4	5	6	7	8	9	10	11	12	13	14	15	16	17	18	19	20	21	22
Kd	Met		His			Arg	Tyr		Val	(Thr)	Ala	Val		Arg	(Pro)					(Pro)	Arg	Phe
Kb	Met	Pro	His		Leu	Arg	Tyr	Phe	Val	(Thr)	Ala	Val		Arg	(Pro)		Leu		—		Arg	Tyr
Kk	Met	Pro	His		Leu	Arg	Tyr	Phe	His		Ala	Val		Ile	Pro		Leu		Lys	Pro	Phe	Ala
Dd	Met	—	His		Leu	Arg	Tyr	Phe	Val	(Thr)	Ala	Val	(Thr)	Arg	Pro		Phe			Pro	Arg	Tyr
Db		Pro			—	Arg	Tyr		—		Ala	Val		Arg	Pro		Leu			Pro	Arg	Tyr

Figure 4–48 Amino acid sequences of the α polypeptides of human and mouse Ia molecules. See legend to Figure 4–44. [Sequence data were obtained from the following sources: human, reproduced from T. A. Springer et al., *Nature* **268**, 213 (1977); I-EC sub-region of mouse, M. McMillan et al., *Proc. Natl. Acad. Sci. USA* **74**, 5135 (1977).]

	1	2	3	4	5	6	7	8	9	10	11	12	13	14	15	16	17	18	19	20
Mouse ECαk	Ile						Ile	Ile		Ala		Phe	Tyr	Leu						
Human p34	Ile	Lys	Glu	Glu	(Arg) Val		Ile	Ile or Leu	Gln	Ala	Glu	Phe	Tyr	Leu	Leu	---	Asn	Tyr	Asp	Phe

Gln   Gly

encode transplantation antigens and certain Ia polypeptides appear to have maintained a close linkage within the major histocompatibility complex over at least the 75 million years during which mouse and man have diverged from one another. This suggests that there are strong selective pressures for maintaining linkage between these genes.

4-14 The 17th chromosome of the mouse has several gene families that apparently control recognition functions of development and immunity

A. The 17th chromosome of the mouse has genetic regions that code for cell-surface molecules involved with neuroectodermal development (T/t locus), immune recognition phenomena (H-2 complex), T-cell differentiation (Qa and Tla complexes), and chronic graft rejection (H-31 and H-32) [Figure 4-49].

The T/t locus, the I region, the S region, the D region, the Qa complex, and the Tla complex each appear to encode two or more gene products. Moreover, the K, D, Qa, and Tla gene products are similar in molecular weight and are associated with β_2-microglobulin, suggesting they may have diverged from a common ancestor. One T/t locus gene product also may be 45,000 in molecular weight and associated with a β_2-microglobulinlike molecule.

B. The *T/t locus* in the mouse is characterized by mutants that affect embryonic development, sperm function, and genetic recombination over a large segment of Chromosome 17.

1. Mutations at the T/t locus fall into two classes, dominant and recessive. All the dominant mutations produce short-tailed heterozygotes (T/+) and are lethal when homozygous (T/T). Recessive mutations produce morphologically normal heterozygotes (t^a/t^b) and interact with dominant T alleles to produce

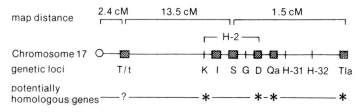

Figure 4-49 A genetic map of Chromosome 17 of the mouse, indicating identified genes (+) or complexes consisting of two or more genes (▨) that code for cell-surface alloantigens. The potentially homologous genes (*) code for gene products of molecular weight 45,000 that associate with β_2-microglobulin. The precise location of the H-31 gene between the H-2 and Tla complexes is unknown.

		genetic crosses			genetic complementation
(a)	parents	T/t^a	x	T/t^a	
	offspring	T/T (die as embryos)	T/t^a tail-less	t^a/t^a (die as embryos)	–
(b)	parents	T/t^a	x	T/t^b	
	offspring	T/T (die as embryos)	$T/t^a\ T/t^b$ tail-less	t^a/t^b morphologically normal	+

Figure 4–50   Complementation of two lethal t alleles, t^a and t^b.

a tail-less phenotype (T/t). Recessive lethal t mutations have been identified in more than 20% of wild mice. Thus there is an enormous, but unknown, selective pressure for these mutants.

2. Mice doubly heterozygous for certain lethal t alleles $(t^a+/+t^b)$ are developmentally and morphologically normal, that is, the mutant alleles complement each other (Figure 4–50). On the basis of such observations, the t mutants can be divided into six complementation groups (Figure 4–51). In the homozygous state (t^a/t^a) mutants in the same complementation group show blocks at a characteristic stage of neuroectodermal development. The t genes appear to code for cell-surface molecules found both on sperm and on cells of certain embryonic tissues at different stages of development. The developmental defect associated with mutant t alleles in a particular complementation group may indicate the developmental stage at which the corresponding wild type allele is expressed (Figure 4–51).

3. The mutant t alleles cause *segregation distortion*. Genetic crosses of the type illustrated in Figure 4–52 show that up to 97% of the progeny of a heterozygous $t/+$ male receive the mutant t allele.

4. The lethal t alleles also appear to suppress crossing over between the T/t locus and the H-2 locus. Indeed, certain t mutants and H-2 haplotypes are in *linkage disequilibrium*, that is, they are inherited together more frequently than would be expected from a separation of 13.5 centimorgans on Chromosome 17. It has been suggested that this suppression of crossing-over permits the H-2 complex and the T locus to behave as a "supergene," that is, to maintain certain combinations of t and H-2 haplotypes.

5. There are several intriguing similarities between the T/t locus and the H-2 complex. Both are found on Chromosome 17. Both appear to encode one or more multigene families and both probably

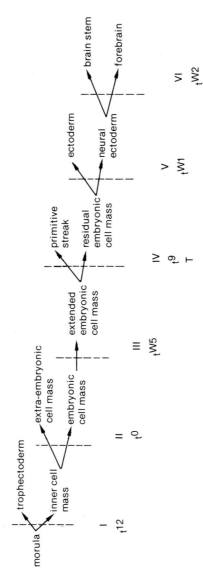

Figure 4–51 The six complementation groups of t mutants and the points at which representative alleles of each group interrupt the development of neuroectodermal structures. The T mutation blocks development at the same stage as t alleles in Group IV. [Adapted from D. Bennett in *Cell Interactions, Third Lepetit Colloquium,* L. G. Silvestri (Ed.), North-Holland Publication Co., Amsterdam, 1972, p. 247.]

$$+/t^a\ (\male)\ \times\ +/+\ (\female)$$

$$\text{segregation} \Big| \text{distortion}$$

$$\text{up to } 97\%\ t^a/+ \text{ offspring}$$

Figure 4–52 A genetic cross indicating segregation distortion in a heterozygous t/+ male mouse.

occupy a large chromosomal region. Both specify cell-surface molecules that are highly polymorphic. Both are in linkage disequilibrium with respect to one another. From these rather general points of similarity, some immunologists have inferred that the T/t locus may represent an embryonic analogue of the H-2 complex; that is, both systems may operate as mediators of cell–cell recognition, the T/t locus primarily in the embryo and the H-2 complex primarily in the adult.

C.   The Qa locus appears to encode at least two cell-surface molecules (Qa-1 and Qa-2) that are present on certain lymphocytes. The Qa-1 molecule only appears to be present on some T_S and T_H cells. Thus the Qa molecules are cell-surface differentiation antigens. Certain of the Qa molecules show a striking general homology to the Class I molecules, in that both are 45,000 in molecular weight and both are noncovalently associated with β_2-microglobulin.

D.   The Tla locus is defined serologically by the TL antigens, which are confined to immature cortical thymocytes. This locus lies 1.5 centimorgans to the right of the H-2 complex. There are three known haplotypes in normal mice (Table 4–11) and four in leukemic cells (Table 4–12) that are defined by four antigens, Tla.1, Tla.2, Tla.3, and Tla.4.

Table 4–11
Tla haplotypes among inbred mice

Tla haplotype	Thymocyte phenotype[a]
a	1, 2, 3, –
b	–, –, –, –
c	–, 2, –, –

[a] indicates that the antigen is not expressed.

Table 4–12
Tla phenotypes and genotypes

Tla haplotypes[a]	Thymocyte Tla phenotype[b]	Leukemia cell phenotype and presumed Tla genotype
a (A)	1, 2, 3, –	1, 2, 3, –
b (C57BL/6)	–, –, –, –	1, 2, –, 4
c (BALB/c)	–, 2, –, –	1, 2, –, –
c (DBA/2)	–, 2, –, –	1, 2, –, 4

[a] in parentheses are given representative inbred strains with the corresponding haplotype.
[b]– indicates that the antigen is not expressed.

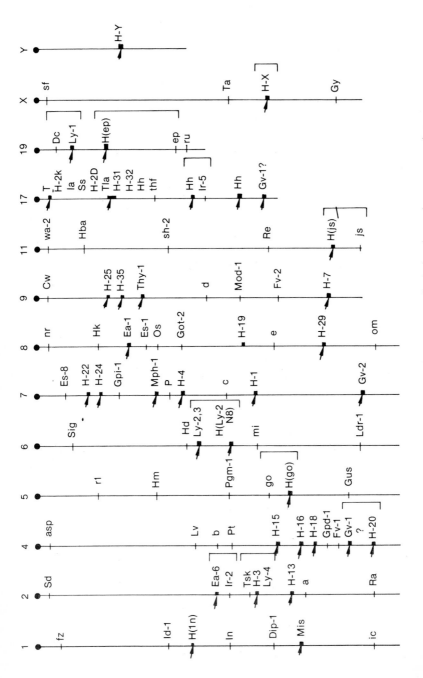

Figure 4–53 A partial linkage map of the mouse, displaying those chromosomes that encode identified membrane cell-surface alloantigens (arrows) and other marker loci. The relative positions of bracketed loci are uncertain. [Adapted from G. D. Snell, J. Dausset, S. Nathenson, *Histocompatibility*, Academic Press, New York, 1976, p. 28.]

1. The fact that Tla.4 is present only in leukemic cells suggests that the Tla locus codes for regulatory gene(s) controlling the expression of the Tla molecules. The genes coding for antigens Tla.1 and Tla.2 are present in all mice, because leukemias from all mouse strains may express these antigens. The Tla.3 and Tla.4 determinants may be coded by alleles at the same locus, since they never appear together in a homozygous mouse. The Ia structural genes might be anywhere in the mouse genome.

2. The Tl antigens can be removed from the cell surface by reaction with antibodies to these antigens. This process has been termed *antigenic modulation.* It has been reported that modulation can be induced by Fab fragments. If this observation is confirmed, antigenic modulation differs from the capping phenomenon, which requires multivalent ligands. Antigens Tla.1, Tla.2, and Tla.3 can be modulated together by anti-Tla.3. Modulation can occur *in vitro* as well as *in vivo,* and can be reversed by removing antisera from the cells.

3. The concentrations of Tla and H-2K antigens on the cell surface are unrelated; however, there is an inverse relationship between the concentrations of Tla and H-2D antigens. This observation is unexplained, but it does suggest either competition for common precursors, competition for common or adjacent membrane sites, or control by a common regulatory mechanism.

4. The Tla molecules show a striking general homology relationship to the Class I molecules. Both are 45,000 in molecular weight and both are noncovalently associated with β_2-microglobulin. These findings raise the possibility that the Tla locus shares a common ancestor with the Class I and Qa genes.

E. Two minor histocompatibility (H) loci, H-31 and H-32, appear to be near the Tla locus (Figure 4–49). Every species of mammal that has been studied possesses a large number of minor H loci, each of which is capable of causing chronic graft rejection. In the mouse there could be as many as several hundred of these loci. Indeed, 35 already have been genetically mapped (Figure 4–53). These loci may control a variety of functions, such as synthesis of enzymes and structural proteins. It is not clear whether any of these loci mediate immunelike recognition phenomena. Perhaps most of the corresponding gene products behave as histocompatibility antigens only because (1) they are polymorphic and (2) they are located on the cell surface. Variant products of these loci are recognized as nonself by the MHC-dependent recognition system, and a cytotoxic reaction can be mounted against these variant cells just as it is against virally infected cells with neoantigens (Essential Concept 1–12). Thus the minor H loci may have emerged as histocompatibility loci with the emergence of the surveillance function of the MHC.

Selected Bibliography

Where to begin

Cunningham, B. A., "The structure and function of histocompatibility antigens," *Sci. Am.* **237,** 96 (1977).

Greaves, M. F., *Cellular Recognition*, Chapman and Hall, Ltd., London, 1975. A brief and well written summary of communication across the plasma membrane and various systems that have been studied in this connection.

Singer, S. J., "Architecture and topography of biologic membranes," in *Cell Membranes: Biochemistry, Cell Biology and Pathology*, G. Weissmann, and R. Claiborne (Eds.), H. P. Publishing Co., Inc., New York, 1975, p. 35. A clear summary of the fluid mosaic model of membrane structure.

General

Cuatrecasas, P., and Greaves, M. F. (Eds.), *Receptors and Recognition*, Chapman and Hall, Ltd., London, 1975. An excellent series of articles on many different aspects of the cell surface.

Klein, J., *Biology of the Mouse Histocompatibility-2 Complex*, Springer-Verlag, New York, 1975. A well written book that clearly introduces the general principles as well as the finer details of the mouse MHC.

McMahon, D., and Fox, C. F. (Eds.), *Developmental Biology*, W. A. Benjamin, Inc., Menlo Park, Calif., 1975. This book contains a series of articles on cellular adhesion and pattern formation.

Snell, G. D., Dausset, J., and Nathanson, S., *Histocompatibility*, Academic Press, New York, 1976. A book that covers every aspect of mammalian histocompatibility.

Weissmann, G., and Claiborne, R. (Eds.), *Cell Membranes: Biochemistry, Cell Biology and Pathology*, H. P. Publishing Co., Inc., New York, 1975. A collection of well written and nicely illustrated articles on various aspects of the cell surface.

Slime-mold cell surfaces

Barondes, S. H., and Rosen, S. D., "Cellular recognition in slime molds: evidence for its mediation by cell-surface species-specific lectins and complementary oligosaccharides," in *Receptors and Recognition*, Cuatrecasas, P., and Greaves, M. F. (Eds.), Chapman and Hall, Ltd., London, 1975. A summary of the evidence for lectinlike receptors in slime molds.

Membrane glycoproteins

Ashwell, G., and Morell, A. G., "Membrane glycoproteins and recognition phenomena," *Trends in Biol. Sci.* **2**, 76 (1977). A brief, up-to-date review of carbohydrates and cell-surface specificity.

Watkins, W. M., "Blood-group substances," *Science* **152**, 172 (1966). An old but well-written paper on the human ABO system.

Cellular adhesion

Glaser, L., "Cell–cell recognition," *Trends in Biol. Sci.* **1**, 84 (1976). A brief review of this area with up-to-date references.

Gottlieb, D. I., Rock, K., and Glaser, L., "A gradient of adhesive specificity in developing avian retina," *Proc. Natl. Acad. Sci. USA* **73**, 410 (1976). This paper employs membrane fragments to study cell-surface specificity.

Moscona, A. A., "Embryonic cell surfaces: mechanisms of cell recognition and morphogenetic cell adhesion," in *Developmental Biology*, McMahon, D., and Fox, C. F. (Eds.), W. A. Benjamin, Inc., Menlo Park, Calif., 1975, p. 19. A summary of evidence for the hypothesis that specific cell surface molecules mediate tissue adhesion.

Cell recognition in invertebrates

Burnet, F. M., "Self-recognition in colonial marine forms and flowering plants in relation to the evolution of immunity," *Nature* **232**, 230 (1972).

Oka, H., and Watanabe, H., "Problems of colony-specificity in compound ascidians," *Bull. Marine Biol. Station Asamush.* **10**, 153 (1960).

Valembois, P., "Cellular aspects of graft rejection in earthworm and some other metazoa," *Cont. Topics Immunobiol.* **4**, 121 (1974).

A series of papers that probe the ancient origins of the immune system.

Major histocompatibility complex: serology, genetics, and function

Bodmer, W. F., "Evolutionary significance of the HLA system," *Nature* **237**, 139 (1972).

Klein, J., "Evolution and function of the major histocompatibility complex: facts and speculations," in *Major Histocompatibility Complex*, Gotze, D. (Ed.), Springer-Verlag, New York, 1977, p. 339.

Schreffler, D. C., and David, C. S., "The H-2 major histocompatibility complex and the I immune response region: genetic variation, function, and organization," *Adv. Immunol.* **20**, 125 (1975).

The Role of Products of the Histocompatibility Gene Complex in Immune Responses, Katz, D. H., and Benacerraf, B. (Eds.), Academic Press, New York, 1976.

"Origins of Lymphocyte Diversity," *Cold Spring Harbor Symp. Quant. Biol.* **41** (1976).

Schreffler, D. C., "The S region of the mouse major histocompatibility complex (H-2): genetic variation and functional role in complement system," *Transplant. Rev.* **32**, 140 (1976).

Zinkernagel, R. M., and Doherty, P. C., "Major transplantation antigens, viruses, and specificity of surveillance T cells," *Contemp. Top. Immunobiol.* **7**, 179 (1977).

A series of excellent reviews and articles that discuss in detail the serology, genetics, and function of the major histocompatibility complex.

Major histocompatibility complex: structure

Silver, J., and Hood, L., "Preliminary amino acid sequences of transplantation antigens: genetic and evolutionary implications," *Contemp. Top. Mol. Immunol.* **5**, 35 (1976).

Strominger, J. L., Mann, D. L., Parham, P., Robb, R., Springer, T., and Terhorst, C., "Structure of HLA A and B antigens isolated from cultured human lymphocytes," *Cold Spring Harbor Symp. Quant. Biol.* **41**, 323 (1976).

Walsh, F. S., and Crumpton, M. J., "Orientation of cell-surface antigens in the lipid bilayer of lymphocyte plasma membrane," *Nature* **269**, 307 (1977).

These three articles and reviews show how the chemical analysis of Class I and II gene products has provided insights into their structure, genetic organization, and evolution.

The T/t complex

Bennett, D., "The T-locus of the mouse," *Cell* **6**, 441 (1975).

Klein, J., and Hammerberg, C., "The control of differentiation by the T complex," *Immunol. Rev.* **33**, 70 (1977).

Jacob, F., "Mouse teratocarcinoma and embryonic antigens," *Immunol. Rev.* **33**, 1 (1977).

These three papers are general reviews of this fascinating mouse chromosomal region.

Miscellaneous references

Edelman, G. M., "Surface modulation in cell recognition and cell growth," *Science* **192**, 218 (1976). Some new hypotheses on phenotypic alteration and transmembranous control of cell-surface receptors.

Hood, L., Huang, H. V., and Dreyer, W. J., "The area-code hypothesis: the immune system provides clues to understanding the genetic and molecular basis of cell recognition during development," *J. Supramol. Struct.* 7 (1977), 531. Some ideas about cell-recognition molecules and how their genes are organized and expressed.

Problems

4–1   Indicate whether each of the following statements is true or false. Explain the error in each statement you consider to be false.
(a)   The plasma membrane is generally impermeable to polar molecules.
(b)   Cholesterol has a molecular shape that is very different from the shapes of other membrane lipids.
(c)   Glycoproteins form spontaneous bilayers in aqueous solution.
(d)   The loose association of peripheral proteins with the plasma membrane makes it difficult to define precisely the outer and inner limits of the cell surface.
(e)   Glycophorin is an integral membrane protein with linearly distributed hydrophilic and hydrophobic domains.
(f)   Most membrane glycoproteins attach their oligosaccharide moieties through serine, threonine, or asparagine residues.
(g)   Lipids may flip-flop across the membrane almost as rapidly as they diffuse in a translational direction.
(h)   Membranes with predominantly saturated fatty acids are more fluid than those with a higher degree of unsaturated fatty acids.
(i)   Microfilaments appear to have direct connections with the plasma membrane and therefore may be involved in cellular movements.
(j)   The heavy chain of the immunoglobulin receptor molecule is known to be identical to that of antibody secreted by that same lymphocyte.
(k)   Slime molds have cell-surface recognition molecules with lectinlike properties.
(l)   When disassociated liver and retinal cells from chick and mouse embryos are mixed together and gently agitated, the two species of liver cells specifically associate with one another, but not with either species of retinal cells.
(m)   Interaction of anti-Le^b antibodies and the Le^b human blood group specificity can be inhibited by a monosaccharide.
(n)   Allogeneic reactions in tunicates lead to union between sex cells and rejection between somatic cells.
(o)   Coelomocytes that aid in graft rejection in earthworms resemble lymphocytes morphologically.

(p)   The major histocompatibility complex has been found in all mammals studied to date.

(q)   The mixed lymphocyte reaction (MLR) and the graft versus host reaction (GVHR) are indicative of a similar phenomenon *in vivo* and *in vitro*, respectively.

(r)   Two congenic strains that differ at the H-2 complex may also differ in genes closely linked to the H-2 complex.

(s)   The H-2 complex has sufficient DNA to code for 10–20 genes 600 nucleotides in length.

(t)   A single D gene product from the mouse may contain multiple public and private serological specificities.

(u)   All vertebrates exhibit the ability to destroy allografts by an acute rejection process.

(v)   The Class I gene products of man, mouse, and guinea pig show amino-acid-sequence homologies.

(w)   The gene products of the K and D alleles of the mouse are examples of complex allotypes.

(x)   The six complementation groups of the T/t locus appear to govern the differentiation of the immune system.

(y)   The Tla locus is multigenic in nature.

(z)   Minor histocompatibility loci encode cell-surface antigens.

4-2   Supply the missing word or words in each of the following statements.

(a)   The three major kinds of membrane lipids are _____, _____, and _____.

(b)   _____ interactions are primarily responsible for the thermodynamic tendency of lipid bilayers to form in aqueous solutions.

(c)   _____ molecules have distinct hydrophobic and hydrophilic regions.

(d)   Membrane proteins can be divided into two categories: _____ and _____.

(e)   _____ confers a significant negative charge on most plasma membranes.

(f)   The two types of carbohydrate linkages to glycoproteins are _____ and _____.

(g)   Oligosaccharide synthesis is not mediated by a template mechanism; instead, _____ are responsible for the enzymatic synthesis of these macromolecules.

(h)   _____ are proteins or glycoproteins isolated from plants that exhibit specificities for monosaccharides.

(i)   _____ are submembranous elements composed of actin that appear to be involved in various cell movements.

(j)   A membrane receptor must carry out three distinct functions: _____, _____, and _____.

(k)   The _____ of the receptor immunoglobulin is attached to the lymphocyte membrane.

(l)   The five distinct blood-group specificities of the Lewis and ABO systems are _____, _____, _____, _____, and _____.

(m)   The monosaccharide that determines the A blood-group specificity is _____.

(n)   Two general mechanisms of specific cellular association are _____ and _____ recognition.

(o)   Graft rejection in earthworms appears to be mediated by cells termed _____.

(p)   The major histocompatibility complex of man is designated _____, and that of the mouse is designated _____.

(q)   _____ mice are genetically identical except for a single chromosomal region.

(r)   A unique combination of alleles at loci within the MHC is termed a _____.

(s)   Regions and subregions of the H-2 complex are defined by _____ events among distinct genes.

(t)   The Class I regions of the MHC code for the classical _____.

(u)   Serological specificities shared by many Class I molecules are said to be _____ specificities.

(v)   The I-J subregion appears to code for an antigen-specific T-cell _____.

(w)   LD is an abbreviation for _____, which provide an assay for Class _____ gene products.

(x)   The primary structures of the transplantation antigens of mice, guinea pigs, and men are _____ to one another.

(y)   _____ allotypes are those that differ by multiple amino acid residues.

(z)   The cell-surface TL antigens become inaccessible upon reaction with specific antibodies. This process is termed _____.

4–3   (a)   Consider Table 4–5 and then suggest a plausible scheme for human blood transfusions between individuals of different blood groups. Who is a universal donor? Who is a universal recipient? Explain.

(b)   What other factors should be considered in blood transfusions apart from the ABO blood groups?

4–4   Which member of each of the following pairs of membrane components will make a membrane more fluid when present as part of the structure?

(a)   (1) $CH_3(CH_2)_7CH = CH(CH_2)_7COO^-$ or (2) $CH_3(CH_2)_{16}COO^-$

(b)   (1) $CH_3(CH_2)_{16}COO^-$ or (2) $CH_2(CH_2)_{14}COO^-$

(c)   (1) $CH_5(CH_2)_{16}COO^-$ or (2) the compound shown in Figure 4–54.

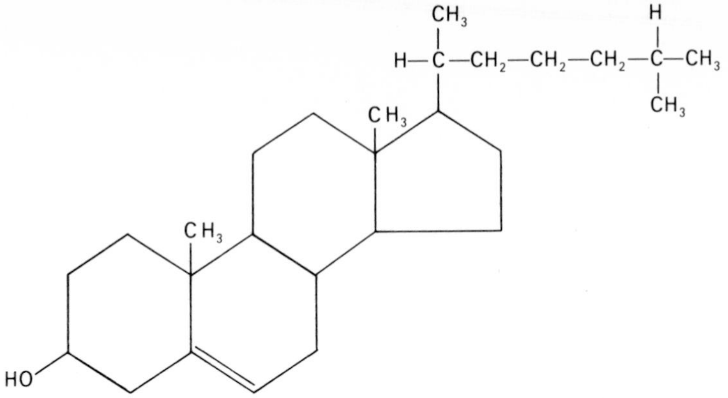

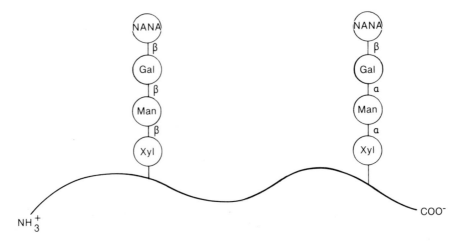

Figure 4—54 The structural formula of a membrane component (Problem 4—4).

Figure 4—55 A hypothetical polypetide chain with two oligosaccharides (Problem 4—5). α and β denote configurations of glycosidic linkages. Abbreviations for monosaccharide residues are explained in the legend to Figure 4—16.

4–5   (a)   Figure 4–55 shows a hypothetical polypeptide chain with two attached oligosaccharides. Assume that the carbohydrate residues are linked through the same hydroxyl groups in both oligosaccharides. How many glycosyl transferases would be necessary to synthesize these chains?

(b)   To which amino acid would these oligosaccharides be linked?

4–6   Why must individuals who exhibit a strong Le[a] specificity on their red blood cells be nonsecretors?

4–7   The carbohydrates shown in Figure 4–56 can be derived from alkaline or acid hydrolysis of various human blood-group substances. Each carbohydrate has the ability to inhibit the hemagglutination test for a specific blood-group specificity. Identify the specificity blocked by each carbohydrate.

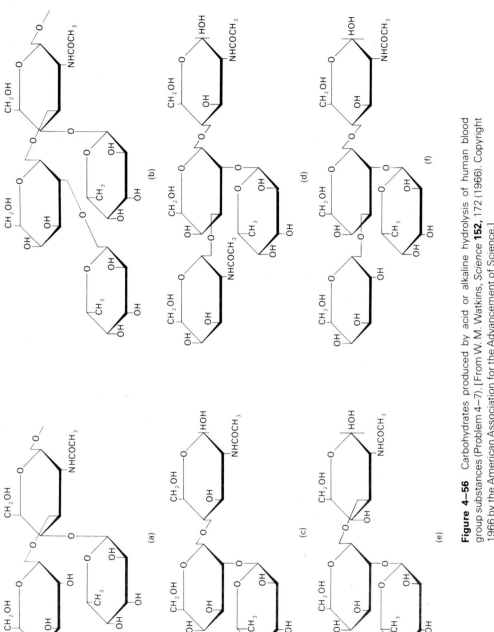

Figure 4-56 Carbohydrates produced by acid or alkaline hydrolysis of human blood group substances (Problem 4–7). [From W. M. Watkins, *Science* **152**, 172 (1966). Copyright 1966 by the American Association for the Advancement of Science.]

4-8 A new alloantigen, S, is discovered on the spleen cells of the A inbred strain of rats, and is missing on the corresponding cells of the B inbred strain. This alloantigen is expressed in (A × B) F_1 individuals and segregates in a classical Mendelian fashion. Two surprising observations are made. (a) Occasional leukemias that arise in the B strain express the S antigen. (b) Rats of the B strain can be immunized with lethally irradiated cells of an S^+ B-strain leukemia; these rats then produce anti-S antibodies which will kill S^+ B-strain leukemia cells *in vitro*. However, when such immunized rats are injected with S^+ B-strain leukemic cells, the rats are killed by the leukemia. Leukemic cells taken from these rats are S^-. However, the S^+ phenotype of these cells reappears upon passage of the tumor through nonimmune hosts. What conclusions can you draw from these observations?

4-9 Suppose that you inject mouse red blood cells into a rabbit and then carry out the analysis shown in Table 4-13.
(a) What is the minimum number of antigenic determinants required to explain these reactions? Use the symbols A, B, C, etc. for antigenic determinants.
(b) What analogies can you draw between these determinants and known cell-surface components?

Table 4-13
An absorption analysis of rabbit anti-mouse red blood cell (RBC) serum (Problem 4-9)

Mouse test cells		Rabbit anti-mouse RBC serum			
			Absorbed with:		
Source	Unabsorbed	RBC	Liver	Kidney	Brain
RBC	+[a]	−	+	+	+
Liver	+	−	−	−	−
Kidney	+	−	−	−	−
Brain	+	−	+	+	−

[a] +indicates a positive reaction between the rabbit anti-mouse RBC serum and mouse red blood cells. − indicates a negative reaction.

4-10 Suppose you prepare an alloantiserum by immunizing an inbred mouse of Strain A with cells "X" from an inbred mouse of a different strain. The absorption analysis of this serum is presented in Table 4-14.
(a) How might you interpret these results in terms of the minimum number of antigenic determinants necessary to explain them? Use the symbols A, B, C, etc. as antigenic determinants.
(b) Which of these antigens do the X cells have? May the X cells have additional antigens? Which of these antigens are present on cells from the host in which the antiserum was raised?

Table 4–14

An absorption analysis of anti-X serum: distribution of the reaction (+ versus −) of the serum with cells of four mice from different inbred strains, 1–4 (Problem 4–10)

| Test cells from each of four inbred strains | Anti-X serum | | | | |
| | | Absorbed with test cells of strain: | | | |
	Unabsorbed	1	2	3	4
1	+	−	+	−	+
2	+	+	−	−	+
3	+	+	+	−	+
4	+	−	−	−	−

(c)   Are the detectable antigens allelic forms of the same structural gene? How would your answer change if mice 1 through 4 were wild mice?

(d)   How may you raise an alloantiserum that is directed specifically against the product of a single genetic locus?

4–11   The rejection of tissue transplants is determined by multiple histocompatibility or H genes. Graft acceptance occurs if all the histocompatibility alleles present on the graft are also present in the host. The H alleles code for alloantigenic cell-surface molecules present on most tissues, which induce an immune response in an allogeneic or xenogeneic host. In an individual heterozygous at an H locus, both gene products are expressed on the cell surface. This phenomenon is termed codominance. From these simple generalizations and the following data it is possible to deduce the five laws of transplantation first summarized in 1941 by the pioneer of mouse transplantation genetics, C. C. Little.

In the following problems, the different histocompatibility loci are represented by H-1, H-2, H-3, etc. Different alleles at one locus are indicated by H-1^a, H-1^b, H-1^c, etc. Suppose that two inbred strains of mice, A and B, with a single histocompatibility difference at the H-2 locus are crossed. The results of transplants to various generations are given in Table 4–15.

(a)   Comment on the acceptance or failure of the following grafts and explain in molecular terms why failure or acceptance occurred: (1) from Strain A to Strain A individuals, (2) from Strain A to Strain B individuals, (3) from Strain A to F_1 individuals, and from F_1 individuals to Strain A, (4) from F_2 or subsequent generations to F_1 individuals, and (5) from Strain A to F_2 individuals, and to individuals resulting from a backcross of F_1 individuals to Strain B.

(b)   When the parents differ at one H locus, what fraction of the

Table 4–15
The expected outcome of transplants made from Strain A to Strain B, and to F_1, F_2, and backcross generations produced by crossing Strain A and Strain B (Problem 4–11)[a]

Generations	Genotypes and outcomes of transplants		
	Strain A	F_1	Strain B
Parental strains (P)	H-2ª/H-2ª(+)		H-2ᵇ/H-2ᵇ(−)
F_1		H-2ª/H-2ᵇ(+)	
F_2	25% H-2ª/H-2ª(+)	50% H-2ª/H-2ᵇ(+)	25% H-2ᵇ/H-2ᵇ(−)
Backcross of F¹ to Strain B		50% H-2ª/H-2ᵇ(+)	50% H-2ᵇ/H-2ᵇ(−)

[a]A plus (+) sign indicates graft acceptance, a minus (−) graft rejection.
[From G. Snell and J. Stimpfling in *Biology of the Laboratory Mouse*, E. L. Green (Ed.), McGraw-Hill, New York, 1966, p. 457.]

F_1 generation is susceptible to tumor grafts from one of the parents? What fraction of the F_2 generation? What fraction of a backcross generation?

(c)   Suppose the parents differ at two H loci. Answer the same questions as for Part (b).

(d)   Can you generalize from Answers (b) and (c) to predict what fraction of F_1, F_2, and backcross individuals will be susceptible to a parental tumor if two inbred strains that differ at n histocompatibility loci are crossed?

(e)   How could this prediction be used to estimate a lower limit for the number of H loci in various inbred strains of mice or in wild mice?

4–12   Suppose that you have generated four congenic strains, three from mating inbred Strains A and B [A.B(1), A.B(2), and A.B(3)] and the fourth from mating inbred Strains A and C [A.C(4)]. Assume that each congenic strain differs from the background strain A at either the H-1 or H-2 locus. Pairs of the congenic lines are crossed and the F_1 generation is challenged with a tumor transplant from the A strain (Table 4–15). This experiment is termed the F_1 *test*.

(a)   What conclusions can you draw about the identity of the histocompatibility loci in various strains?

(b)   Table 4–16 is an actual analysis of congenic strains by the F_1 test. What conclusions can you draw about the identity of the H loci in the two congenic strains?

(c)   Given a known congenic strain A.B that carries the H-1ᵇ allele in an A background, how can an F_1 test be used to determine whether the H-1 allele in a new congenic strain A.U is the same as or different from the H-1ª allele in the background strain?

Table 4–16
Analysis of CR lines B10.C(41N) and B10.C(47N) by the F_1 test[a] (Problem 4–12)

		Test F_1's			Simultaneous controls	
Experiment	Known parent	Difference from C57BL/10	Unknown parent	Fraction dying	Strain	Fraction dying
					C57BL/10	50/50
					B10.C(47N)	0/27
1	B10.LP	H-3	B10.C(41N)	10/10	B10.LP	0/10
2	B10.BY	H-1	B10.C(41N)	0/10		
3	B10.129(5M)	H-1	B10.C(41N)	0/10	B10.129(5M)	0/10
4	B10.129(5M)	H-1	B10.C(47N)	10/10		
5	B10.C(41N)	H-1	B10.C(47N)	10/10	B10.C(41N)	0/10
6	B10.D2	H-2	B10.C(47N)	10/10		
7	B10.LP	H-3	B10.C(47N)	10/10	B10.LP	0/19
8	B10.129(21M)	H-4	B10.C(47N)	10/10	B10.129(21M)	0/19

[a]Strains run as controls with each group always including the susceptible congenic partner. C57BL/10, and usually one or both of the CR strains used as parents in any given cross. All mice were preimmunized with three injections of C57BL/10 thymus and challenged with a C57BL/10 transplantable leukemia. CR denotes congenic resistant. [From G. Snell and J. Stimpfling in *Biology of the Laboratory Mouse*, E. L. Green (Ed.), McGraw-Hill, New York, 1966, p. 457.]

4–13   Class I cell-surface molecules can be analyzed by serological techniques. For example, if cells from a mouse of background Strain A (H-2^a) haplotype are injected into mice congenic at the H-2 complex (A.B), the congenic mice make antibodies against the antigenic determinants encoded by the H-2^a complex that are different from those encoded by the H-2^b complex. Appropriate cross absorptions can then render the antiserum specific for one (monospecific) or a few H-2 determinants. This is one way that a series of specific alloantisera have been raised against various H-2 specificities. The antigenic determinants present on the most common H-2 chromosomes from inbred strains of mice are given in Table 4–9.
(a)   Which H-2 chromosome in Table 4–9 encodes the most public antigenic determinants? The least? Which polypeptide (K or D) carries the most? The least?
(b)   What explanation can you offer for the presence of multiple antigenic determinants on a single polypeptide?
(c)   Explain the distinction between private and public H-2 specificities.
(d)   What does the existence of identical or cross-reactive specificities shared between the D and K regions of the H-2 complex suggest about the evolution of these regions?

4–14   The H-2 K and H-2 D Class I molecules are integral membrane proteins that are difficult to purify. These alloantigens constitute somewhat less

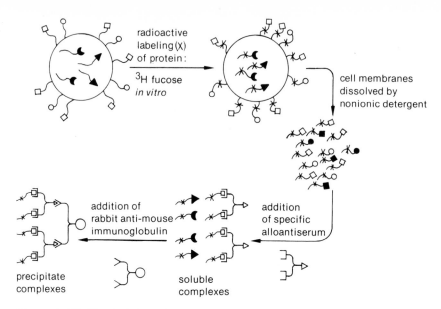

Figure 4–57 The isolation of specific membrane molecules by indirect immuno-precipitation (Problem 4–14).

than 1% of the protein in the membranes of mouse spleen cells. A partial purification has been achieved by *indirect immunoprecipitation.* This technique employs specific alloantisera to isolate alloantigens, as depicted in Figure 4–57. Class I molecules are radiolabeled by incubation of living spleen cells *in vitro* with tritiated fucose. The membranes of the radiolabeled cells then are solubilized by incubating with the nonionic detergent NP-40. This detergent solubilizes the membrane without destroying the antigenic determinants on the alloantigens. The soluble spleen cell extract is incubated with a specific unlabeled mouse alloantibody, for example anti-H-2K^a. This alloantibody combines with its complementary alloantigen, but the complex does not precipitate. Precipitation is achieved by adding goat anti-mouse gamma globulin, which combines with the mouse alloantibody and precipitates the entire complex. When the complex is run on SDS polyacrylamide gels, the specific H-2K or H-2D product appears as a single tritiated peak of about 45,000 daltons.

Consider the following experiment. Spleen cells from F_1 mice (H-2^a/H-2^b heterozygous) are labeled with ^{3}H-fucose. Alloantisera that detect private specificities of the four H-2 gene products present are used: specificity H-2.4 to detect the H-2D^a gene product, specificity H-2.11 to detect the H-2K^a gene product, specificity H-2.33 to detect the H-2K^b gene product, and specificity H-2.2 to detect the H-2D^b gene product (see Table 4–9). The ^{3}H-fucose-labeled antigen preparation is solubilized with NP-40 and divided into five portions (*A–E*). *A* is reacted with a control antiserum that can detect none of the specificities known to exist in this heterozygous cell type. *B* is reacted with antiserum to H-2.2; *C* with an antiserum to H-2.4; *D* with an antiserum to H-2.11; and *E* with an antiserum to H-2.33. Goat anti-mouse gamma globulin is added, and the precipitates that form are removed from the supernatant solutions. In the next phase of this experiment, the supernatant solutions from *A*, *B*, *C*, *D*, and *E* each are subdivided into five portions and retested for the presence of radioactive material reactive with the five antisera. The results of this second set of alloantigen–antibody precipitin assays are presented in Figure 4–58, which shows the polyacrylamide gel patterns obtained from these precipitates.

(a)   What can you deduce from Figure 4–58 about the molecular structure of the various private alloantigens on the cell surface of spleen cells from a heterozygous mouse? Explain your reasoning.

(b)   What does this finding indicate about the expression of the genes that code for these alloantigens in heterozygous mice?

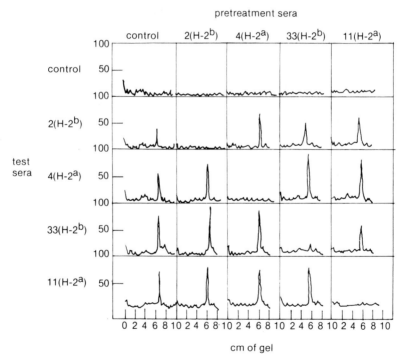

Figure 4–58 The analysis by immunoprecipitation of antigen extracts solubilized with NP-40 (Problem 4–14). This figure shows the SDS-polyacrylamide gel patterns of precipitates from the reactions of test antisera (shown on the *left* of the figure) with the supernatant fraction remaining after reaction with the pretreatment antisera (shown across the *top* of the figure) and removal of the resulting precipitate. The cpm of ³H-fucose labeled antigen are plotted along the ordinate of each graph. [From S. Cullen *et al.*, *Proc. Natl. Acad. Sci. USA* **69,** 1394 (1972).]

4–15   (a)   The techniques originally developed for the study of the H-2K and H-2D products of the major histocompatibility complex of the mouse can be employed to search for other cell-surface antigens (see Problem 4–14). For this purpose inbred strains of mice that are recombinant at the H-2 complex have been particularly useful (Table 4–17). An antiserum was made by injecting spleen cells from A.TL mice into A.TH mice. These inbred strains are congenic at the H-2 complex. The haplotypes of these and other relevant inbred strains are given in Table 4–17. By indirect immunoprecipitation, the A.TH anti-A.TL antiserum was used to isolate cell-surface molecules radioactively labeled with ^{125}I from spleen cells of a B10.D2 mouse. The antigens isolated were electrophoresed on SDS polyacrylamide gels to separate molecules on the basis of their molecular weight. The gels were then cut into thin slices and counted for radioactivity, as shown in Figure 4–59. Suggest the probable identity of the peaks that range in molecular weight from 28,000 to 35,000.

(b)   A second antiserum was made by injecting cells from B10.D2 mouse spleens into (B10 × A) F$_1$ hybrids. Figure 4–60 shows the gel pattern obtained when the antigens from radioactively labeled B10.D2 cell membranes were isolated using this antiserum. Against what antigens would you expect the (B10 × A) F$_1$ anti-B10.D2 antiserum to be directed?

(c)   How does your reasoning in (b) check with the data in Figure 4–60?

(d)   The technique of using antisera made in congenic strains to immunoprecipitate specific antigens requires awareness of some important limitations. Suggest several limitations in this technique.

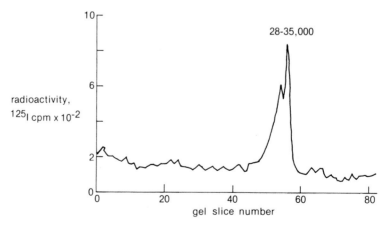

Figure 4–59   SDS-polyacrylamide gel electrophoresis of molecules isolated from B10.D2 spleen cells by indirect immunoprecipitation using A.TH anti-A.TL antiserum (Problem 4–15). Numbers above peaks indicate molecular weights. [Courtesy of J. Silver.]

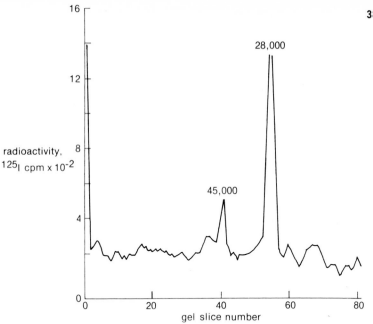

Figure 4–60 SDS-polyacrylamide gel electrophoresis of molecules isolated from B10.D2 spleen cells by indirect immunoprecipitation using (B10 x A) F_1 anti-B10.D2 antiserum (Problem 4–15). Numbers above peaks indicate molecular weights. [Courtesy of J. Silver.]

Table 4–17
H-2 haplotypes of various recombinant inbred mouse strains (Problem 4–15)

Strain	H-2 haplotype	Region of H-2 complex			
		K	I	S	D
A	a	k	k	d	d
B10	b	b	b	b	b
B10.D2	d	d	d	d	d
A.TH	th	s	s	s	d
A.TL	tl	s	k	k	d

4–16 Reciprocal immunizations of congenic mouse strains allow one to raise specific antisera with which to study the genetic organization of the H-2 complex. Three specific antisera raised in three congenic strains of C57BL mice carrying the H-2b, d, or k haplotypes, respectively, were tested against cells from each congenic strain as shown in Table 4–18. In some experiments, the antisera were first absorbed with lymphocytes carrying the indicated haplotype.

(a) What is the minimum number of specificities detected by these antisera?

(b) Which specificities are associated with each haplotype?

Table 4–18
Absorption experiments with anti-H-2 antisera and cells from three different haplotypes (Problem 4–16)

Antiserum	Haplotype of cells used for absorption	Haplotype of "target" cells		
		b	d	k
d-anti-k	—	+a	0	+
	b	0	0	+
b-anti-d	—	0	+	+
	k	0	+	0
k-anti-b	—	+	+	0
	d	+	0	0

a+ indicates a serological reaction; 0 indicates no reaction.

(c) Are specificities shared?

(d) Assume that these specificities all are present on K-region gene products. If so, how would you reconcile this fact with the immunochemical evidence that the K region of each haplotype codes for a single, distinct cell-surface molecule?

(e) Cells from (b × d) F_1 progeny reacted with both the b-anti-d antiserum absorbed with k cells and the k-anti-b antiserum absorbed with d cells. What does this result indicate about expression of these antigens?

(f) The (b × d) F_1 mice were backcrossed with d mice. Cells from half the backcross mice reacted with both absorbed antisera ("F_1-like" mice); cells from the other mice reacted only with the absorbed b-anti-d antiserum. Explain.

(g) One thousand backcross "F_1-like" mice received (b × d) F_1 skin grafts. Every mouse except one accepted the graft. The exceptional mouse, X, subsequently rejected another F_1 graft, this time even more vigorously. Suggest an explanation for these observations.

(h) Suggest a way to test your hypothesis in Part (g).

4–17 In order to examine the hypothesis that the T/t complex codes for a sperm cell-surface antigen, sperm from a T/t^{w2} individual (see Figure 4–51) were used to immunize wild type (+/+) male mice (antiserum). In addition, sperm from a BALB/c mouse congenic for the T^J allele were used to immunize ordinary BALB/c mice (Antiserum 2). Antisera 1 and 2 were absorbed with recipient-type sperm to remove sperm autoantibody.

(a) Various tissues were used to absorb Antiserum 1 to determine whether the T/t^{w2} specificity is found on tissues other than sperm. The absorbed antisera were then reacted with BALB/T^J sperm in the presence of complement. If antibodies combine with sperm in the presence of complement, the sperm are killed; therefore this reaction is called a *cytotoxicity test*. The dead sperm are detected by their inability to exclude the dye trypan blue. The results of various absorption tests are given in Figure 4–61. Assume differences such as that between control and BALB sperm-absorbed sera in Figure 4–61a are caused by nonspecific absorption. What would you conclude from these four experiments?

(b)   Consider the experiments in Table 4–19. What is the importance of using the congenic strain $BALB/T^J$ in Table 4–19? Explain the results observed.

(c)   In view of the probable cellular location of the T/t^{w2} gene products, how may they play a role in segregation distortion? Is the T/t^{w2} allele likely to be expressed in the diploid state of early sperm development, or in the haploid state?

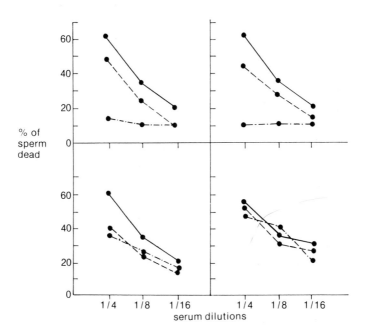

Figure 4–61   The tissue representation of antigen T determined by absorption of $+/+$ anti-T/t^{w2} serum with various cell types and subsequent testing on BALB/T^J sperm (Problem 4–17). Control (—): no absorption except for routine preabsorption with $+/+$ testicular cells to remove sperm autoantibody. (a) absorbed with BALB sperm (---); absorbed with BALB/T^J sperm (-•-). (b) absorbed with BALB testicular cells (---); absorbed with BALB/T^J testicular cells (-•-). (c) absorbed with BALB brain cells (---); absorbed with BALB/T^J brain cells (-•-). (d) absorbed with T/t^{w2} lymphocytes and thymocytes (---); absorbed with $+/+$ lymphocytes and thymocytes (-•-). [From D. Bennett et al., *Proc. Natl. Acad. Sci. USA* **69**, 2076 (1972).]

Table 4–19
Cytotoxicity tests with serum[a] of BALB male mice immunized with BALB/T sperm; T-specificity was confirmed by tests on epididymal sperm of mice of selected genotypes (Problem 4–17)

Sperm tested	Result of cytotoxicity test (% sperm dead)
BALB/T^J	60
BALB/T^J	41
BALB/T^J	50
T/+	75
T/+	45
BALB	<20
BALB	<20
+/+	<20
+/+	<20

[a]Serum dilution: 1/4.
[From D. Bennett et al., Proc. Natl. Acad. Sci. USA **69,** 2076 (1972).]

4–18   The mutant t alleles are found in high frequencies in wild mouse populations. These populations are highly polymorphic at the T/t locus, which differs in this respect from most loci at which recessive lethal alleles are found. In the heterozygous state, most mutant t alleles suppress crossing-over throughout a large region of Chromosome 17. The high frequency of heterozygous t/+ mice in wild populations suggests that the mutant t alleles may confer a physiological advantage that outweighs their lethality in the homozygous state and that has led to the evolution of preferential t allele transmission by males as a mechanism for maintaining these alleles in the population. Can you suggest a possible physiological advantage to crossover suppression on Chromosome 17 that may create a selective pressure for maintenance of mutant t alleles?

4–19   Six groups of individuals are distinguishable on the basis of the ABO and Lewis (Le^a or Le^b) red-cell phenotype and the A, B, H, Le^a, and Le^b activities present in secretions (See Figure 4–22). Table 4–20 presents results of serological tests on red blood cells (RBC) and secretions from these six groups.
(a)   Predict the probable genotype for each group (H or h/h; Le or le/le; Se or se/se).
(b)   Why is Le^b not expressed in Group 2?
(c)   Why is Le^b not expressed in Group 5?
(d)   What blood-group specificities cannot be present in the secretions of individuals with se/se genotype?
(e)   Individuals of Group 4 have in their secretions substances that are closely related chemically to the A, B, H, and Le^a substances.

Table 4–20

Red-cell phenotypes in six groups of individuals[a] (Problem 4–19)

Group	Probable genotype	Antigen detectable on RBC			Specificities detectable in secretions		
		ABH	Le[a]	Le[b]	ABH	Le[a]	Le[b]
1	?	+++	−	++	+++	+	++
2	?	+++	+++	−	−	+++	−
3	?	+++	−	−	+++	−	−
4	?	+++	−	−	−	−	−
5	?	−	+++	−	−	+++	−
6	?	−	−	−	−	−	−

[a] +++, strong specific activity; +, weak specific activity; −, no activity; ABH +++ indicates A+H, B+H, or just H.

What may these substances be?

(f)   Will the A and/or B genes be present in some individuals of Groups 5 and 6? Why?

4–20   Embryonic tissues can be dissociated by mild proteolysis or other treatments to yield suspensions of single cells that will reaggregate and eventually reproduce many of the features of the original tissue. When aggregates are prepared from cells derived from two different tissues, these cells will eventually segregate into two homotypic aggregates. Little is known about the molecules that mediate these cell–cell interactions. Plasma membrane fractions have been prepared from neural retina and cerebellum to determine what effect, if any, they have on the formation of homotypic aggregates. Cell aggregation is measured by determining the fall in the single-cell count over the time period of the experiment. The effects of membrane fragments on the aggregation of retinal cells and cerebellar cells are shown in Figures 4–62 and 4–63, respectively.

(a)   What effects do the plasma membrane preparations have on the aggregations of retinal and cerebellar cells?

(b)   Figure 4–64 measures the binding of ^{3}H-retinal plasma membranes to retinal and cerebellar cells. What is observed?

(c)   What general conclusions can you draw from the results observed in Figures 4–62, 4–63, and 4–64?

(d)   What is the effect of trypsin on inhibition of aggregation (Figure 4–65)?

(e)   Retinal membranes also have been isolated from 7-, 8-, and 9-day embryos and examined for their ability to inhibit the aggregation of 7-, 8-, and 9-day retinal cells (Figure 4–66a). Likewise tectal membranes have been isolated from 8- and 9-day embryos and examined for their ability to block the aggregation of 7-, 8-, and 9-day-old tectal cells (Figure 4–66b). What conclusions can you draw from the results?

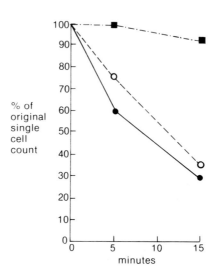

Figure 4–62 Effects of membrane preparations on retinal cell aggregations (Problem 4–20). 1.5 × 10⁵ neural retinal cells were incubated in 3 ml of medium with no additions ●; with cerebellar fraction B-1 (0.1 mg of protein) ○; or with retinal fraction B-1 (0.1 mg of protein) ■. The percent remaining single cells is plotted as a function of time. [From R. Merrell and L. Glaser, *Proc. Natl. Acad. Sci. USA* **70,** 2794 (1973).]

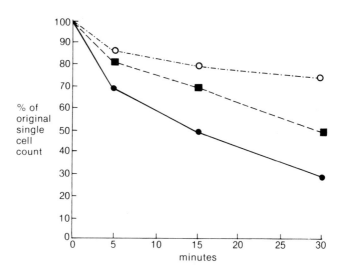

Figure 4–63 Effects of plasma membrane preparations on cerebellar cell aggregation (Problem 4–20). Conditions are identical to those of Figure 4–62, except that cerebellar cells are used. ●, no addition; ■, 0.1 mg of retinal fraction B-1; ○, 0.1 mg of cerebellar fraction B-1. [From R. Merrell and L. Glaser, *Proc. Natl. Acad. Sci. USA,* **70,** 2794 (1973).]

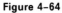

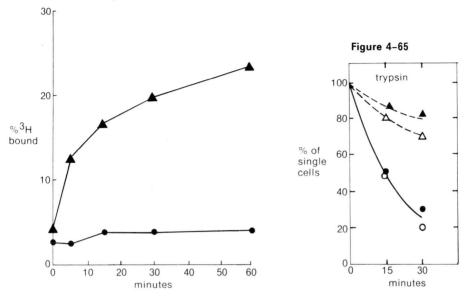

Figure 4–64 The binding of radioactive membranes to cells (Problem 4–20). 6×10^5 cells were incubated in 3 ml of medium with ^{3}H glucosamine-labeled retinal fraction B-1 (20 μg of protein, 15,000 dpm). At each time point the aggregation was stopped by 3-fold dilution; cells with attached membranes were collected by centrifugation. The pellet was washed, dissolved, and counted. ●, cerebellar cells; ▲, retinal cells [From R. Merrell and L. Glaser, *Proc. Natl. Acad. Sci. USA* **70,** 2794 (1973).]

Figure 4–65 The effect of trypsin on membrane activity (Problem 4–20). A suspension (0.1 ml) of 8-day retinal membranes (0.1 mg of protein) was incubated for 10 minutes at 37°C with trypsin. Soybean trypsin inhibitor was added and the membranes were assayed for their ability to inhibit aggregation of 8-day retinal cells. ○, no addition; ▲, intact membranes (0.1 mg protein); ●, trypsin-treated membranes; △, membranes treated with a preincubated mixture of trypsin and trypsin inhibitor. [From D. I. Gottlieb *et al., Proc. Natl. Acad. Sci. USA,* **71,** 1800 (1974).]

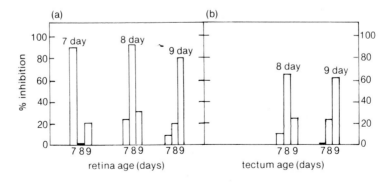

Figure 4–66 The effect of embryonal age on membrane specificity (Problem 4–20). All experiments were carried out with membranes prepared from whole neural retina, obtained from 7-, 8-, or 9-day-old embryos. The membranes were used to inhibit aggregation of either retinal or tectal cells of the ages indicated. [From D. I. Gottlieb *et al., Proc. Natl. Acad. Sci. USA,* **71,** 1800 (1974).]

4–21   Lethal irradiation of mice destroys primarily cells associated with the blood-cell system. The irradiated animals generally die within a period of weeks. However, lethally irradiated recipients can be "protected" by injection with bone-marrow cells; protected animals will survive for extended periods of time. If the protecting bone marrow comes from an F_1 donor (i.e., progeny of a cross between the recipient and another inbred strain), the irradiated recipient is a hemopoietic chimera with blood cells that express the phenotypes of both the donor's parents. Frequently such chimeras show permanent acceptance of skin grafts from either parental type.

Suppose that you carried out the following set of experiments. You protected lethally irradiated recipients of inbred mouse strain C57BL/6 with (C57BL/6 × A) F_1 hematopoietic cells. Animals you grafted one week later with skin from either A or F_1 accepted the grafts. However, animals you grafted similarly 11 weeks later all rejected the grafts. Subsequent tests showed that the lymph node cells and erythrocytes in the recipients were exclusively of the donor type. What would you suggest is the basis for the graft rejection after 11 weeks? Propose an explanation for the finding that the F_1 hematopoietic cells are not tolerant to skin grafts of an identical genotype.

4–22   The T-cell receptor has remained elusive, even though immunologists have made a concerted effort to characterize this molecule for the past five years. One promising approach has been taken recently using the inbred rat strains Lewis and DA. T cells are purified by passage over a column of inert beads coated with rabbit anti-rat gamma globulin. The immobilized antibody in the column binds B cells, but does not retain T cells. The flow-through T-cell preparation obtained in this manner contains <2% B cells. F_1 hybrid rats (DA × Lewis) are immunized with Lewis column-purified T cells. A pool of the resulting immune serum, designated 1003, is obtained from five (DA × Lewis) F_1 rats and then absorbed with normal F_1 hybrid spleen and lymph nodes to remove possible autoimmune antibodies. The specificity of Serum 1003 is shown in Table 4–21.

(a)   What is the specificity of Serum 1003? With what component(s) on the cell surface must Serum 1003 react? Is it reacting with V regions or C regions? Explain.

(b)   The binding of Serum 1003 by Lewis spleen cells and Lewis purified T cells can be measured by first reacting these cells with Serum 1003 and then reacting the cells with [125] I-labeled rabbit anti-rat antibodies. The results of these measurements are given in Table 4–22. Which cells bind Serum 1003? What does this finding indicate?

(c) F_1 hybrid antisera produced against parental antibodies to the F_1 alloantigens will, in the presence of complement, prevent parental T lymphocytes from functioning in a GVHR. This test was carried

Table 4–21
The specificity of Serum 1003[a] (Problem 4–22)

Indirect hemagglutination		Gel diffusion	
Target	Titer	Target serum	Line
SRBC–Lewis normal IgG	Neg	Lewis normal	–
SRBC–Lewis anti-DA IgG	2^{16}–2^{18}	Lewis anti-DA	+
SRBC–Lewis anti-BN IgG	Neg	Lewis anti-BN	–
SRBC–DA normal IgG	Neg	DA normal	–
SRBC–DA anti-Lewis IgG	Neg	DA anti-Lewis	–
SRBC–(DA × L) F_1 normal IgG	Neg	(DA × L) F normal	–

[a]Lewis anti-DAIgG and DA anti-Lewis IgG were obtained by immunization of the appropriate mice using skin grafts to present the antigens. For the hemagglutination test these immunoglobulins were coupled to sheep RBC. L (Lewis), DA, and BN are different inbred rat strains.
[From H. Binz and H. Wigzell, *J. Exp. Med.* **142,** 197 (1975). © 1975 by the Rockefeller University Press.]

Table 4–22
The binding of Serum 1003 by Lewis spleen cells and Lewis purified T cells as measured by ^{125}I-labeled rabbit anti-rat Ig (Problem 4–22)

Lymphoid cells[a]	Incubated with	Uptake of ^{125}I rabbit anti-rat Ig[b] (mean cpm of quadruplicates ± standard error)
L–S	Serum 1003	16,878 ± 1,274
L–S	Normal rat serum	7,712 ± 1,018
L–T	Serum 1003	12,756 ± 700
L–T	Normal rat serum	6,869 ± 534
L–Thp	Serum 1003	1,269 ± 106
L–Thp	Normal rat serum	1,105 ± 44
DA–S	Serum 1003	9,119 ± 1,513
DA–S	Normal rat serum	8,578 ± 489
DA–T	Serum 1003	6,350 ± 457
DA–T	Normal rat serum	5,580 ± 552
DA–Thp	Serum 1003	566 ± 53
DA–Thp	Normal rat serum	498 ± 55
F_1–S	Serum 1003	4,622 ± 306
F_1–S	Normal rat serum	4,818 ± 112
F_1–T	Serum 1003	3,346 ± 490
F_1–T	Normal rat serum	3,927 ± 523
F_1–Thp	Serum 1003	528 ± 41
F_1–Thp	Normal rat serum	415 ± 33
BN–T	Serum 1003	4,196 ± 58
BN–T	Normal rat serum	5,393 ± 78
BN–Thp	Serum 1003	480 ± 42
BN–Thp	Normal rat serum	342 ± 28

[a]S denotes a mixture of spleen and lymph node cells; T denotes T lymphocytes prepared by fractionation of spleen and lymph node cells over anti-Ig bead columns; Thp denotes thymocytes which have been passed over anti-Ig columns.
[b]Input per tube: 5×10^5 cpm of ^{125}I rabbit anti-rat Ig.
[Adapted from H. Binz and H. Wigzell, *J. Exp. Med.* **142,** 197 (1975). © 1975 by the Rockefeller University Press.]

Table 4–23
Reaction of Serum 1003 in GVHR (Problem 4–22)

Cells injected[a]	Host	Injected cells pretreated with:[b]	Mean of "Lewis" lymph node weights[c]	Mean of "DA" lymph node weights[c]	Mean of "BN" lymph node weights[c]	Mean log ratio ± standard error
L DA	(L × DA) F₁	(L × DA) F₁ NS + C' (L × DA) F₁ NS + C'	70.7 ± 8.6	70.2 ± 7.6		−0.01 ± 0.02[d]
L DA	(L × DA) F₁	Serum 1003 + C' Serum 1003 + C'	11.2 ± 0.9	73.2 ± 5.03		0.81 ± 0.02
L BN	(L × BN) F₁	(L × DA) F₁ NS + C' (L × DA) F₁ NS + C'	33.7 ± 5.3		32.2 ± 2.5	−0.01 ± 0.05[d]
L BN	(L × BN) F₁	Serum 1003 + C' Serum 1003 + C'	31.5 ± 3.7		31.9 ± 4.3	−0.00 ± 0.07[d]

[a] 5×10^6 spleen and lymph node cells were injected into each foot pad.
[b] NS denotes normal serum; C' denotes complement.
[c] Mean weights of four nodes (mg).
[d] Not significantly different from 0.
[e] Significantly different from 0 ($p < 0.01$).
[Adapted from H. Binz and H. Wigzell, *J. Exp. Med.* **142**, 197 (1975). © 1975 by The Rockefeller University Press.]

out for Serum 1003 with the results given in Table 4-23. Is Serum 1003 capable of preventing GVHR? If so, what is the specificity of the 1003 antiserum? What are the implications of these observations?

(d) What are the implications of these studies for T- and B-cell receptors? According to this study, how are the genes that code for T-cell receptors related to those that code for B-cell receptors?

Answers

4-1   (a)   True

(b)   False. Cholesterol, phospholipids, and glycolipids all have a cylindrical shape (see Figure 4–9).

(c)   False. Few if any glycoproteins have the shape and solubility properties required for spontaneous bilayer formation.

(d)   True

(e)   True

(f)   True

(g)   False. The flip-flop of lipids across the membrane is about 10^9 times slower than translational diffusion.

(h)   False. Unsaturated fatty acids are "kinked" and therefore increase membrane fluidity.

(i)   True

(j)   False. It is not known whether the heavy chains for receptor immunoglobulin and secreted molecules are identical.

(k)   True

(l)   True

(m)   False. The Le^b specificity is produced by the action of two gene products, H and Le, which add two sugar residues to the precursor oligosaccharide (see Figure 4–22). Consequently, Le^b–anti Le^b interaction may be blocked by an appropriate disaccharide, but not by a monosaccharide.

(n)   True

(o)   False. The coelomocytes of earthworms appear to resemble macrophages morphologically.

(p)   True

(q)   False. MLR and GVHR probably result from the same phenomenon, but the MLR occurs *in vitro* and the GVHR *in vivo*.

(r)   True

(s)   False. It contains sufficient DNA to code for hundreds of genes 600 nucleotides in length.

(t)   True

(u) False.   Acute graft rejection is an advanced immunological trait found only in some fish, some amphibia, birds, and mammals.

(v) True

(w) True

(x) False.   The T/t locus appears to govern the differentiation of neuroectodermal structures (Figure 4–51).

(y) True

(z) True

4–2 (a) phospholipids, glycolipids, and cholesterol

(b) Hydrophobic

(c) Amphipathic

(d) integral and peripheral

(e) Sialic acid (or N-acetylneuraminic acid)

(f) N-glycosidic and O-glycosidic

(g) glycosyltransferases

(h) Lectins

(i) Microfilaments

(j) recognition, transduction, and initiation of effector mechanisms

(k) C-terminal domain (see Figure 4–1c)

(l) A, B, O, Le^a, Le^b

(m) N-acetyl-D-galactosamine

(n) complementary and self-self

(o) coelomocytes

(p) HLA, H-2

(q) Congenic

(r) haplotype

(s) recombination (or crossover)

(t) transplantation antigens

(u) public

(v) suppressor factor

(w) lymphocyte-activating determinants, II

(x) homologous

(y) Complex

(z) antigenic modulation

4–3 (a) It is best to transfuse blood between individuals of identical ABO genotype. However, O individuals are universal donors because they have neither A nor B antigens; therefore, their cells will not be agglutinated by anti-A or anti-B antibodies when transfused into individuals with other ABO genotypes. AB individuals can accept red blood cells from any donor because they lack antibodies and the ability to make antibodies to the A and B antigens.

(b) A mismatch of other blood-group specificities could lead to a transfusion reaction (agglutination and lysis of the foreign cells). The presence of natural antibodies to these antigens can be checked simply by determining whether serum from the recipient agglutinates donor cells.

4–4 Components a(1), b(2), and c(2) will make a membrane more fluid. The compound shown in Figure 4–54 is cholesterol.

4–5 (a) Six glycosyl transferases would be necessary to synthesize the oligosaccharides shown in Figure 4–55. Separate transferases would be required for: (1), addition of the initial xylose residues of both oligosaccharides; (2) and (3), addition of the mannose residues in α and β linkage, respectively; (4) and (5), addition of the galactose residues in α and β linkage, respectively; and (6), addition of the N-acetylneuraminic acid (sialic acid) residues to both oligosaccharides.

(b) Xylose residues in oligosaccharides always are linked to glycoproteins through O-glycosidic bonds to the hydroxyl group of a serine residue (Table 4–2).

4–6 Individuals who exhibit strong Le^a specificity must lack the fucose transferase coded by the H gene, which normally converts the Le^a specificity to the Le^b specificity (Figure 4–22). Lack of H gene activity, in turn, indicates an se/se (nonsecretor) genotype (Essential Concept 4–2E4).

4–7 Each carbohydrate will block agglutination of the blood-group substances whose structure it most closely resembles. See Figure 4–22 for the structures of the blood-group substances.

(a) Le^a (d) A
(b) Le^b (e) H
(c) H (f) B

4–8 (a) The gene that specifies the S^+ antigen must be present in S^- as well as S^+ strains of rats. Its phenotypic expression must be under the control of one (or more) additional gene(s) whose function is altered in certain S^- strain leukemias so that the S^+ antigen can be expressed.

(b) Apparently antibody specific to the S^+ antigen can modulate its expression, so that in the presence of antibody S^+ leukemias become S^-. When the anti-S antibody is removed, these same tumors can revert back to the S^+ phenotype. This process, called antigenic modulation, is observed in the TL system (Essential Concept 4–14D).

4–9 (a) Three classes of antigenic determinants on mouse RBC's are indicated. One class (A) is present on all test cells; a second class (B) is present only on RBC's and brain cells; and the third class (C) is present only on RBC's.

(b) The A antigens could be H-2 determinants. The C antigens could be blood-group antigens. There is no known cell-surface marker with the B distribution.

4–10 (a) The cells from Mouse 1 have antigenic determinant A; the cells from Mouse 2 have antigenic determinant B; the cells from Mouse 3 have antigenic determinants A and B; the cells from Mouse 4 lack these antigenic determinants.

(b) The X cells have both determinants, A and B, since the antiserum was raised against X cells. The X cells could have additional antigens that could be detected by absorption tests with cells from other inbred strains of mice. The host has neither of these antigens, otherwise it could not have generated an immune response to them.

(c)   These antigens could not be alleles because both are present in inbred Mouse 3 which presumably is homozygous for all genetic loci.

Wild mice could be heterozygous; hence it would be impossible to determine whether these antigens are alleles without breeding studies to follow their genetic segregation.

(d)   Construct a congenic mouse strain of the 1.2 type (i.e., with the locus of interest from inbred Mouse 2 superimposed on the background of inbred Mouse 1). Then immunize a 1 mouse with 1.2 cells.

4-11   (a)   (1) Grafts within inbred strains are successful. Syngeneic grafts between individuals of the same sex always succeed because the H-2 alleles in graft and host are identical. Because all the graft antigens are self-antigens of the host, the host cannot mount an immune response to any of them. (2) Grafts between inbred strains with different H-2 alleles are not successful. Allogeneic grafts always fail because the H-2 alleles are different in the graft and the host. Consequently the host will mount an immune response against the alloantigens of the graft. (3) Grafts from either inbred parent strain to the F_1 hybrid succeed, but grafts in the reverse direction fail. When the graft is from the parent to F_1, the H-2 determinants on the graft are all present in the host and, accordingly, are not immunogenic. In contrast, the F_1 graft has an H-2 allele, $H-2^b$, which is not present in Strain A; therefore the corresponding alloantigen is rejected. (4) Individuals from the F_2 and subsequent generations of mice can be heterozygous or homozygous for the H-2 alleles. In either case a heterozygous F_1 recipient will have both of the H-2 alleles present in any F_2 graft, and therefore will not reject it. (5) Grafts from (either) inbred parent strain are accepted by some members of the F_2 generation and rejected by others. The same is true for backcross individuals as recipients. In both cases rejections occur in those homozygous recipients that lack the parental H-2 allele expressed in the graft. The foregoing five answers have been termed the five laws of transplantation.

(b)   All F_1 individuals are susceptible to a parental tumor graft. Three quarters of the F_2 generations are susceptible to such a graft. One half of a backcross generation is susceptible to such a graft.

(c) F_1: all susceptible
F_2: $(3/4)^2 = 9/16$ susceptible
backcross: $(1/2)^2 = 1/4$ susceptible

(d) F_1: all susceptible
F_2: $(3/4)^n$
backcross: $(1/2)^n$

(e)   To determine a lower limit on the number of H loci in a given population one could cross two mice and raise a large F_2 generation, and then determine what fraction (x) of grafts from one parent are successful in the F_2 generation. Since $x = (3/4)^n$, n can be readily evaluated. If this process is repeated with a number of inbred strains or with wild mice, an estimate can be made of the number of H loci that differ in each parental combination.

4-12 (a)   If the two congenic strains are identical, the F_1 reduplicates their genotype and likewise their resistance to tumors of the background strain (Table 4–16, Experiment 2). If the two congenic strains are not identical, the two genotypes complement each other and produce a susceptible hybrid (Table 4–16, Experiment 1). A special case arises when the two congenic lines come from different initial crosses. Here the two lines may differ from the common partner at the same locus, but by different alleles. Accordingly, the hybrid will not have all of the A strain H alleles, and therefore will be resistant (Table 4–16, Experiment 3). However, if A.B(3) and A.C(4) differed from strain A at different loci, the hybrid would be susceptible. The F_1 test is very useful for identifying shared H loci among congenic strains with the same background.

(b)   See Table 4–24.

Table 4–24
Conclusions from the F_1 tests in Table 4–16 (Answer 4–12)

(1) B10.C(41N) is not H-3	(5) B10.C(47N) is not H-1
(2) B10.C(41N) is H-1	(6) B10.C(47N) is not H-2
(3) B10.C)41N) is H-1	(7) B10.C(47N) is not H-3
(4) B10.C(47N) is not H-1	(8) B10.C(47N) is not H-4

(c)   You have three strains of mice:

tissue donor	known parent	unknown parent
A	A.B	A.U
(A) H-1^a	(A) H-1^b	(A) H-1^u

Cross A.B $\times$ A.U. If u = a, the F_1 will be susceptible to a tumor from A. If not, the F_1 will be resistant.

4-13 (a)   The d chromosome encodes 21 known antigenic determinants. The z chromosome encodes 6. The D^d gene product has 14 antigenic specificities. The D^z gene product has just one.
(b)   The K and D alleles encode gene products that differ from one another by multiple structural differences that can be detected serologically.
(c)   In general, the private specificities are encoded only in either the D or K region of one of the known H-2 chromosomes. Hence these specificities can be used to identify particular haplotypes. In contrast, the public specificities are encoded in more than one H-2 chromosome, and sometimes in both the D and K regions (e.g.,

specificities 1, 3, 5, 35, and 36 in Table 4–9). The private specificities elicit very high titer antisera, whereas the public specificities tend to elicit less specific antisera of lower titer.

(d)   The presence of shared serological specificities suggests that the K and D genes arose from a common ancestor by gene duplication. The alternative hypothesis to explain structural similarities, the convergent evolution of genes of independent origin, is considered less likely because of the requirement for parallel evolution.

4–14   (a)   Precipitation of solubilized spleen cells from a mouse heterozygous at the H-2 complex with alloantisera to any one of the four private alloantigens completely removes that alloantigen but none of the other three. This observation suggests that each of the four alloantigens is present on different glycoproteins, each about 45,000 in molecular weight.

(b)   The K and D gene products are *codominantly* expressed in heterozygous individuals, so that each cell carries four different H-2 gene products: two from the K locus and two from the D locus.

4–15   (a)   The A.TH anti-A.TL antiserum should be directed only against I and S region cell-surface gene products, which represent the only known differences between the two congenic strains A.TH and A.TL (see Table 4–17). The S region does not encode any known cell-surface molecules. Therefore, the 28,000 to 35,000 molecular weight components are probably Ia molecules. Their precipitation with the A.TH anti-A.TL sera indicates that the I region of the d haplotype has serological specificities that crossreact with the I region of the k haplotype (see Table 4–17). Thus the Ia molecules of different haplotypes have cross-reacting serological specificities similar to those of the K and D gene products (Table 4–9).

(b)   The (B10 × A) anti-B10.D2 antiserum should be directed against cell-surface molecules encoded by the K and I regions of the d haplotype, since these molecules represent the only antigenic differences between a B10.D2 and a (B10 × A) F_1 hybrid mouse (Table 4–17).

(c)   An Ia-like molecule (28,000) and a K molecule (45,000) are seen on the gel in Figure 4–60. Thus the experimental data agree very well with theoretical expectations.

(d)   Several precautions must be considered when defining the specificities of antisera produced with congenic pairs of mice. First, the number of genes in the H-2 complex almost certainly exceeds the number of available genetic markers. This means that independently derived recombinants that appear identical by the limited number of genetic markers currently available may differ in genes for which no genetic markers are available. Accordingly, the antiserum raised against the lymphocytes of one recombinant may have antibodies directed against cell-surface molecules that are absent in a second apparently identical recombinant strain. Second, congenic strains may retain genes that are outside the H-2 complex, but closely linked to it, and for which there are no genetic markers. Therefore the use of lymphocytes from such a strain may result in antisera that are directed against the products of a non-H-2 gene. Third, one must be careful of antisera raised against cell-surface molecules encoded by viruses present in the immunizing cells. Fourth, one may raise antibodies to differentiation antigens expressed only on a subset of cells (e.g., B_α cells), and their detection depends on the concentration of these cells in the test sample. Finally, one must be certain that the immunoprecipitate contains cell-surface molecules detected by the primary antiserum, rather than aggregated γ-globulins in general, and that the cell-surface antigens detected are actually coded by the H-2 genes in question.

4–16   (a)   The data in Table 4–18 can be explained by three antigenic specificities, which could be designated A, B, and C.
(b)   If the A and B specificities are assigned to the k haplotype, then the d haplotype has B and C specificities and the b haplotype has A and C specificities.
(c)   Each specificity is shared by two haplotypes.
(d)   These antigens appear to be public specificities that are present on the K gene products of several haplotypes (Table 4–9).
(e)   The absorbed antisera are specific for the K gene products of the b and d haplotypes, respectively. Hence the gene products must be codominantly expressed on the cells of F_1 hybrid mice.
(f)   Half the backcross mice should be b/d heterozygotes and the other half should be d homozygotes. Cells from the heterozygotes should react with both absorbed antisera, whereas cells from the homozygotes should react only with absorbed b-anti-d antiserum.
(g)   The X mouse must have had a mutation in the H-2 complex of one choromosome that led to alteration of a cell-surface Class I molecule. Thus this mouse would reject as foreign (b × d) F_1 skin grafts, because it differs from the donor mouse in one of its b or d haplotype Class I gene products.
(h)   One approach to testing the hypothesis in (g) is the following. Construct a congenic C57Bl.X mouse strain. Attempt to raise alloantiserum against the mutant gene product. If you are successful, use this antiserum with the indirect immunoprecipitation procedure to isolate the mutant molecule. Do peptide-map and microsequencing studies on the K molecules from the x, b, and d haplotypes to determine whether the K gene product from X differs from its counterparts in either d or b by a single amino acid substitution.

4–17   (a)   The sperm and testicular cells from BALB/T^J males have the T/t^{w2} mutant surface antigen whereas sperm and testicular cells from BALB males, lymphocytes and thymocytes from T/t^{w2} or +/+ males, and brain cells from BALB and BALB/T^J males do not have this antigen.

(b)   The congenic BALB/T^J mice differ genetically from the normal BALB mice by a single gene, the T^J allele. This single genetic difference is sufficient to cause the antiserum raised against BALB/T^J sperm to kill the homologous congenic sperm cells but not the heterologous BALB/c sperm cells. The mutant cell-surface specificity is shared by sperm from T/+ individuals, but not by sperm from +/+ individuals.

(c)   The T allele probably specifies an antigen on the surface of sperm. Presumably the altered transmission ratios produced by t alleles of the + locus are due to the properties of the sperm surface coded by these alleles, for it is highly probable that if T mutations alter a surface component, then + and t alleles at this locus also code for cell-surface components. This hypothesis also predicts that the constitution of the sperm surface must reflect in part the *haploid* genotype of the sperm. If the final constitution of the sperm surface were determined at a precursor diploid stage, it would be unlikely for a recessive allele in a heterozygous individual to cause preferential transmission of the recessive allele. Such an effect of a recessive allele on germ-cell function is called a haploid gene effect or postmeiotic gene effect.

4-18   Most lethal t alleles cause marked suppression of crossing-over between the T/t locus and the tf locus, and extending to the H-2 region. The effect of this suppression is that alleles at many different loci are inherited together, including alleles at loci that code for cell-surface determinants, such as T/t and H-2. If these determinants are members of a cooperative system important for cell recognition and morphogenesis, then certain combinations of alleles may function more effectively than others. The advantage conferred by t alleles may result from their ability to lock favorable allele combinations together and insure their inheritance as single units.

4-19   (a)   Group   1   H*, Le, Se
                       2   H, Le, se/se
                       3   H, le/le, Se
                       4   H, le/le, se/se
                       5   h/h, Le, Se or se/se
                       6   h/h, le/le, Se or se/se

*H can be H/H or H/h; Le can be Le/Le or Le/le; Se can be Se/Se or Se/se.

(b)   Le^b is not expressed in Group 2 individuals because the se/se genotype blocks the activity of the H fucose transferase, which is necessary for the formation of the Le^b specificity.

(c) Le^b is not expressed in Group 5 individuals because the H fucose transferase is not synthesized in individuals of h/h genotype.

(d)   H, A, B, and Le^b

(e)   They appear to be the precursor oligosaccharides unmodified by any of the transferases (see Figures 4–21 and 4–22 and Table 4–6).

(f)   The A and/or B genes are present in some of these individuals. They cannot be expressed because the H transferase is necessary to produce the precursor groups on which the A and B transferases act.

4–20   (a)   The plasma membranes from neural retina almost totally inhibit retinal cell aggregation (Figure 4–62) and have a much smaller inhibitory effect on cerebellar cell aggregation (Figure 4–63). Cerebellar membranes inhibit the aggregation of cerebellar cells, but have virtually no effect on the aggregation of retinal cells.

(b)   The retinal plasma membranes bind significantly to retinal cells and only slightly to cerebellar cells.

(c)   The specific site responsible for cellular recognition in embryonic cells can be retained in isolated plasma cell membranes. This recognition site appears to be highly specific for cell type. It binds rapidly to homotypic cells.

(d)   Trypsin abolishes the inhibitory effects of plasma membranes on the aggregation of homotypic cells. The effect of the enzyme depends upon its proteolytic activity, because trypsin in the presence of a specific proteolytic inhibitor does not abolish membrane inhibition activity. Trypsin presumably exerts its effect by destroying cell-surface protein molecules.

(e)   The surface specificity responsible for cell aggregation changes rapidly during development, either due to changes in cell types or to changes in the surfaces of preexisting cells.

4–21   The skin from the A or F donors apparently contains cells that express a differentiation antigen that is not recognized as self by the hemopoietic cells. This skin antigen must be quite antigenic, because the chimeras reject A skin almost as rapidly as if there were an H-2 incompatibility. The rejection must be carried out by donor cells (F_1), for there is no evidence that any recipient cells survive. Therefore the donor cells must have lost tolerance to their native skin alloantigen during residence for 11 weeks in the new host, which lacks that allele. This observation implies that the immune system can remain tolerant to differentiation alloantigens expressed in the same animal only so long as these alloantigens are continuously exposed to the immune system. Removal of the immunocompetent cell population to another host may result in the termination of self-tolerance to alloantigens not expressed on the hemopoietic cells. Accordingly, this approach may be used to demonstrate new types of differentiation alloantigens.

4–22   (a)   Serum 1003 reacts against Lewis anti-DA immunoglobulin. Thus it must react against the T-cell receptors of Lewis lymphocytes that are directed against the allogeneic cell-surface antigens of DA. Presumably Serum 1003 is reacting with V regions, because a variety of controls in Table 4–21 are negative.

(b)   The peripheral T cells from Lewis appear to bind Serum 1003, although there is no obvious explanation of the high level of binding of normal rat serum. This observation suggests that a significant fraction of nonimmunized Lewis T cells have receptors for the alloantigens of DA.

(c)   Serum 1003 blocks the GVHR when Lewis cells are injected into a (L × DA) F_1, but does not block the reaction of DA cells injected into the (L × DA) F_1. In addition, Serum 1003 does not block the reaction of BN cells injected into a (L × BN) F_1. Thus the Serum 1003 appears to be specific for Lewis cells. In particular, in the presence of complement, it can destroy Lewis cells that mediate the GVHR. This observation suggests that Serum 1003 is directed against Lewis T-cell receptors for DA alloantigens.

(d)   This study suggests that the V regions of T-cell receptors and B-cell antibodies are very similar, if not identical. The observations raise the possibility that the B- and T-cell receptors share at least some of the same V genes, even though the C genes may be different.

5 CANCER BIOLOGY AND IMMUNOLOGY

This chapter begins by describing the properties of cancer cells and of the agents that transform normal cells into malignant tumors. The subsequent sections deal with immune-related aspects of cancer: tumor-specific cell-surface changes that act as antigens to the host, the role of the immune system in immunosurveillance and elimination of cancers, the mechanisms by which cancers escape immunosurveillance, and the future of immunological approaches to the therapy, diagnosis, and prevention of cancer.

Essential Concepts

5-1   Cancer cells divide when they should not

A.   Normal cell growth is regulated *in vivo* so that the proportion of proliferating cells in an organ increases or decreases to maintain a balance between the rates of cell division and cell loss, thereby maintaining constant organ size. Cancer cells do not respond to such regulation, consequently a higher proportion of their descendants continue to proliferate (Figure 5–1) and can give rise to large masses called tumors.

A tumor (designated by the suffix *-oma*) is a swelling that may be due to cancer, inflammation, or infection. A tumor caused by cellular proliferation is called a neoplasm (new growth). Neoplasms that invade surrounding tissues and ultimately spread throughout the body are called *malignant neoplasms,* or *cancers.* Neoplasms that form noninvasive tumors, which do not spread to distant sites, are called *benign neoplasms.* Tumors that arise from epithelial cells are called *carcinomas* (Figure 5–2), and those that arise from stromal or mesenchymal elements are called *sarcomas* (Figure 5–3).

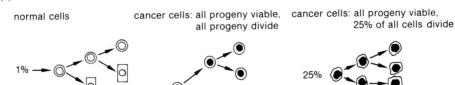

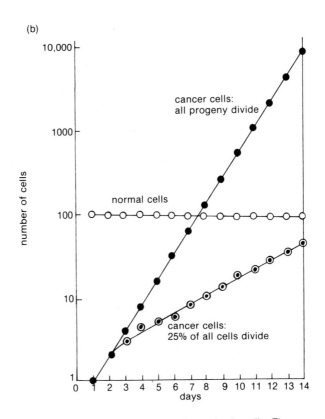

Figure 5–1 The growth kinetics of normal and neoplastic cells. The example shown considers 100 cells in a typical organ. Normally 99 of these cells will be differentiated and nondividing, and the remaining one will be a dividing stem cell. At each division the stem cell gives rise to a daughter stem cell and a differentiated cell, as diagramed in (a). The resulting rate of increase in cell number just compensates for the rate of cell loss from the tissue, so that the total number of viable cells remains constant [(b), open circles]. If one of the 100 cells becomes a cancer cell of which all progeny are viable dividing cells as diagramed in (a), middle figure, then the number of cancer cells in the tissue will increase exponentially [(b), solid circles]. If one of the 100 cells becomes a cancer cell of which only 25% of the progeny give rise to two dividing daughters with each division, as diagramed in (a), right figure, then the number of cancer cells will increase more slowly [(b), open circles with solid centers].

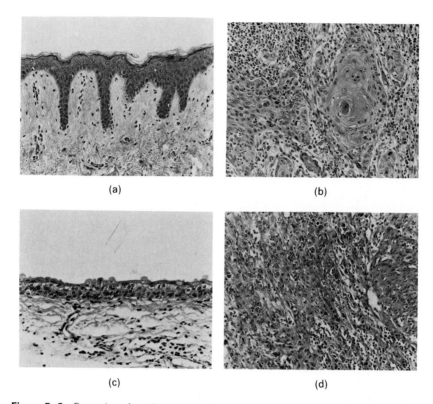

(a)

(b)

(c)

(d)

Figure 5–2 Examples of carcinomas and their normal counterparts. (a) A section of skin with normal epidermis showing orderly maturation from a row of basal cells to layers of thin, dead surface cells, which form a protective layer. (b) Invasive skin carcinoma composed of cells with frequent mitoses. Disorderly maturation is exhibited by the whorls of cells in the center of a mass of tumor cells, rather than on the surface as seen in normal epidermis. (c) Normal lining cells of the bladder (transitional epithelium) consisting of lower layers of cuboidal-shaped cells and a single top layer of flattened cells. (d) Malignant transitional cell carcinoma arising in the lining of the bladder. The cells are invading the underlying tissue as cohesive, but irregular, masses. [Photographs courtesy of R. Rouse.]

B. There are two phases in the growth of any solid tumor: a first phase in which cells gain nutrients by diffusion from the surrounding intercellular fluids, and a second phase in which the tumor appears to induce proliferation of host blood vessels that nourish the tumor mass. Most cancer cells possess more active membrane transport systems than those of normal cells for uptake of amino acids, sugars, nucleosides, and so on. Despite this competitive advantage, the maximum size to which a tumor can grow without a vascular supply appears to be a spheroid about 1 mm in diameter. Beyond this size, availability of nutrients to interior cells limits their proliferation and eventually can cause their death. However, most tumors greater than 1 mm in diameter

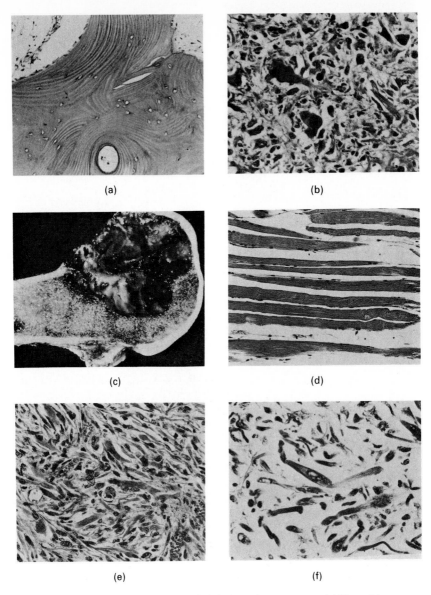

(a)

(b)

(c)

(d)

(e)

(f)

Figure 5–3 Examples of sarcomas and their normal counterparts. (a) Normal bone, consisting of regular layers of calcified matrix. Very few cells are present; they include individual bone cells (osteocytes) within spaces and a row of bone-forming cells (osteoblasts) on the surface. (b) The histologic appearance of a malignant osteosarcoma, showing increased cellularity, with numerous large wild-looking cells. In some areas the cells are laying down irregular, uncalcified bone matrix (upper left corner). (c) A gross photograph of an osteosarcoma, in a typical location, at the end of the femur. The malignant neoplasm can be seen invading the medullary cavity as well as eroding the cortex of the bone. Extensive bleeding and tissue death is common in these tumors. (d) Normal skeletal muscle with small, regular nuclei on the outer surfaces of the fibers. Cross striations are visible in most of the fibers. (e) The histologic appearance of a malignant rhabdomyosarcoma (sarcoma of rod-shaped [rhabdo] muscle [myo] cells), consisting of cells with centrally located, large, abnormally shaped nuclei. Some of the cells exhibit cross striations in their cytoplasm. (f) A higher-power view of a rhabdomyosarcoma, showing a cell with prominent cross striations. [Photographs courtesy of R. Rouse and P. Horne.]

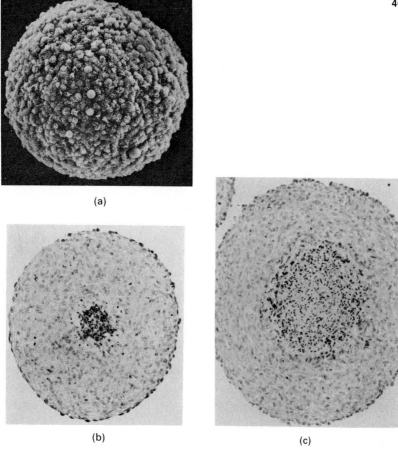

Figure 5–4 Multicellular tumor spheroids. (a) A scanning electromicrograph of a large spheroid of a breast cancer in mice. (b) A cross section of the spheroid in (a). The central core of dark cells represent a zone of cell death due to lack of nutrients. (c) A larger spheroid with a larger necrotic core. [Courtesy of R. M. Sutherland.]

appear to release *angiogenesis factors,* which stimulate growth of host blood vessels. These new vessels penetrate the outer cell layers of the tumor. Subsequent tumor growth ensues by rapid proliferation of these outer layers, leaving behind an interior core of dead and dying cells (Figure 5–4). The actual growth rate of a tumor depends on the fraction of cells that are in the mitotic cycle, the average cell-cycle time, and the cell loss fraction.

5–2 Cancer cells invade other tissues

A.   The spread of cancer cells from the original transformed focus to distant organs is termed *metastasis.* The property of metastasis appears to be related to the nature of the original transformed focus, and is inherited by the progeny of the metastatic cells. The first stage of metastasis is the invasive extension of cancer cells into surrounding tissues. The second stage is the invasion of a vessel wall and the entry of cancer cells into either the lymphatic or the blood vascular system (Figure 5–5).

1.   Lymphatic vessels drain all intercellular fluid spaces in the body, conducting both particulate matter and plasma fluid into lymph nodes (Essential Concept 1–5). Cancer cells that break free from a tissue or invade a lymphatic vessel almost always become trapped in the meshwork of a draining lymph node. If these cancer cells proliferate, the result is abnormal enlargement of the lymph node (lymphadenopathy). Continued cancer cell proliferation may result in release of cancer cells into the efferent lymphatic vessel leading from the lymph node to the next lymph node up the chain. Eventually, cancer cells may enter a large collecting lymphatic such as the thoracic duct, which empties directly into the larger veins leading to the heart. Thus unchecked lymphatic metastases can lead to escape of cancer cells into the bloodstream.

2.   Cancer cells also may invade blood vessels (Figures 5–5 and 5–6), and thereby enter the bloodstream directly. Cancer cells that enter the bloodstream and lodge in distant sites are called hematogenous (born from the blood) metastases.

3.   Metastatic cancer cells that come to rest in small vessels begin a reverse invasion of the vessel wall leading to the

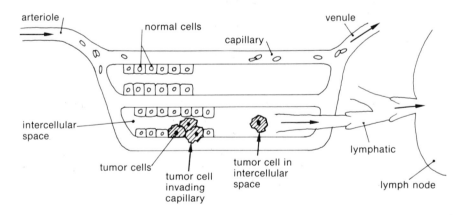

Figure 5–5 A diagrammatic view of the routes of tumor-cell invasion and the implications of these routes for the sites of distant metastases. Tumor cells that break off the original focus into the intercellular space enter afferent lymphatics and lodge in draining lymph nodes. Tumor cells that invade adjacent blood vessels enter the bloodstream and are distributed throughout the body.

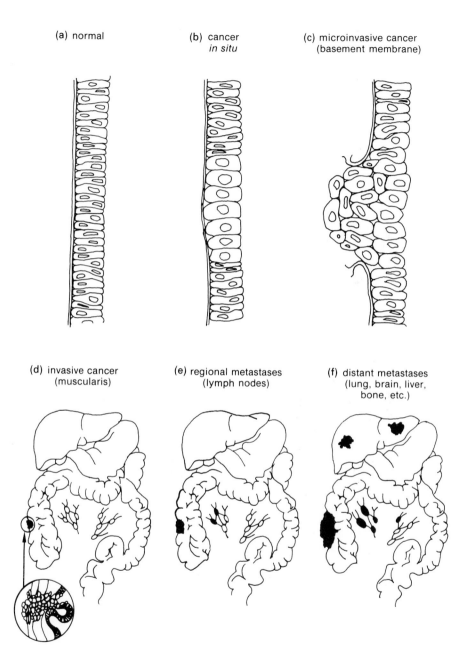

(a) normal

(b) cancer
    in situ

(c) microinvasive cancer
    (basement membrane)

(d) invasive cancer
    (muscularis)

(e) regional metastases
    (lymph nodes)

(f) distant metastases
    (lung, brain, liver,
    bone, etc.)

Figure 5–6   Successive stages in the development of a cancer of the colon (lower intestine). Going from left to right with time, an abnormal focus of cells invades the deeper muscular layer of the intestinal wall, spreads to local lymph nodes via the tissue lymphatics, and then to the liver following entry into blood vessels. [Adapted from N. Berlin, *Hosp. Pract.* **10(1),** 83 (1975).]

extravascular tissue spaces. The result is a new focus of cancer cells that may be far from the original site.

B.   Some metastatic cancers appear to spread almost exclusively via the lymphatics, whereas others also spread through the blood vascular system. Knowledge of the patterns of spread is important for therapeutic intervention.

1.   Some cancers have a predictable route of lymphatic metastasis. Such metastases can be diagnosed microscopically (Figure 5-7); for example, breast cancers that arise in the lateral portion of the breast spread via draining lymphatics to lymph nodes in the armpit (axilla), whereas those arising in the medial portion of the breast usually spread to a chain of lymph nodes under the ribs next to the breastbone, or sternum (Figure 5-8).

2.   Hematogenous metastases settle throughout the body, often in essential organs, which cannot be removed without lethal consequences. The pattern of these metastases is sufficiently random that they usually escape localized therapeutic maneuvers

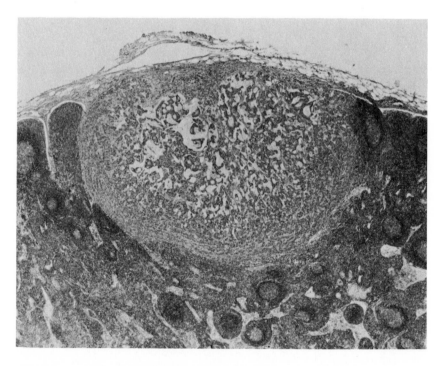

Figure 5-7   Lymph node metastasis. The central light area is a metastatic breast cancer that has formed abnormal apithelial structures. The dark surrounding tissue is the lymph node cortex with prominent secondary follicles. The light zones in the lower one fifth of the photograph are medullary sinuses. [Photographs courtesy of R. Warnke and P. Horne.]

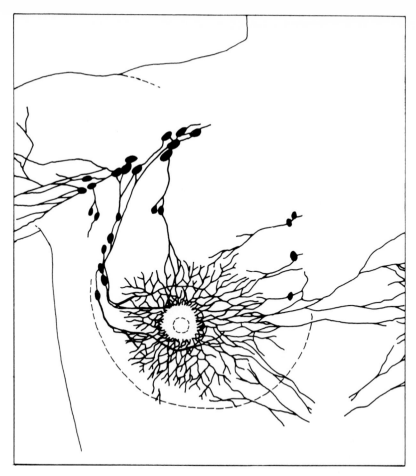

Figure 5–8 A diagram of the lymphatic drainage of the breast. Lymph nodes in the axilla drain the lateral portion of the breast, while lymph nodes just under the ribs next to the sternum drain the medial portion of the breast.

such as radiotherapy or surgery. Thus the consequences of hematogenous metastases usually are graver than those of lymphatic metastases. The frequency of metastases increases with the age of the cancer; the tendency to metastasize depends upon tumor size and the inherent invasive potential of the cancer (Figure 5–9).

5–3   The development of cancer cells may involve change or activation of the cellular genome

Carcinogenesis, the process by which cancers arise, is still poorly understood. The conversion of a normal cell to a cancer cell is called *transformation*. A transformed cell will produce only transformed

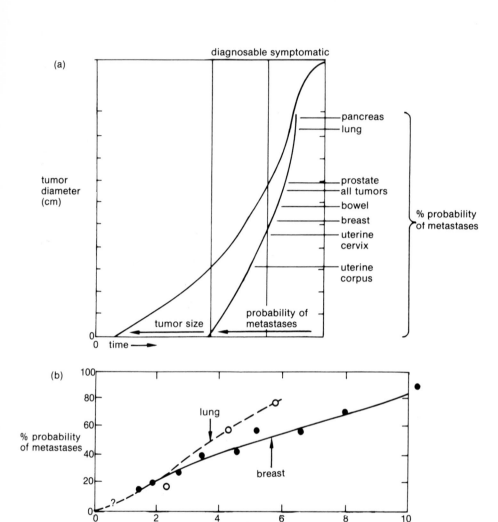

Figure 5–9 The relationship between primary tumor size and metastasis. Most cancers are diagnosed only when they become symptomatic. By that time the probability that metastases are present is 66% (for all tumors). The correlation between tumor size and probability of metastases has been shown for carcinoma of the breast and lung. For asymptomatic breast cancers smaller than 1 cm, the probability of metastases approaches zero, but it rises rapidly from 20% for palpable tumors of 2 cm or more to over 80% for tumors of 10 cm or more. For lung cancers, the probability of metastasis increases even faster, from about 20% for a 2-cm tumor to almost 80% for a 6-cm tumor. [Adapted from N. Berlin, *Hosp. Pract.* **10(1)**, 83 (1975).]

progeny, thereby giving rise to a clone of cancer cells. By the time any cancer is diagnosed, it has had a history much longer than the subsequent lifespan of the cancer, and of the host, if no therapy is attempted. The two principal theories of carcinogenesis hold that the preclinical development of a cancer involves a *progression* of transformations, giving rise to subclones of increasing malignancy.

1.   The *somatic mutation theory* states that somatic genetic changes are responsible for transformation, and that development of the malignant phenotype proceeds from a series of somatic mutations that lead first to moderately decreased tumor doubling times, and ultimately to complete loss of growth control.

2.   The *selective gene activation theory* holds that transformation results from the inappropriate expression of normal cellular genes. This hypothesis predicts that the transformed phenotype should be reversible, and that cancer cells possess only the full set of normal genes. Tumor progression could involve sequential activation of different genes, and somatic mutations would be incidental rather than causative in the development of highly malignant subclones.

3.   By the time they are clinically detectable, most cancers appear monoclonal, that is, as if they were derived from a single cell. This finding could be consistent with either of the two hypotheses for carcinogenesis. Either mutation or selective gene expression might lead to small changes in cell cycle time, susceptibility to growth control, nutritional requirements, or antigenicity. Such changes could give a particular subclone such a competitive advantage that it would grow to dominate the tumor (clonal dominance).

5-4   Some chemical and physical agents reproducibly cause cancer

A.   Epidemiological studies of cancer first suggested that substances in the environment could be responsible for carcinogenesis (Table 5-1). Tests in experimental animals showed that indeed some substances, for example cigarette smoke, are carcinogenic (Figure 5-10). Purification and fractionation of these substances sometimes led to loss of carcinogenic activity. Selective recombination of fractions, sometimes from separate sources (such as coal tar and cigarette smoke), restored activity. Such studies defined two classes of compounds active in chemical carcinogenesis: *carcinogens* and *promotors* (Table 5-2)

1.   Carcinogens act acutely on target cells, and cause an irreversible change in, or selective activation of, the cellular genome. This event is necessary but not sufficient for the neoplastic transformation of the affected cell.

Table 5–1

The progressive increase of bladder tumors with increasing length of exposure to aromatic amines[a] among 78 distillery workers

Length of latent period (years)	Length of exposure in years:					
	up to 1	1	2	3	4	5 & over
	(percentage of workers with tumors)					
Up to 5	0	0	0	0	0	0
10	0	0	0	0	0	11
15	0	17	22	0	10	45
20	4	17	22	40	30	69
25	9	17	22	70	70	88
30	9	17	48	70	80	94

[a]The statistics are given for bladder tumors among 78 men engaged under conditions of heavy exposure in the distillation of 2-naphthylamine and benzidine, two highly carcinogenic dyestuff intermediates. The group of workers who were exposed for only 4 years did not show a response for the first 10 years of observation, but after 20 years their bladder tumor incidence was up to 30%, and by 30 years it was as high as 80%. For the workers exposed for 5 years or more the incidence observed in 30 years went up to 94%. [Courtesy of National Cancer Society.]

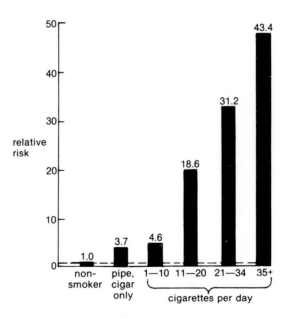

Figure 5–10   The relative risk of incurring lung cancer among nonsmokers and various groups of smokers. Those who smoke more than 35 cigarettes per day, for example, are more than 43 times as likely to develop cancer as those who do not smoke. [Courtesy of National Cancer Society.]

Table 5–2
Some common carcinogens and promotors

Class of compound	Carcinogens	Typical source	Promotors	Typical source
Polycyclic aromatic hydrocarbons	3,4-Benzpyrene (BP)	Coal tar; cigarette smoke; soot	Phorbolmyristate acetate (PMA)	Croton oil
	Methylcholanthrene (MC)	Coal tar; cigarette smoke; soot	Natural hormones	Ovary, adrenal, etc.
	Aflatoxin B_1	Aspergillus flavus (a fungus that grows on grains and peanuts)		
Aromatic amines	Dimethylaminobenzene (butter yellow; DAB)			
	2-Acetylaminofluorene (AAF)			
Food preservatives	Nitrates convert secondary amines to nitrosamines	Preserved meats such as frankfurters		
Azo dyes		Dye industry		
Irradiation	X ray	Military; nuclear reactors; medical diagnosis		
	Ultraviolet	Sun		
Other chemicals	Asbestos	Insulating material		
	Bis (2-chlorethyl) sulfide (mustard gas)	Military		
	Vinyl chloride	Plastics industry		
Drugs	Diethylstilbesterol	Medical therapy		

2. Promotors stimulate cell division of particular target cells. At least two cell division cycles are required for malignant transformation of carcinogen-treated cells. Promotor action is reversible, and is not by itself carcinogenic. It must occur after carcinogen treatment to cause transformation.

B.   Direct application of most carcinogenic substances to target cells *in vitro* does not lead to malignant transformation, even in the presence of appropriate promotors. These carcinogenic substances are modified metabolically *in vivo* to become *ultimate carcinogens*. The crucial modification usually takes place in the liver, where detoxifying enzymes first convert the substance to a highly reactive intermediate and then esterify this intermediate with glucuronides (Figure 5–11). This modification renders the substance biologically inactive and susceptible to kidney tubule-cell transport systems, which excrete the substance into the urine. The highly reactive intermediates are ultimate carcinogens. They may reach carcinogenic levels if their rate of production exceeds their rate of glucuronidation. For example, people with abnormally high levels of aryl hydrocarbon hydroxylases have a greatly increased risk of some types of cancer.

C.   Although the mode of action of ultimate carcinogens in transformation is not yet established, there is increasing evidence that most if not all these compounds are potent mutagens. This generalization is the basis for the *Ames test*, a simple inexpensive screening procedure that can detect low levels of environmental carcinogens by their ability to increase the frequency of known mutational events in a bacterium such as *Salmonella.*

The physical agents that cause cancer, such as ultraviolet and irradiation also are highly mutagenic, acting directly on nucleic acids to cause genetic changes. Therefore it seems likely that carcinogenic agents act on DNA to cause transformation, but whether their primary effect is through mutation or alteration of gene expression remains unresolved.

5–5   Genes that induce the malignant phenotype can be demonstrated in both DNA and RNA tumor viruses

A.   Certain DNA and RNA viruses, termed *oncogenic*, can transform the cells they infect and thereby induce tumor formation. There are several varieties of oncogenic DNA viruses, ranging from very simple to very complex. A classification of these viruses and the neoplasms they induce is given in Table 5–3. The simplest viruses, SV40 and polyoma, have been analyzed most completely, and are therefore most useful for elucidating general principles. Both of these viruses can undergo alternative routes of infection. In some kinds of host cell,

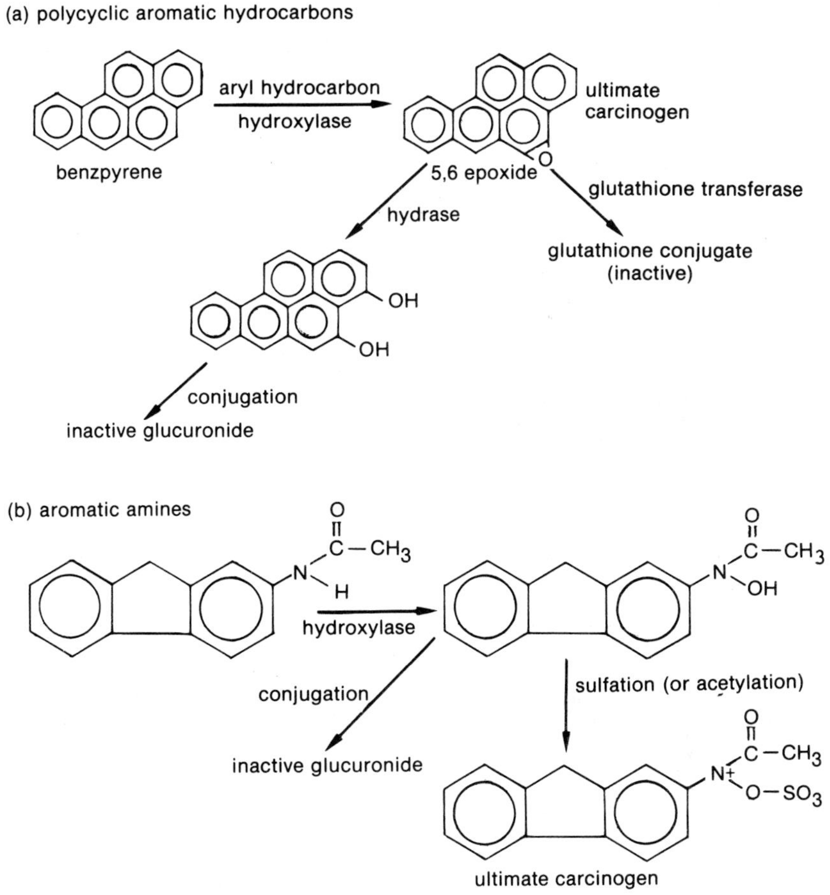

(a) polycyclic aromatic hydrocarbons

(b) aromatic amines

Figure 5-11   The metabolism of some carcinogens in the liver (see text).

called *permissive,* the virus appropriates the cell's synthetic machinery, produces nearly 10^6 progeny virus particles per cell, and then causes cell *lysis* with release of the new virus. In other, so-called *nonpermissive* host cells, some viral genes are expressed, but the infection then aborts and the host cells survive. A small fraction of these cells undergo malignant transformation. The transformed cells retain one or a few viral genomes, integrated covalently into the host genome. It is not known whether any of the DNA oncogenic viruses (except papilloma virus) cause cancer in humans.

B.   Oncogenic RNA virus (*oncornavirus*) infections differ from DNA tumor virus infections in several respects. A unique set of enzymes

Table 5–3
Some DNA oncogenic viruses and their properties

Class	Virus	Genome size (molecular weight)	Host cell for productive infection	Host cell for *in vitro* malignant transformation
Papova	SV40 (Simian virus 40)	3×10^6	Monkey	Human, mouse, hamster
	Polyoma (poly = many, oma = tumors)	3×10^6	Mouse	Mouse, hamster, rat
	Papilloma (causes the benign skin tumors called warts)	5×10^6	?	Rabbit, human
Adenoviruses	Several types (e.g., adenovirus-12)	25×10^6	Human	Hamster, rat, human
Herpes	Herpes saimiri	100×10^6	?	Monkey
	Lucke carcinoma	100×10^6	?	Frog
	Marek's disease	100×10^6	?	Chicken
	Epstein–Barr virus (EBV)	100×10^6	Human (infectious mononucleosis)	Human? (Burkitt's lymphoma)

coded for and carried by all oncornaviruses provides for the synthesis of a double-stranded circular DNA copy of the RNA genome, called the *provirus*, which becomes inserted into the host cell genome (Figure 5–12) with concomitant transformation of the host cell. Oncornavirus-infected cells continually produce progeny virus by a budding process at the cell membrane. During budding the viral core is in the shape of an inverted C; hence these viruses are called C-type viruses (Figure 5–13). A classification of the several varieties of oncornaviruses and the neoplasms they produce is shown in Table 5–4. Like DNA tumor viruses, oncornaviruses have not been demonstrated to cause cancer in humans.

The structural glycoproteins of the cell membrane budding site, which become the envelope glycoproteins of the virus, are coded by the viral genome. The molecules apparently organize into a cell membrane complex which largely, if not completely, excludes host cell membrane proteins. This budding site appears to be recognized specifically by cytoplasmic viral core assemblies that contain the virion RNA. Budding occurs by evagination of the core-membrane complex, ending with a separation of viral and cellular membranes (Figure 5–14).

Uninfected host cells also contain and sometimes express genes which are closely related to these viral genes. In some tissues these

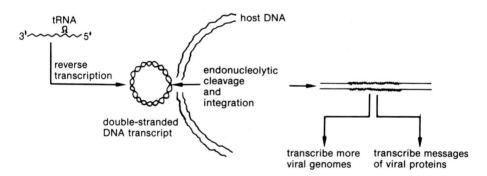

Figure 5–12 Events in the reverse transcription and integration of oncornavirus genes into host genomes. The enveloped virus penetrates into the target-cell cytoplasm. Using an enzyme called *reverse transcriptase*, which it codes for and carries with it, the virus begins the transcription of its RNA nucleotide sequence template into a complementary DNA nucleotide sequence. The reaction requires a primer, a host-cell transfer RNA (tRNA), which binds to a complementary sequence near the 5' end of the viral RNA. A single-strand DNA is copied to the 5' end of the viral RNA, and then synthesis continues, beginning at the 3' end of the viral RNA. During this process the used viral RNA template is digested or removed, and a second-strand DNA copy is made using the reverse transcribed DNA as a template. The result is a double-stranded closed-circular proviral DNA copy of the viral RNA information. In cells susceptible to infection by this virus, the DNA provirus apparently integrates into a unique site in host chromosomal DNA, where it may act as a site of transcription of new viral RNA's and individual gene messages.

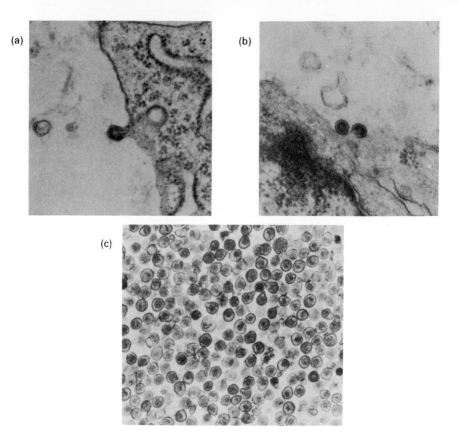

Figure 5–13 The budding of an oncornavirus. In (a) the virion bud is in the characteristic C-configuration, whereas in (b) one completed virion is adjacent to a nearly completed particle. In (c) a concentrate of these viruses is shown. [Photographs courtesy of O. Witte and D. Rice.]

Table 5–4
A list of oncornaviruses and their effects

Name	Susceptible species	Type of tumor induced
Rapidly transforming viruses:		
Rous sarcoma virus	Chickens; other aves	Sarcomas
Moloney sarcoma virus	Rodents	Sarcomas
Friend focus forming virus	Rodents	Erythro and myelomonocytic tumors
Abelson leukemia virus	Rodents	Hematopoietic tumors; B-cell tumors?
Simian sarcoma virus	Simians	Sarcomas
Slowly transforming viruses:		
Avian leukosis virus	Chickens	Lymphoid leukemia
Gross leukemia virus	Rodents	T-cell leukemias
Radiation leukemia virus	Rodents	T-cell leukemias
Friend lymphatic leukemia virus	Rodents	T-cell leukemias
Moloney leukemia virus	Rodents	T-cell leukemias
Feline leukemia virus	Cats; baboons?	Leukemias
Bovine leukemia virus	Cattle	Leukemias
Mouse mammary tumor virus	Rodents	Mammary carcinomas

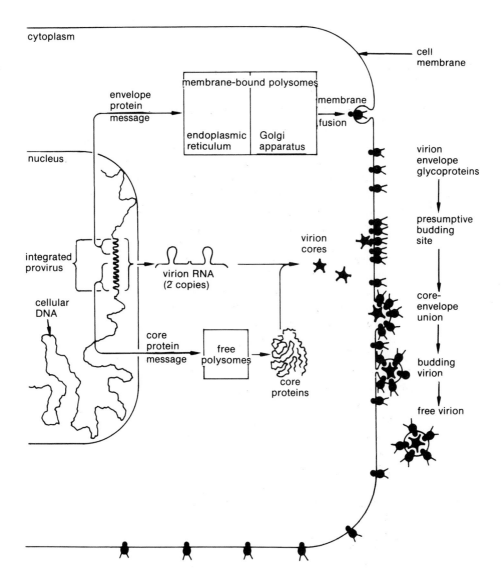

Figure 5-14 Cellular formation of oncornavirus budding sites. Virion mRNA's of two classes, core and envelope, are transcribed from integrated vital DNA copies. A core polyprotein is produced from core mRNA in the free polysome fraction, and this is cleaved into several distinct proteins which combine with virion RNA to form the virion cores. Simultaneously, envelope mRNA is translated in polysomes bound to membranes of endoplasmic reticulum. This envelope precursor polyprotein is glycosylated, cleaved to its functional subunits, and inserted into the plasma membrane of the cell at presumptive budding sites. Core assemblies bind to the inner surface of presumptive budding sites and evaginate through them, with eventual separation of viral and cellular membranes.

gene products are reliable cell-surface markers of a particular differentiation stage of the cells expressing them; in other tissues these molecules are secreted.

5-6 Three kinds of methods currently are employed for treatment of cancer in humans

Two of the commonly used therapeutic approaches are localized, and one is systemic.

1. The primary method of localized cancer therapy is surgical removal of cancerous organs and tissues. This approach obviously requires a precise knowledge of the location and extent of the cancer, because only limited amounts of tissue can be excised.

2. The second method of localized therapy is the application of ionizing radiation (radiotherapy) to the site of known primary and suspected metastatic sites. The radiation results in irreparable damage to cellular DNA; those cells that enter the next cell cycle are unable to complete mitosis and die (mitotic death). A few cell types, such as lymphocytes, die without mitosis within hours after absorbing a lethal dose of irradiation (interphase death). Radiotherapy also requires precise knowledge of tumor location and extent. This treatment is most useful against tumors of lymphoid origin with known metastatic patterns, such as Hodgkin's Disease, which now can be cured in up to 80% of all cases. Radiotherapy is also useful where an important structure must be cleared of cancer cells, but subsequently can function without extensive cell division. For example, radiotherapy for laryngeal carcinoma leaves the patient with intact, functioning vocal cords, whereas the surgical approach usually does not.

3. The third method of cancer treatment is chemotherapy, the systemic administration of cytotoxic drugs. These drugs are designed to affect proliferating cells preferentially by interfering with pyrimidine and purine metabolism, DNA synthesis, or the process of mitosis (Figure 5-15). Because these drugs are accessible to all cells, malignant and normal, their major limitation is that they kill normal cells.

4. With one or more of these therapeutic approaches, a number of cancers now can be cured that were incurable ten years ago. However, these cures may only be partially effected by the therapeutic treatment. Many oncologists believe that all cancer therapies act to reduce the tumor cell load to a size that host defense mechanisms can handle. In any case, curative cancer therapy must have as its goal the removal of all cancer cells, because a single cancer cell left unimpeded will multiply to kill the patient.

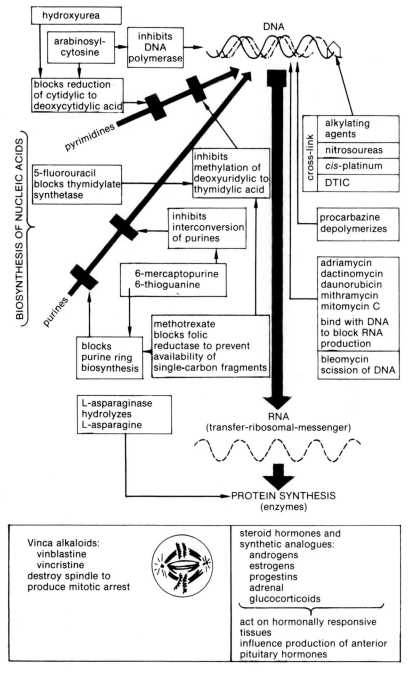

Figure 5–15 The actions of currently used anticancer chemotherapeutic agents. Three classes of agents are depicted: those that interfere with DNA synthesis or replication, those that affect the mitotic spindle and therefore arrest cells at metaphase, and those that act on tissues that require or are inhibited by steroid homones. [Adapted from I. Krakoff, *Ca—A Cancer Journal for Clinicians* **27(3),** 130 (1977).]

5–7   Most cancers are antigenic in their host of origin

A.   In 1908 the famous biologist Paul Ehrlich postulated that cancer cells arise frequently, and that they bear membrane changes that could be recognized as foreign antigens by the host. He further stated that the cellular immune response may in most cases be sufficient for cancer cell rejection. Fifty years later Lewis Thomas postulated that the development of cell-mediated immunity in evolution was driven by the need for *immunological surveillance* of newly arising neoplasms.

B.   To demonstrate that cancer cells are in fact antigenic, one must show that they can induce an immune response in the host of origin, and that the response is specific for the cancer cells. If most cancer cells are antigenic, one must assume that tumor formation is the result of an immunoresistant cancer, or that the immune response itself is ineffective. If so, it may be very difficult to demonstrate immunity of a host to its own tumor. Experimentalists in the early twentieth century attempted to circumvent this problem by removing the tumor from the original host and transplanting tumor cells to a second animal of the same species. In every case these tumors indeed began to grow and then were rejected. However, we now know that because these investigators did not use inbred strains, the immune responses observed were against the transplantation antigens of the donor animal rather than against tumor-specific antigens. Only with the development of inbred strains of mice and rats did it become possible to ascertain the existence of tumor-specific antigens.

1.   Tumor antigenicity and host immunity to tumors was first demonstrated by a three-stage experiment (Figure 5–16). A carcinogen-induced cancer was excised completely from its original host, and then varying numbers of tumor cells were transplanted to syngeneic hosts. The number of transplanted cells that reproducibly induced tumors in the recipient hosts was determined. Retransplantation of this number of tumor cells from the secondary hosts to the original host usually resulted in no tumor growth. This phenomenon was *specific* for the original tumor. Adoptive transfer of lymphocytes from the original host to genetically identical naive hosts conferred specific resistance to the original tumor. This transfer of immunity required the transfer of live lymphocytes, subsequently identified as T lymphocytes.

2.   With the advent of sensitive techniques, such as immunofluorescence and radioimmunoassay, for assaying antibodies specific to tumor antigens, it was demonstrated that tumor-bearing hosts had both a cell-mediated and a humoral immune response to their own tumor antigens. The resulting humoral antibodies were used in cross-absorption studies to compare large numbers

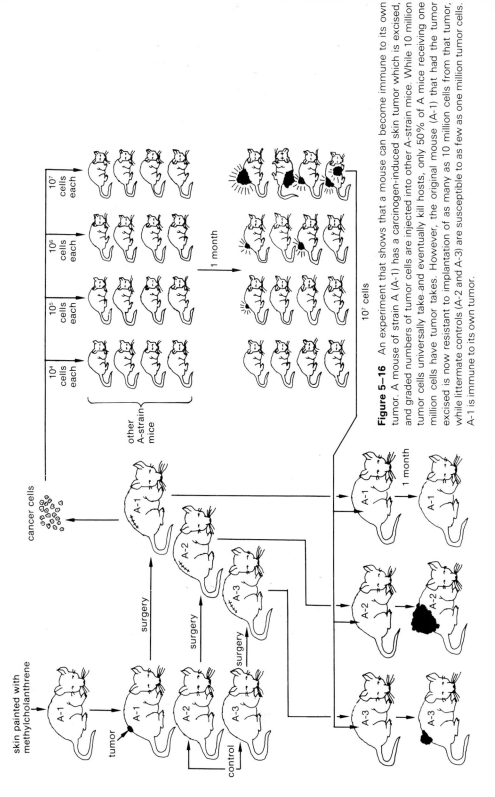

Figure 5–16 An experiment that shows that a mouse can become immune to its own tumor. A mouse of strain A (A-1) has a carcinogen-induced skin tumor which is excised, and graded numbers of tumor cells are injected into other A-strain mice. While 10 million tumor cells universally take and eventually kill hosts, only 50% of A mice receiving one million cells have tumor takes. However, the original mouse (A-1) that had the tumor excised is now resistant to implantation of as many as 10 million cells from that tumor, while littermate controls (A-2 and A-3) are susceptible to as few as one million tumor cells. A-1 is immune to its own tumor.

skin painted with methylcholanthrene

cancer cells

surgery

surgery

surgery

tumor

control

1 month

10^7 cells

10^4 cells each

10^5 cells each

10^6 cells each

10^7 cells each

other A-strain mice

1 month

of tumors and normal cells. Thus it was possible to identify tumors with *cross-reacting antigens,* tumors with *tumor-unique antigens,* and tumors with antigens common to a subset of normal cells (*differentiation antigens*).

C.   In theory, apparent tumor-specific antigens could be new determinants or simply very rare normal determinants. Most tumors are populated predominantly by a single clone of cells, all of which share the cell membrane properties of the original transformed cell. Some of the surface determinants of each normal cell may be unique, or shared by only a few other cells. If so, the concentration of these unique determinants will be far too low to trigger either an immunogenic or tolerogenic response. However, if such a cell gives rise to a transformed clone of identical cells, its surface molecules may provoke an immune response even if no new determinants are present. Thus a carcinogen-induced transformation may produce a change in the cell surface, or simply may select for expansion of a rare subset of preexisting cells bearing unique cell-surface determinants (Figure 5–17).

D.   In experimental situations, four classes of tumor antigens are found. The first class is called oncofetal antigens. These antigens are found on the surfaces of cancer cells, but also are expressed during a specific phase of embryonic differentiation.

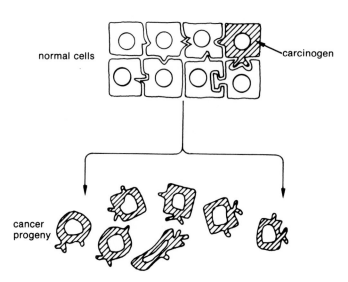

Figure 5–17 A clonal selection hypothesis to describe carcinogen-induced tumor-specific antigens. Several distinct cell types in a tissue adhere to each other by cell-specific surface properties. The carcinogen selectively transforms one of these types. The clonal progeny resulting from this transformation bear the same cell-specific determinants, but these cancer cells show a wide variety of morphological characteristics (pleomorphism). Because these malignant progeny no longer have complementary cells to adhere to, they tend to grow away from the original focus.

1. An important example is the carcinoembryonic antigens of the colon (CEA). This set of antigens is found on the surfaces of all tumor cells derived from the gastrointestinal tract or derivatives of the fetal gastrointestinal tract, such as pancreas, liver, and gall bladder. These antigens, which appear to be glycoproteins, have been demonstrated to be present on only a small subset of normal adult cells, so that the total body concentration of CEA normally is extremely small.

2. Another important example is alpha-fetoprotein (αFP), normally secreted by yolk sac and fetal liver epithelial cells, and also produced by malignant yolk sac and liver cells. Although αFP is a secreted product, anti-αFP immune responses restrict growth of these neoplasms. Careful analysis has revealed that αFP is not solely a tumor antigen in adults, but is normally expressed by the proliferating fraction of liver cells.

E. The second class of tumor-specific antigens is those induced by chemical carcinogens. Each carcinogen-induced tumor expresses unique cell-surface antigens. When a single mouse is skin-painted with the carcinogen methylcholanthrene at several different sites, each of the resulting carcinomas will express cell-surface antigens that are identical on all cells within the tumor but different from the antigens expressed by the other methylcholanthrene-induced tumors. The following experiment suggests that in at least one case these antigens are unlikely to be normal cell-specific determinants.

Mouse epithelial cells from the prostate were cloned *in vitro*, and several progeny cells from the same clone were independently transformed by carcinogen *in vitro*. The tumor-specific cell-surface antigens were identical among the progeny of any given transformed cell, but the tumor-specific antigens of each transformed clone were unique. Other chemical carcinogens also show induction of diverse tumor-specific antigens. These findings are important for at least two reasons.

1. At the biological level it is important to know whether chemical carcinogens somehow select for rare cells, each of which when cloned expresses a unique surface antigen present on the original cell just prior to transformation, or whether transformation *invariably* results in a genetic event that is expressed as a new cell-membrane antigen. If the second alternative is true, it will be important to establish whether neoplastic transformation is dependent upon the membrane alteration. If so, transformation could be postulated to have its primary effect on cell–cell interactions or cell-membrane functions, which as a secondary consequence promote cell proliferation.

2. There is also an important clinical consequence of the finding that carcinogens induce unique tumor-specific antigens. If each

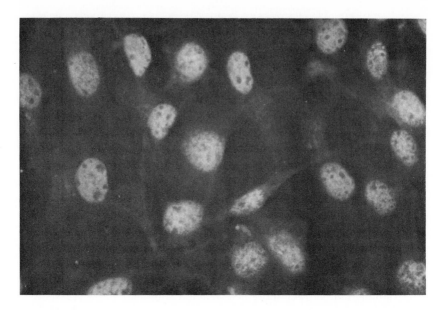

Figure 5–18 The detection of nuclear (T) antigens by immunofluorescence in cells infected with SV40. [Courtesy of C. Croce and K. Huebner.]

new carcinogen-induced tumor bears only unique tumor-specific determinants, then it will be difficult if not impossible to prepare in advance a stockpile of specific immunologic reagents for tumor detection or treatment.

F.   The third class of tumor-associated antigens comprises those induced by oncogenic DNA viruses. Each of these viruses induces unique nuclear and cell-surface antigens in cells that it transforms. For a particular virus these antigens are always the same, regardless of differences in the tissue, the animal, or even the species in which the transformation occurs. Thus both the nuclear (T) antigens and surface (S) antigens are diagnostic of the virus (Figure 5–18).

It is not yet certain whether the surface antigens are coded by the viral genome, or are present already on cells selected in the transformation process. Because the induced antigens are the same from tissue to tissue and species to species it would seem likely that they are specified by the virus. However, an alternative explanation is suggested by experiments in which normal cells from several different species were treated with a proteolytic enzyme to remove the outer glycoprotein coat of the cell membrane. The cells remained viable, but now exhibited previously hidden surface antigens, presumably glycolipid in nature. Among these antigens was that typical of SV40-transformed cells. Thus the surface antigens induced by DNA tumor viruses could be normal cell-membrane components that somehow are exposed as a result of transformation. The nuclear T antigen of SV40, however, is known to be a viral gene product. Both the T antigen and the cell-surface antigen are distinct from antigens of the viral protein coat, which are not detectable in transformed cells. The three major candidates for human DNA virus-induced tumors, Burkitt's lymphoma, nasopharyngeal carcinoma, and cancer of the cervix of the uterus (the virus candidates are various herpes viruses), do express tumor-associated cell-surface antigens, which are the same on all tumors of a particular type.

G.   The fourth class of tumor-associated antigens is those induced by oncornavirus transformation. Like the DNA tumor viruses, each RNA tumor virus induces specific antigens that are the same, regardless of differences in the host cell. By contrast, most, if not all, oncornavirus-specific tumor antigens are viral protein antigens. Some of these proteins represent precursors of virus budding sites on the transformed cell membrane (Figure 5–14). These antigens may have *group-specific* determinants in common with all viruses of a certain group, for example mouse leukemia viruses, *type-specific* determinants shared by only a few closely related viruses, for example Gross and Radiation leukemia viruses, and unique virus-specific determinants. These determinants may be present on various virion polypeptides; at least one cell-surface antigen is an internal virion protein.

Most of the leukemogenic oncornaviruses induce neoplasms that express normal differentiation antigens as well. In the mouse, one differentiation antigen, TL, may be anomalously expressed by thymic lymphomas from a mouse strain that normally does not express TL antigens on its thymocytes. Thus the control of TL expression somehow can be interfered with by oncornavirus-induced transformation. In the special case of the murine oncornavirus-induced cell-surface antigens, the virion envelope protein may express virus-unique determinants, as well as determinants common to host differentiation antigens, in keeping with the homology between certain host genes and virion envelope genes.

5-8   Cancer cells are attacked by the cellular immune system

A.   The first experiment clearly to define the role of antibodies and cells in the immune response to cancers was carried out in the late 1940's. Cancer cells were placed into a cell-impermeable chamber with pores 0.2 μ in diameter that allowed molecules, but not cells to enter and exit. When the chambers were placed into hosts immune to the cancer cells, the cells survived and multiplied, although high concentrations of cancer-specific antibodies diffused into the chamber and bound to the cells. However, when the experiment was repeated with a chamber that contained pores large enough for cells to enter, the cancer cells were destroyed, and host lymphoid cells could be found infiltrating the tumor mass. These experiments provided the first evidence that most tumors are not susceptible to attack by antibodies alone or by antibodies plus complement, but that they are susceptible to attack by killer cells. Three kinds of killer cells may be involved in cell-mediated immunity to tumors: T_c cells, the cells responsible for antibody-dependent cell-mediated cytotoxicity (ADCC), and natural killer (NK) cells. In most cancers, the T_c response is dominant (see Essential Concept 1–12). However, leukemias are quite sensitive to natural killer cells, to antibody and complement, and to antibody-dependent cell-mediated cytotoxicity. In general, cancers of the hematolymphoid system are sensitive to both humoral and cellular immunity, whereas all other cancers are susceptible to cellular immunity only.

If the T-cell immune system is important for elimination of newly arising tumors, then animals and humans deficient in this system should be highly susceptible to induced tumors and also should have a high incidence of spontaneous tumors.

1.   Animals deprived of their thymus early in life are indeed extremely susceptible to various oncogenic viruses. For example, when neonatally thymectomized mice are exposed to Moloney sarcoma virus or polyoma virus, the animals suffer a high incidence of tumors that grow more rapidly than the tumors induced at low incidence in nonthymectomized littermate controls. Furthermore, the tumors from thymectomized animals are more highly antigenic on a per cell basis than the tumors in nonthy-mectomized littermates. These results, and those described in the preceding section, fulfill a postulate of the immunosurveillance hypothesis, that is, that the immune system responds to the antigens of endogenous neoplasms.

2.   Another postulate of the hypothesis, that the cellular immune system has evolved to protect against a high rate of spontaneously arising neoplasms, is more controversial. As improvements in animal husbandry have allowed congenitally athymic animals to survive longer, it has been found that they do not have a high incidence of death from cancer. Further experiments are needed to determine whether these animals have a thymus-independent immune response that is sufficient for immunosurveillance, whether there is a nonimmune surveillance mechanism for removal of antigenic or newly arising tumor cells, or whether the assumption that tumors frequently arise by mutation simply is not true.

3.   Immunologically deficient humans suffer a strikingly high incidence of cancer. For example, nearly 10% of children with

congenital immunological deficiency disease develop cancer. However, these cancers are principally derived from cells of the lymphoid system, and it is not certain whether the high rate of neoplasia is due to lack of immunosurveillance, or to pathological consequences of the lymphoid system imbalance.

4. The best documented examples of increased tumor incidence in immunosuppressed hosts come from patients treated with immunosuppressive drugs for allogeneic kidney transplants. These patients have an eighty-fold increased risk of developing cancer; about 60% of their cancers are of epithelial origin and about 40% of lymphoid origin. Again, it is unclear whether these cancers reflect the patient's immunodeficient state, or result from a pathological lymphoid disorder. The results are further complicated by the observation that the frequencies of the various epithelial neoplasms that develop in these patients do not correspond to the frequencies found in other groups of patients matched for age, sex, and geographical location. For example, immunosuppression causes little increase in the incidence of breast cancer or lung cancer, whereas it causes large increases in the incidence of other epithelial neoplasms.

In summary, there is circumstantial evidence to support the immunosurveillance hypothesis, but the theory has not been conclusively tested. Still lacking is knowledge of all the immune mechanisms that could be involved, and proof that cancers arise spontaneously at a high frequency.

5-9   Some cancer cells escape immunological surveillance

A.   Whatever the general validity of the immunosurveillance hypothesis, by the time a tumor is diagnosed most cancer patients demonstrate both cellular and humoral immunity directed specifically at cell-surface antigens of the tumor cells. How then do these tumor cells survive in what should be a hostile environment? Tumor growth under these conditions has been termed immunological escape. Tumor transplantation experiments have shown that in some cases low doses of cancer cells "sneak through" to form tumors, whereas somewhat higher doses will not. Growth of small tumors is progressive despite evidence of an active host immune response. In other cases, termed concomitant immunity, a large primary tumor grows quite well, yet antigenic metastases are rejected by the host. In these cases, a small number of tumor cells is handled by the immune system, whereas a large number is not. Several different mechanisms of immunologic escape have been found in research on experimental tumors; these studies form the basis for our current understanding of human tumor immunology.

1. *Immunological tolerance:* Animals injected very early with tumors or high concentrations of tumor-associated antigens before the development of full immunological competence maintain a specific unresponsiveness to these tumors if they are transplanted into the animals later in life. This phenomenon appears to be identical to that of immunological tolerance described in Essential Concept 1–14.

2. *Immunoselection:* Rare variant cells that have lost the original surface antigens occur in large tumor cell populations. In the face of an immune response against the antigenic tumor cells, the variants selectively grow to dominate the tumor. These cells may bear a different set of antigens and may in turn induce their own specific immune response. The immune response does not induce antigenic change; it merely selects for cells that have undergone antigenic change independently.

3. *Antigenic modulation:* This interesting phenomenon provides an example of how understanding the basic biology of microorganisms leads to an important clinical insight. In the 1940's Beale and Sonneborn observed that treatment of paramecia with antibodies specific for their ciliary antigens leads to cessation of movement. However, if the paramecia are metabolically active, they soon begin to swim again, even in the continued presence of antibody. Further examination reveals that they have lost the antigens formerly present on their cilia and are expressing a new set of antigens. In the presence of antibody to the new antigens, modulation may occur again, with either reexpression of the first antigens or expression of another new set of antigens. These ciliary antigens all are determined by nuclear genes of the paramecium.

Similar antigenic modulation has been demonstrated in two systems of mouse leukemic cells. Thymic leukemias induced in some mouse strains by thymotropic murine leukemia viruses express TL antigens. Transfer of these thymic leukemia cells to hosts immune to TL antigens does not stop progressive growth of the tumor. Analysis of the leukemia cells growing in these recipient hosts reveals no cell-surface TL antigens. In tissue culture as well, when anti-TL antibody is added to TL-positive leukemia cells they also lose the TL antigens, and within a few hours 100% of the cells are TL-negative. In the absence of anti-TL antibodies, the TL antigens usually reappear, indicating that both the controlling genes and the structural genes for the TL antigens remain intact in the modulating cells and in their descendants.

Immunoglobulin molecules on the surfaces of B cells and B-cell leukemias also are subject to antigenic modulation. In this case, it has been demonstrated directly that the original antigenic molecules are removed from the cell surface by endocytosis and/or shedding following capping by anti-Ig.

4. *Immunostimulation:* In the 1950's it was first suggested that some aspect of the immune response against a tumor may actually trigger cancer cells into more rapid or extensive proliferation. Recently it has been demonstrated in a few tumor systems that a weak immune response may indeed promote increased outgrowth of antigenic tumor cells. The mechanism of this stimulation is not known.

5. *Immunosuppression:* There are at least two ways in which immunosuppression can occur in a cancer patient. The most common is iatrogenic immunosuppression, that is, immunosuppression caused by agents used to treat the cancer. Most anticancer agents, including ionizing radiation, and cytotoxic drugs, have as side effects the destruction of lymphocytes and other cells important in the generation and maintenance of immunity.

In some cancers the tumors themselves seem to release immunosuppressive factors. The most striking example of this phenomenon is Hodgkin's disease, in which a small tumor in a single lymph node releases or induces the release of immunosuppressive factors that have a powerful effect on the entire cell-mediated immune system. Patients with Hodgkin's disease have a poor delayed hypersensitivity response and are abnormally sensitive to intracellular parasitic infections such as tuberculosis and Herpes virus infections.

6. *Immunological enhancement:* In some cases animals that have been preimmunized with allogeneic grafts of disrupted cells from a certain tumor and then subsequently challenged with the same tumor will support its growth and eventually die. Nonimmunized animals challenged with the same tumor will allow it only brief growth and then reject it. Several experiments suggest a diversity of mechanisms to explain this paradoxical finding.

Immunological enhancement of tumor allograft growth may be accomplished by passive transfer of serum from an immunized host to a syngeneic nonimmune host, even if antiserum injection is delayed until as late as seven days after tumor implantation. This result suggests that enhancement is due to blockade of the effector mechanisms that normally promote tumor rejection (Figure 5–19). However, immunological enhancement also is observed if tumor cells precoated with enhancing antibodies are injected, suggesting that enhancement can operate by altering the initial sensitization mechanism. Experiments with an *in vitro* model system support the existence of serum blocking factors

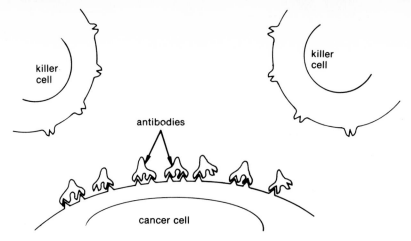

Figure 5–19 The blockade of effector (killer) cell function by competing antibodies directed against the same target-cell antigens that the killer cells recognize.

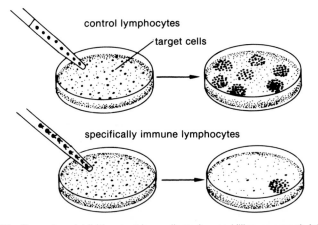

Figure 5–20 The colony inhibition test is predicated upon killing or growth inhibition of tumor cells by specifically immune lymphocytes. By comparing the number of colonies formed when immune lymphocytes are used with the number when control lymphocytes are used, the percentage of tumor cells killed or inhibited by the immune lymphocytes can be derived. [Adapted from K. E. and I. Hellström, "Immunologic defenses against cancer," in *Immunobiology*, R. A. Good and D. W. Fisher (Eds.), Sinauer Associates, Stamford, Conn., 1971, Chapter 21.]

that interfere with effector cell mechanisms. Growth of tumor cells in tissue culture normally is inhibited by lymphocytes from the tumor-bearing host (Figure 5–20). This lymphocyte effect can be blocked by addition of serum from the tumor-bearing host (Figure 5–21) but not by serum from hosts with another tumor type. This result could be due to blockade of tumor target-cell antigenic determinants by anti-tumor antibodies, which would prevent attack by immune lymphocytes. If so, these

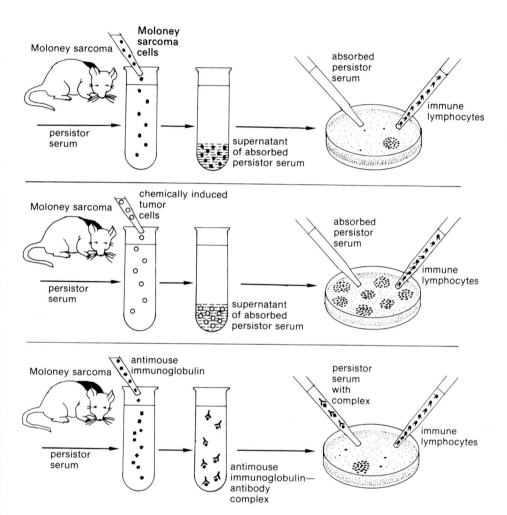

Figure 5–21 Two types of experiment provide evidence that the serum factors protecting persistent tumors contain specific antibodies. When persistor serum from an animal with a Moloney sarcoma is absorbed with Moloney sarcoma cells, the serum loses its ability to protect tumor cells (top). When cells from a different type of tumor (chemically induced) are used, the protective effect of the serum is unchanged (middle). The protective effect also is lost when goat anti-mouse immunoglobulin is added, which complexes and removes serum antibody (bottom). [Adapted from K. E. and I. Hellström; see Figure 5–20 legend.]

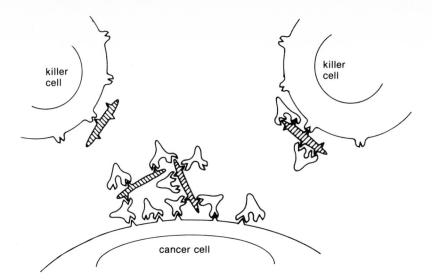

Figure 5–22 Two models of blocking-factor action. Antigen (shaded) or antigen–antibody complexes form lattices which may obscure target-cell antigenic determinants and/or killer-cell receptors.

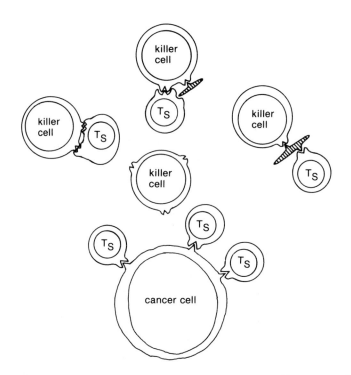

Figure 5–23 How suppressor T cells may block tumor immunity. T_s cells may affect T_c cells by having receptor specificity for T_c-cell idiotype, or for the combination of antigen with T_c idiotype, or for antigen alone. Alternatively, T_s cells may suppress by direct action on the tumor target cell, and thus have receptor specificity for tumor antigens.

experiments appear to indicate a basic antagonism between humoral and cell-mediated immunity to tumors. Alternatively, the serum-blocking factors could be solubilized tumor-cell antigens, which either alone or complexed with anti-tumor antibodies inhibit immune lymphocytes by blockade or elimination reactions (Figure 5–22).

In some cases of immunological tolerance as well as immunological enhancement, the dominant influence in specific inhibition of the immune response appears to be suppression, that is, suppressor T cells or products of suppressor T cells. Thus it is possible that specific suppression also plays some role in the enhancement of tumor growth by inhibition of immune responses (Figure 5–23).

5-10   Immunological approaches to the therapy, diagnosis, and prevention of cancer may be important in cancer management

A.   Given the complexity of immune responses in patients with clinically detectable tumors, what are the prospects for development of cancer immunotherapy? It is clear that humans usually have both a humoral and a cell-mediated immune response to their own tumor antigens, but that for some reason this response is not always effective.

1.   Cell-mediated immunity provides the best defense against most cancers. However, attempts to increase the number of killer T cells and antibody-dependent killer cells in a patient may result in expansion of inhibitory cell clones as well. Moreover, because the dimensions of the blocking-factor problem are not yet understood, it is not clear that increased clones of killer cells could compete with the blocking system.

2.   Adoptive transfer of immunity to human cancer antigens from one patient to the next by transfer of live lymphocytes could be exceedingly dangerous because of the probable GVHR to the recipient's transplantation antigens. Such a response affects several of the body's important organ systems, and is often fatal. Until it is possible to separate lymphocytes specific for normal cell targets from those specific for tumor cells this approach to immunotherapy will not be possible.

3.   An approach currently being tested is called adjuvant immunotherapy. In this method the tumor is inoculated with BCG, an attenuated mycobacterium that is related to the tubercle bacillus and is an intracellular parasite of macrophages. The resulting immune response leads not only to the destruction of intracellular forms of BCG, but also to a massive increase in the number and activity of the phagocytic cells. BCG in combination with most immunogens heightens the immune response. In mice it slightly but significantly increases the immune response to tumors. BCG may act either as an immunological adjuvant by increasing the immunogenicity of the antigens it is mixed with, or by increasing the activity of the macrophage system. This increased activity could be nonspecific, or it could involve an increase in either natural killer cells or in the cells responsible for antibody-dependent cell-mediated immunity. Thus far the effect of BCG on human tumors seems limited to those accessible to injection or infection with BCG; distant metastases and internal tumors usually are unaffected. BCG is potentially dangerous because increasing the immunogenicity of tumor cell antigens could increase the levels of blocking factors or suppressor cells as well as the cell-mediated immune response against a tumor.

4.   Antibody therapy of tumors also is impractical at this time. Injections of tumor-specific antibody into tumor-bearing hosts would be helpful only for leukemias, in which the cells are sensitive to antibody-triggered immunological destruction rather than to immunological enhancement, which otherwise is the most likely consequence of passive antibody transfer. Triggering antibody-dependent cell-mediated immunity would be another hypothetical approach, but this possibility will be impractical until more is known about the requirements for effective antibody in the triggering process.

In summary, the current prospects for development of an effective cancer immunotherapy are not promising.

B.   By contrast, immunodiagnosis of cancer is likely to be an important addition to the clinician's armamentarium. Many tumors release specific cell-surface antigens into the bloodstream, and these antigens can be detected by radioimmunoassay (see the appendix to Chapter 2). There are three important limitations to this type of assay: first, antigen must be available in highly purified form so that the radioimmunoassay will be specific; second, the determinants must retain antigenicity when radiolabeled with iodine; and third, the antigen must be free to enter the circulation in tumor bearing hosts.

Immunoassay also can be used to measure levels of serum antibody to a specific tumor antigen. Assays that detect antibody action on whole tumor cells *in vitro* may be used, so that it is unnecessary that purified antigen be available or that the tumor release antigen into the circulation. It is necessary only that antibody responses be related in some way to the presence or absence of tumor antigens in the host.

C.   Immunological techniques also could be useful in cancer prevention. If it ever becomes possible to identify infectious agents, such as oncornaviruses that induce tumors bearing virus-specific antigens, then the possibility of vaccination with attenuated forms of these agents could be considered. However, as pointed out in Essential Concept 5–9, induction of an immune response to a tumor-associated antigen may result in immunological enhancement rather than in protective immunity. Extensive animal testing would be required to determine the potential benefits and risks of such an approach before it could be applied to humans. Whereas immunodiagnosis and immunotherapy would be applied to patients with poor prognoses, vaccination would be carried out on a healthy population. Large-scale vaccination could not be justified unless the risk of inducing disease was proven to be virtually nonexistent.

Selected Bibliography

Where to begin

Cairns, J., "The cancer problem," *Sci. Am.* **233**, 64 (1975) A general review of cancer biology, with emphasis on possible environmental causes of cancer.

Koprowski, H. (Ed.), *Neoplastic Transformation: Mechanisms and Consequences,* Pergamon Press, Berlin, 1977. A recent comprehensive review written for nonexperts.

Biology of cancer cells

Holley, R. W., "A unifying hypothesis concerning the nature of malignant growth," *Proc. Natl. Acad. Sci. USA* **69**, 2840 (1972). An argument for the possibility that the crucial change in a malignant cell is an alteration in the cell-surface membrane that results in increased internal concentrations of nutrients that regulate cell growth.

Nowell, P. C., "The clonal evolution of tumor cell populations," *Science* **194,** 23 (1976).

Friedman, J. M., and Fialkow, P. J., "Cell marker studies of human tumorigenesis," *Transplant. Rev.* **28,** 17 (1976). The preceding two articles are on the question of monoclonal versus multiclonal origins of cancers, including a discussion of the factors involved in the progression of tumors of low malignancy into tumors of high malignancy.

Nicolson, G. L., and Poste, G., "The cancer cell: dynamic aspects and modifications in cell-surface organization," *N. Engl. J. Med.* **295,** 197 (1976). A current review of cell-membrane changes associated with specific properties of cancer cells.

Chemical and physical agents that cause cancer

Berenblum, I., "The two-stage mechanism of carcinogenesis in biochemical terms," in *The Physiopathology of Cancer* **1,** 393 (1974). A discussion of the evidence for carcinogens and promotors.

Heidelberger, C., "Chemical carcinogenesis," *Annu. Rev. Biochem.* **44,** 79 (1975). A comprehensive survey of the field, including consideration of carcinogens (and their metabolic activation) *in vivo* and *in vitro,* and discussion of their possible modes of action.

Favus, M. J., Schneider, A. B., Stachura, M. E., Arnold, J. E., Ryo, U. Y., Pinsky, S. M., Colman, M., Arnold, M. J., and Frohman, L. A., "Thyroid cancer occurring as a late consequence of head-and-neck irradiation," *New Engl. J. Med.* **294,** 1019 (1976). A clinical study on the incidence of irradiation-induced thyroid cancer in a selected subset of patients.

Mutational and nonmutational models for the origin of cancer

Knudson, A. G., Hethcote, H. W., and Brown, B. W., "Mutation and childhood cancer: a probabilistic model for the incidence of retinoblastoma," *Proc. Natl. Acad. Sci. USA* **72,** 5116 (1975). An epidemiological perspective on the interaction of heredity, environment, and mutation in the genesis of a cancer of the retina.

Mintz, B., and Illmensee, K., "Normal genetically mosaic mice produced from malignant teratoma cells," *Proc. Natl. Acad. Sci. USA* **72,** 3585 (1975). This paper details an elegant series of experiments which demonstrate that teratocarcinoma cells can revert completely to the normal phenotype, given the right conditions.

Rubin, H., "Carcinogenicity tests," *Science* **191,** 241 (1976).

Ames, B. N., "Reply," *Science* **191,** 241 (1976). Are carcinogens mutagens, and if so, does their mutagenicity explain their mode of action in malignant transformation? Two distinguished scientists from the University of California, Berkeley, debate the issue.

Oncogenic viruses

Weissman, I., and Baird, S., "Oncornavirus leukemogenesis as a model for selective neoplastic transformation," in Koprowski, H. (Ed.). *Neoplastic Transformation: Mechanisms and Consequences,* p. 135, 1977.

Following are three Nobel Prize lectures for 1975:

Dulbecco, R., "From the molecular biology of oncogenic DNA viruses to cancer," *Science* **192,** 437 (1976).

Baltimore, D., "Viruses, polymerases, and cancer," *Science* **192,** 632 (1976).

Temin, H. M., "The DNA provirus hypothesis," *Science* **192,** 1075 (1976).

Gross, L., "The role of C-type and other oncogenic virus particles in cancer and leukemia," *N. Engl. J. Med.* **294,** 724 (1976).

Klein, G., "The Epstein–Barr virus and neoplasia," *N. Engl. J. Med.* **293,** 1353 (1975).

Green, M., "Viral cell transformation in human oncogenesis," *Hospital Practice* **10,** 9, 91 (1975).

The preceding three articles describe the borderland between animal oncogenic virus studies and human cancers.

Tooze, J., *The molecular biology of tumor viruses,* Cold Spring Harbor Laboratory (1973). A clear and authoritative volume on cancer viruses and cancer biology.

Immunosurveillance of cancer: The beginnings of tumor immunology

Ehrlich, P., "Uber den jetzigen Stand der Karzinomforschung," in *The Collected Papers of Paul Ehrlich,* Vol. II, Pergamon Press, London, 1957, p. 550. Cited here is the famous 1908 speech by Ehrlich setting the stage for the study of tumor immunology.

Thomas, L., "Reactions to homologous tissue antigens in relationship to hypersensitivity," in *Cellular and Humoral Aspects of the Hypersensitive States,* Lawrence, H. S., (Ed.), Hoeber-Harber, New York, 1959, p. 529.

Burnet, F. M., "The concept of immunological surveillance, *Prog. Exp. Tumor Res.* **13,** 1 (1970).

The preceding are two restatements of the Ehrlich hypothesis, with a more elaborate discussion of the possibility that development of immunosurveillance provided the selective pressure for evolution of cellular immunity.

Tumor Antigenicity

Prehn, R. T., and Main, J. M., "Immunity to methylcholanthrene-induced sarcomas," *J. Natl. Cancer Inst.* **18,** 769 (1957). In this landmark study it was demonstrated that hosts may show specific immunity to carcinogen-induced tumors, that such tumors express the same tumor antigens through hundreds of cell generations, and that each carcinogen-induced tumor possesses unique tumor antigens. Twenty years later we know little more about these tumors.

Klein, G., "Tumor antigens," *Annu. Rev. Microbiol.* **20,** 223 (1966). Antigens induced by oncogenic viruses are common from tumor to tumor induced by a particular virus.

Alexander, P., "Foetal 'antigens' in cancer," *Nature* **235,** 137 (1972). A review of the known oncofetal antigen systems.

Boyse, E. A., and Old, L. J., "Some aspects of normal and abnormal cell-surface genetics," *Annu. Rev. Genet.* **3,** 269 (1969). Differentiation antigens, tumor antigens, and an extensive discussion of the TL antigen.

Gold, P., and Freedman, S. O., "Specific carcinoembryonic antigens of the human digestive system," *J. Exp. Med.* **122,** 467 (1965). This paper (and a companion paper in the same journal issue) demonstrates that oncofetal antigens are expressed in humans.

Cellular and humoral participants in immune responses to tumors

Algire, G. H., Weaver, J. M., and Prehn, R. T., "Growth of cells *in vivo* in diffusion chambers. I. Survival of homografts in immunized mice," *J. Natl. Cancer Inst.* **15,** 493 (1954). A classical paper that demonstrated the primacy of cell-mediated immunity over humoral immunity in the rejection of tumor transplants.

Hellström, K. E., and Hellström, I., "Immunologic defenses against cancer," in *Immunobiology,* Good, R. A., and Fisher, D. W., (Eds.), Sinauer Associates, Stamford, Conn., 1971, Chapter 21. A review of *in vitro* assays which revealed cell-initiated immunity to human tumor antigens, and its inhibition by serum blocking factors.

Kiessling, R., Petranyi, G., Kärre, K., Jondal, M., Tracey, D., and Wigzell, H., "Killer cells: a functional comparison between natural, immune T-cell, and antibody-dependent *in vitro* systems," *J. Exp. Med.* **143,** 772 (1976). A survey of known killer cell types that suggests that all three such systems may be operative in tumor rejection.

Relationship of immunosurveillance to killer-cell and immune-cell systems

Miller, J. F. A. P., Ting, R. C., and Law, L. W., "Influence of thymectomy on tumor induction by polyoma virus in C57Bl mice," *Proc. Soc. Exp. Biol. Med.* **116,** 323 (1964). The T-cell system operates to regulate DNA virus-induced tumors.

Prehn, R. T., "The immune reaction as a stimulator of tumor growth," *Science* **176,** 170 (1972). But immune cells also can augment tumor growth!

Möller, G., and Möller, E., "The concept of immunological surveillance against neoplasia," *Transplant. Rev.* **28,** 3 (1976).

Schwartz, R. S., "Another look at immunologic surveillance," *N. Engl. J. Med.* **293,** 181 (1975).

The preceding two reviews question the immunosurveillance theory.

Immunological escape by tumor cells

Kaliss, N., "The survival of homografts in mice pretreated with antisera to mouse tissues," *Ann. N. Y. Acad. Sci.* **64,** 977 (1957). An important early paper on the phenomenon and mechanism of immunological enhancement.

Hellström, K. E., and Hellström, I., "Lymphocyte-mediated cytotoxicity and blocking serum activity to tumor antigens," *Adv. Immunol.* **18,** 209 (1974). Antigen–antibody complexes as blocking factors.

Klein, G., "Immunological surveillance against neoplasia," *Harvey Lecture Series* **69,** 71 (1975).

Melief, C. J. M., and Schwartz, R. S., "Immunocompetence and malignancy," in *Cancer, a Comprehensive Treatise,* Becker, F. F., (Ed.), Plenum Press, New York, 1975, Vol. I, p. 121.

The preceding two articles are reviews of immunological escape and host–tumor interactions leading to tumor growth.

Problems

5-1   Indicate whether each of the following statements is true or false. Explain the error in each statement you consider to be false.

(a)   Cancer cells generally divide more rapidly than normal cells.

(b)   The daughters of a cancer cell generally have identical morphological and metabolic characteristics.

(c)   Every tumor appears to have one or more tumor-associated antigens on its cell surface.

(d)   Tumor-associated antigens that are expressed earlier in development as fetal membrane components cannot induce an immune response in the adult animal because of the lack of immunologic responsiveness to self-components (tolerance).

(e)   The spread of cancer viruses from one organ to another, causing *de novo* cancer induction in the second organ, is called metastasis.

(f)   The site of metastatic spread via lymphatics usually is predictable, whereas the site of metastatic spread via the bloodstream usually is unpredictable.

(g)   Rapidly transforming oncornaviruses contain a gene that codes for the malignant phenotype when expressed in host cells.

(h)   Chemical carcinogens and x rays act by introducing new genetic information into the cell.

(i)   At the time of clinical diagnosis, most cancers consist of several independent clones of malignant cells, presumably due to the multicentric origins of most cancers.

(j)   Most oncogenic RNA viruses have an RNA-dependent DNA polymerase that permits the transfer of information from RNA to DNA.

(k)   The fact that many cancers undergo several progressions in their malignant behavior is proof of the somatic mutation hypothesis of carcinogenesis.

(l)   Each chemically induced tumor appears to have a unique tumor-associated antigen.

(m)   The lymphocytes from a patient dying of malignant melanoma usually can destroy his own tumor cells *in vitro*.

(n)   The lymphocytes from one patient with malignant melanoma usually can destroy *in vitro* the tumor cells from a second patient with this same disease.

(o)   Osteogenic sarcoma with a single diagnosed lung metastasis is most likely to be cured by surgery alone.

5–2   Supply the missing word or words in each of the following statements.

(a)   Tumors with little cellular adhesiveness tend to _____ to distant sites rapidly.

(b)   The three conventional forms of cancer therapy are _____, _____, and _____.

(c)   Most anticancer drugs _____ the immune system.

(d)   _____ infections occur in permissive cells, whereas _____ infections occur in nonpermissive cells infected by polyoma.

(e)   _____ viruses appear to cause most spontaneous virus-induced cancers in animals.

(f)   DNA copies of the RNA virus genome are made by the enzyme _____ _____.

(g)   Cigarette smokers who have an exceptionally high risk of developing lung cancer may have abnormally _____ levels of the aryl hydrocarbon hydroxylase enzymes.

(h)   The rapid loss of a cell-surface tumor antigen upon contact with specific antibody is called _____ _____.

(i)   The cellular immune system may have evolved as a _____ system for cancer.

(j)   Tumor-associated antigens that result in immune rejection usually are located in the cancer cell _____ _____.

(k)   _____ _____ appear to be composed of humoral antibodies and tumor-associated antigens.

(l)   Ultimate carcinogens cause irreversible changes necessary for neoplastic transformation, but transformation also requires the subsequent action of another class of substances, termed _____.

5–3   As an epidemiologist, how would you interpret the following data taken from a recent journal article? In 1963 a study was initiated on 370 unionized asbestos insulation workers, all of whom had been working for at least twenty years. Previous analysis of members of the union between 1943 and 1963 had shown lung cancer deaths to be 6.8 times as frequent as expected from statistics on the general population. Among the 370 men, there were 87 who had no history of cigarette smoking. By April 1967, there had been no death from lung cancer in this group. By contrast, 24 of the 283 with a history of regular cigarette smoking had died of lung cancer, although only less than three such deaths had been expected, given their smoking habits.

5-4   The entire SV40 genome usually is integrated into the host genome during transformation. The virus can be induced by fusion of the transformed cell with a permissive cell, leading to cell lysis and the release of mature infectious virions. Offer a possible explanation for this observation.

5-5   Polyoma virus infection occurs naturally in adult mice without apparent ill effect. However, when injected into newborn mice the virus causes several different tumors. Can you offer an explanation for this surprising behavior?

5-6   Leukemia is a cancer of blood-forming cells, and usually is restricted to one or another blood-cell type. The diagnosis and treatment of leukemia requires an understanding of leukemic cell growth kinetics. For most of the life history of a leukemia the number of leukemic cells increases exponentially with time, usually doubling in number with each cell cycle. The cell-cycle time, designated TC, is the interval between mitoses. In leukemias that originate in or home to the bone marrow, a total body load of at least 10^{10} leukemic cells ($\sim$10 g of tumor cells) must be present before an experienced pathologist can diagnosis leukemia by microscopic analysis of a sample of bone marrow. A total body load of 10^{11} leukemic cells must be present before diagnosis can be made by an examination of the blood, and 10^{12} cells generally must be present before a patient becomes aware that he is ill because of either bleeding or infection, caused by leukemic replacement of platelets or polymorphonuclear leukocytes, respectively. Nearly 10^{13} cells must be present before leukemic infiltration of vital organs causes death.

     The elimination of leukemic cells by chemotherapeutic agents also is roughly an exponential function of dose; for example, if 10 mg of Drug A eliminates 90% of the leukemic cells, then 20 mg will eliminate 99%, 30 mg will eliminate 99.9%, and so on. However, at a certain dose of any drug the side effects become so severe that treatment with that drug must be stopped. Suppose that you are a clinical oncologist treating a leukemia patient who has come to you with bleeding gums. You treat him initially with 30 mg of the Drug A described above, and despite a few days of nausea and diarrhea (due to death of gastrointestinal tract cells) his gums clear up. However, he returns

Table 5–5
Properties of six drugs used for chemotherapy of leukemia (Problem 5–6)

Drug	Dose to eliminate 90% leukemic cells	Limiting dose because of side effects	Type of side effects
A	10 mg	30 mg	Gastrointestinal
B	5 mg	20 mg	Gastrointestinal
C	100 mg	200 mg	Bone marrow depression
D	0.5 mg	1.0 mg	Gastrointestinal
E	50 mg	200 mg	Peripheral neuritis (tingling and pain)
F	10 mg	20 mg	Lymphocytopenia (infections)

after 20 days, when his gums again have started to bleed. Assume that the leukemic cells in this patient always double their number with each cell cycle.
(a)   What is the average cell-cycle time for this patient's leukemia?
(b)   How long before the first diagnosis did this patient's leukemia arise?
(c)   In diagnostic chest x rays, you notice that a spot has appeared in the patient's lungs, and you correctly assume that it is a solid leukemic tumor. How long will it take for the tumor to increase in diameter from 10 mm to 40 mm?
(d)   You have at your disposal the drugs listed in Table 5–5. Choose the optimal treatment for your patient, and explain the rationale for it.
(e)   Assuming that all cells are accessible to the chemotherapeutic agents, how many leukemic cells will remain following your treatment? How long will the patient be in remission without symptoms?
(f)   In a case similar to this one, the patient did not have a recurrence of bone-marrow-diagnosable leukemia for five years. Give two possible explanations for this striking remission.

5–7   How would you explain the following results?
(a)   An antiserum raised against unfertilized mouse eggs in a xenogeneic host (of another species) is cytotoxic to SV40-transformed mouse cells but not to normal adult mouse cells.
(b)   The serum from mice immunized with syngeneic SV40-transformed cells is not cytotoxic to mouse eggs, but it does contain antibodies directed against a tumor-specific surface antigen that appears in response to virus infection.

5–8   In 1963 L. J. Old and his co-workers produced antisera in C57Bl/6 mice by immunization with spontaneous leukemias from (A × C57Bl/6) F_1 mice. These antisera were cytotoxic *in vitro* for cells of several

Table 5–6
Tla phenotypes and genotypes (Problem 5–8)

Prototype strain	Tla phenotype of normal thymocytes	Phenotype of leukemic cells and presumed Tla genotype of mouse
A	1, 2, 3, –	1, 2, 3, –
C57Bl/6	–, –, –, –	1, 2, –, 4
BALB/c	–, 2, –, –	1, 2, –, –
DBA/2	–, 2, –, –	1, 2, –, 4

C57Bl/6 leukemias and for normal thymocytes from A and C58 strains. The antigen was designated TL, and the locus coding for the antigen was called the Tla (*t*hymus *l*eukemia *a*ntigen) locus. TL was shown to be a complex consisting of four antigens, Tla.1, Tla.2, Tla.3, and Tla.4. Normal inbred strains of mice fall into three groups based on the presence of these antigens, and leukemia cells fall into four groups (Table 5–6).

(a)   The three *normal* Tla phenotypes (haplotypes) behave as alleles at a single locus that maps about 1.5 centimorgans from the H-2D locus. However, two observations in Table 5–6 suggest that the Tla antigens are not coded by three simple alleles at one locus. What are these observations? Offer a genetic model to explain them.

(b)   One striking observation has been made regarding mice immunized against Tla antigens and containing high titers of cytotoxic Tla antibodies. Such mice might be expected to resist syngeneic Tla-positive leukemias, but they do not; they are readily killed by such tumors. Moreover, the tumors recovered from such immunized hosts lose their sensitivity to Tla antisera *in vitro* and lose their ability to absorb cytotoxic Tla antibodies. However, this loss is only temporary, because a single passage of the tumors in nonimmunized syngeneic hosts allows the tumor to regain its ability to adsorb cytotoxic Tla antibodies. How would you explain these observations? The phenomenon they illustrate is formally similar to another cell-surface phenomenon described for receptor immunoglobulins. What is it? How would you test whether the two phenomena are mediated by similar mechanisms?

5–9   Suppose that you are a cancer immunologist studying the role of the immune response to two highly malignant fibrosarcomas from Patients A and B. The cancer cells grow well in tissue culture, and the cultured cells are proven to be malignant by various tests. Serum, blood lymphocytes, and normal fibroblasts from Patients A and B are readily obtainable. You conduct several tests in tissue culture with patient lymphocytes, serum, tumor cells, and normal target cells, adding serum to target cells at time zero and then adding lymphocytes four hours later, according to the experimental design indicated in Table 5–7. One

Table 5–7
Immunologic analyses of tumor cells from two fibrosarcoma patients (Problem 5–9)

Experiment	Lymphocytes added from patient	Serum added from patient	Tumor target cells from patient	Number of tumor colonies growing
I	—	—	A	100
	—	A	A	97
	A	—	A	12
	A	A	A	98
II	—	—	B	101
	B	—	B	13
	A	—	B	98
III	B	—	A	15
	—	B	A	96
	B	A	A	99
	A	B	A	12

to three days later, you obtain the results shown in the table. In all possible combinations, growth of normal fibroblast colonies from Patient A and Patient B was unaffected by the addition of serum or lymphocytes or both from these patients.

(a)   By which of the following possibilities could one explain the continued growth of tumor in Patient A: lack of an anti-tumor immune response, immunological tolerance, immunostimulation, immunoselection, immunological enhancement, or antigenic modulation? Discuss each possibility.

(b)   What can you conclude concerning individual specific and cross-reacting tumor-associated antigens on tumors from Patients A and B, the ability of lymphocytes from each of these patients to recognize each of these antigens, and the specificity of serum factors from each of these patients?

5–10   As a young physician interested in immunology, you have a brilliant idea. One common type of leukemia is a cancer of the lymphocyte. Why not irradiate these leukemia patients with a dose of x rays sufficient to destroy all their lymphocytes (i.e., normal and leukemic cells) and then give them an adoptive transfer of spleen cells from another individual? The host's immune system is destroyed so there should be no graft rejection. All the leukemic cells are destroyed, hence the cancer should be cured. An older colleague finds your proposal highly amusing. Why?

5–11   Some cancer cells express tumor-specific molecules that make the tumor antigenic to its host. One such tumor is a cancer called Moloney sarcoma

(MS), which is induced by an RNA cancer virus, MSV (Moloney sarcoma virus). Transplantation of this tumor to syngeneic hosts leads to tumor growth and then regression. If the tumor is retransplanted to MS regressors there is no tumor growth. Another tumor, EMT6, is a breast cancer that does not share tumor antigens with MS, and is only weakly antigenic to its hosts.

(a)   Serum from normal mice or from MS regressors was transfused into normal mice just prior to transplantation with MS on one side and EMT6 on the other. The transfusion did not affect the incidence or the growth rate of either tumor in these hosts. What conclusions can you draw from this result?

(b)   The minimal number of viable EMT6 cells that will transplant a tumor to 100% of recipient hosts is 1.5×10^4 cells. Single-cell suspensions of EMT6 and MS were prepared and injected alone or intermixed into the skin of normal or MS-regressor (MS−R) hosts. The incidence of tumor growth is shown in Table 5-8. All hosts had tumors biopsied on Day 24, and all tumors from Group C were identified microscopically as EMT6. Consider Table 5-8, Parts A and B, and compare the growth of EMT6 and MS in Groups 1-3. What conclusions

Table 5-8

Tumor incidence of EMT6 and MS transplanted into normal or MS-immune syngeneic hosts (Problem 5-11)

Group	Tumor	Host	Days after inoculation: 8	15	24
A. Growth of EMT6 in normal and MS-immune hosts					
1	EMT6[a]	N[b]	3/7[c]	7/7	7/7
2	EMT6	MS-R[b]	0/10	6/10	5/10
3	EMT6	MS-R[d]	0/10	6/10	6/8
B. Growth of MS in normal and MS-immune hosts					
1	MS[a]	N	7/7	7/7	3/7
2	MS	MS-R	0/10	2/10	1/10
3	MS	MS-R[d]	1/10	0/10	0/8
C. Growth of EMT6 alone or intermixed in MS-immune hosts					
2	EMT6	MS-R	0/10	6/10	5/10
5	Mixture[a]	MS-R	1/10	7/10	8/10
3	EMT6	MS-R[d]	0/10	6/10	6/8
3	Mixture	MS-R[d]	1/10	5/10	6/8

[a] 1.5×10^4 viable (6×10^4 total) EMT6 cells were inoculated into syngeneic hosts, alone or intermixed with 3×10^6 total (6×10^5 viable) MS cells. At other sites, 3×10^6 total (6×10^5 viable) MS cells were injected into these hosts.
[b] N = untreated BALB/c mice; MS-R = Moloney sarcoma regressor mice.
[c] Incidence of tumor-positive mice/total number mice given injections.
[d] In addition to EMT6 and MS flank injections, a third site was injected with the same number of both tumor lines intermixed.
[From I. Weissman, *J. Natl. Cancer Inst.* **51**, 443, 1973.]

Table 5–9
Specific chromium release from C57Bl and BALB/c Moloney lymphoma tumor cells attacked by anti-MSV lymphocytes from different strains (Problem 5–12)

Anti-MSV spleen cells from	H-2 genotype	Lymphoma target cells from:	
		C57Bl (H-2b/b)	BALB/c (H-2d/d)
		(percent release)	
BALB/c	d/d	7	17
C57Bl	b/b	34	7
(BALB/c × C57Bl) F$_1$	b/d	39	16
[a]BALB.B	b/b	45	8
[b]B10.D2	d/d	7	24

[a]BALB mice with the H-2^b trait of C57Bl mice.
[b]C57Bl mice with the H-2^d trait. [From E. Gomard, V. Duprez, Y. Henin, and J. P. Levy, *Nature* **260,** 706, (1976).]

Table 5–10
Specific chromium release from C57Bl and BALB/c tumor cells attacked by (BALB/c × C57Bl) F$_1$ lymphocytes (Problem 5–12)

Immunization by	Moloney target cells from:	
	C57Bl	BALB/c
	(percent release)	
MSV inoculation	38	16
	13	8
	36	21
BALB/c Moloney lymphoma cells	6	34
	4	26
	0	12
C57Bl Moloney lymphoma cells	7	0
	13	0
	12	0

[From E. Gomard, V. Duprez, Y. Henin, and J. P. Levy, *Nature* **260,** 706 (1976).]

Table 5–11
Blocking of anti-MSV T-cell-induced cytolysis by preincubation of target cells with anti-H-2 antibodies (Problem 5–12)

Antisera	Specific chromium release by BALB.B Moloney lymphoma target cells (percent)
BALB/c normal serum	18
BALB/c anti C57Bl	0
BALB/c anti-C57Bl absorbed in BALB.B	17
BALB/c anti-C57Bl absorbed in B10.D2	4
BALB/c anti-BALB.B	0
C57Bl anti-BALB/c	19
AKR anti-Thy-1.2	19

[From E. Gomard, V. Duprez, Y. Henin, and J. P. Levy, *Nature* **260,** 706 (1976).]

can be drawn and what hypotheses can you propose to explain the data?

(c)   Consider Table 5–8, Part C. Discuss the results in terms of effector cell function and specificity. What can you say about the role in this reaction of T-cell lymphokines such as lymphotoxin?

5–12 Immunity to Moloney tumor antigens can be tested *in vitro*, using Moloney lymphoma cells as targets. A research group compared the anti-Moloney immune responses, using lymphocytes and target cells from different strains of mice. They carried out these assays at a time following immunization, when T_c cells were the only killer cells that could recognize and eliminate Moloney target cells. The data from these experiments are shown in Tables 5–9, 5–10, and 5–11. [The tables are from E. Gomard, V. Duprez, Y. Henin, and J. P. Levy, *Nature* **260**, 706 (1976).]

(a)   What conclusions can you draw from Tables 5–9 and 5–10?

(b)   Discuss Table 5–11 in terms of T_c cell receptor specificity.

Answers

5–1   (a)   False.   Many normal cells divide more rapidly than most cancer cells (e.g., cells of the gastrointestinal tract and bone marrow). Tumor growth occurs primarily because cancer cell division is not regulated.

(b)   True

(c)   True

(d)   False.   If fetal components disappear before the maturation of the immune response (in most animals at or near birth), these components will be recognized as foreign in later life. Indeed, to maintain a state of tolerance or lack of immunologic reactivity, components generally must be exposed to the immune system throughout the individual's life.

(e)   False.   Metastasis is the property of cancer *cells* to move from one site to another, resulting in tumor cell colonization of the second site.

(f)   True

(g)   True

(h)   False.   They modify the existing genetic information or operate in an epigenetic manner. The only carcinogens known to introduce new genetic information into cells are viruses.

(i)   False.   For most types of cancer at the time of diagnosis, most cancer cells in one patient are members of a single clone. Although this observation has been taken as evidence for the unicentric origin of most cancers, it in fact only provides evidence that a single clone is dominant.

(j)   True

(k)   False.   Although the somatic mutation hypothesis *predicts* tumor progression, epigenetic theories such as selective gene activation and inactivation also are consistent with the phenomenon of tumor progression.

(l)   True

(m)   True

(n)   True

(o)   False.   The finding of a bloodborne metastasis rules out the possibility of cure by surgery alone, as other micrometastases at unpredictable sites are surely present. Systemic chemotherapy and surgical or radiotherapeutic removal of the primary tumor are currently the only treatments of this disease pattern.

5–2   (a)   metastasize
    (b)   surgery, radiation, and chemotherapy
    (c)   suppress
    (d)   Lytic, temperate (transforming)
    (e)   RNA tumor
    (f)   reverse transcriptase (RNA-dependent DNA polymerase)
    (g)   high
    (h)   antigenic modulation
    (i)   surveillance
    (j)   plasma membrane
    (k)   Blocking factors
    (l)   promotors

5–3   This study appears to provide an example of the multiple factor etiology of lung cancer. Smoking alone should have caused 3 deaths, not 24. None of the 87 asbestos workers with no history of smoking died, hence it was not the asbestos alone. However, smoking and asbestos exposure in combination had an apparent multiplicative effect. The journal article goes on to conclude that asbestos workers who smoked had a risk of dying from lung cancer eight times larger than that of smokers of the same age who had had no asbestos exposure, and 92 times larger than the risk of an individual who neither worked with asbestos nor smoked. A similar multiple-factor effect has been demonstrated for smoking and uranium exposure.

5–4   One possible explanation may be that the transformed cell lacks a factor that permits the expression of late viral genes. The permissive cell supplies this factor and initiates the lytic pathway.

5–5   Adult mice are immune to polyoma. Under normal laboratory conditions mice presumably are exposed to polyoma after the immune system has matured to the point of being able to generate an adequate response. In contrast, newborn mice with an immature immune system cannot generate an effective immune response rapidly enough to prevent malignant tumor growth.

5–6   (a)   Because the patient arrived with bleeding gums, it is reasonable to assume a tumor load of $\sim 10^{12}$ cells. Drug A should eliminate 99.9% of them, leaving $\sim 10^9$ cells. These cells multiply to give 10^{12} cells again in 20 days. If each cell gives rise to 2 dividing progeny, and n is the number of doublings, then $(10^9)(2^n) = 10^{12}$, and $n \cong 10$. Thus 10 cell cycles take place in 20 days, and the cell-cycle time (TC) is 2 days.

(b)   At first diagnosis the patient had $\sim 10^{12}$ cells. If the leukemia began as a single cell (10^0), then $(10^0)(2^n) = 10^{12}$, and $n \cong 40$. Forty cell cycles would take 80 days, assuming that the TC of two days is constant, that the cells multiplied exponentially throughout, and that there were no cells lost.

(c)   Because solid tumors grow roughly as spheroids, a 4-fold increase in diameter corresponds to a 64-fold increase in volume, and thus a 64-fold increase in cell number. Thus $2^n = 64$; $n = 6$ cell cycles, and 12 days should be required for the specified increase in tumor diameter.

(d)   Three principles should be followed in chemotherapy. (1) Simultaneous treatment with different drugs is preferential to sequential treatment, which allows clonal expansion of tumor cells between doses. More important, tumor resistance results from selection of drug-resistant variants, and the frequency of multiply resistant variants will be the product of the frequencies of singly resistant variants. For example, if the frequency of a singly resistant variant is 10^{-5}, then the probability of a variant that is resistant to 2 drugs simultaneously is 10^{-10}. (2) Drugs used in combination should be those that do not lead to similar side effects. Thus in this case one cannot use any combinations of drugs A, B, and D, because they all damage gastrointestinal cells. (3) The preferred drugs are those with the highest therapeutic index, which is the ratio of toxic drug dose to effective drug dose. One should choose the drug that offers the best therapeutic index, regardless of its potency on a per milligram basis. Therefore the best choice among A, B, and D is B, and the optimal treatment is concurrent administration of B, C, E, and F at their highest tolerable doses (20 mg for B, 200 mg for C, 200 mg for E, and 20 mg for F).

(e)   If each drug acts independently and additively on the leukemic cell population, then the treatment recommended in (d) should reduce the leukemic cell load from 10^{12} to 10^0 cells, that is, to a single cell. Assuming that recurrence of symptoms requires a 10^{12} cell tumor load, symptoms would recur after 80 days [see Part (b)].

(f)   This remission could be explained if some of the drugs acted synergistically rather than in an additive fashion, or if the total tumor cell load was reduced to a level at which host defense mechanisms, such as immunity, could eliminate the remaining leukemic cells.

5–7   The simplest interpretation is that SV40 transformation leads to the appearance in the cell membrane of both a fetal antigen to which adult mice are tolerant and a new tumor-specific surface antigen. Thus multiple new membrane components may be induced by neoplastic transformation.

5-8   (a)   No Tla antigens are expressed on normal thymocytes in C57Bl/6 mice, but three of the Tla antigens are expressed on their leukemia cells. Similarly, only Tla.2 is expressed on normal thymocytes in BALB/c and DBA/2, but additional Tla specificities are expressed on their leukemic cells. This observation suggests that each of the four strains carries at least three of the four Tla structural genes, that the Tla complex includes elements that control the expression of these genes, and that the structural genes are "derepressed," or induced, during leukemogenesis. Alternatively, these structural genes could be expressed in only a small subset of normal cells (e.g., up to 5% of C57Bl/6 thymocytes could be Tla.1,2,4 and not be detectable using Old's assay), and these cells could be preferentially inducible by leukemogenic oncornaviruses.

(b)   This observation is an example of antibody-induced removal of surface antigens, called antigenic modulation. It is similar to the loss of B-cell surface immunoglobulins in the presence of anti-immunoglobulin antibodies, the phenomenon called capping. Most capped immunoglobulins are lost from the cell surface, some by shedding (exocytosis), and some by internalization (endocytosis). The capping of cell-surface immunoglobulins has a well-defined series of steps (ring → patch → cap) and is prevented by metabolic inhibitors and microtubular inhibitors, implying an active energy-dependent process involving the intracellular cytoskeletal system. One could test the sensitivity of TL antigenic modulation to metabolic and microtubular inhibitors. One apparent difference is that antigenic modulation of TL antigens is induced by monovalent Fab fragments, whereas the capping of immunoglobulins is not.

5-9   (a)   Experiment I demonstrates that Patient A's lymphocytes will prevent outgrowth of A tumor-cell colonies, whereas his serum has no direct effect on A tumor-cell growth. However, addition of A's serum to A tumor target cells before addition of lymphocytes blocks the immune effect of the lymphocytes on the tumor cells. Therefore, the patient *has* developed an antitumor immune response, ruling out the lack of immune responsivity, immunological tolerance to tumor antigens, and immunoselection of nonantigenic variants as explanations for continued tumor growth. Since neither arm of the immune response stimulates the growth of more A tumor colonies *in vitro*, it seems unlikely that immunostimulation is occurring *in vivo*. The specific inhibitory action of patient serum on cell-mediated tumor immunity could be the result of antibody-induced antigenic modulation. If so, one could predict that tumor cells taken directly from Patient A would be nonantigenic, and would reexpress tumor antigens only after tissue culture in the absence of patient serum or lymphocytes. Another likely possibility is the phenomenon of immunological enhancement, wherein tumor antigens are continually expressed, but serum blocking factors impede specific cell-mediated immunity.

(b)   It is likely that tumors from Patients A and B share some surface antigens, and that Tumor A has some unique antigens as well. For example, lymphocytes from Patient B recognize and react against both A and B tumor cells, but not against A and B normal cells. The most reasonable explanation is that these lymphocytes become sensitized to the cross-reacting antigens in B's tumor. Further evidence for this reaction comes from the ability of A serum to block the reaction of B's lymphocytes on A's tumor cells.

A's lymphocytes, however, appear to react only to noncross-reacting tumor antigens in tumor A; they do not react against B's tumor cells, and B's serum will not block the reaction of A lymphocytes on A tumor cells. Two points are not clear: (1) it is possible that A's lymphocytes fail to react to B's tumor cells because of a possible lack of associated recognition, and (2) we know nothing about B's humoral response to his tumor.

5–10   Your colleague is amused for several reasons. First, to irradiate and eliminate all leukemia cells one would have to irradiate the patient's *whole body* with a tumoricidal dose of irradiation. Even if all leukemic cells were sensitive to x-ray-induced interphase death, a whole-body dose of ~2000 rads would have to be given to eliminate 10^{11-12} leukemic cells; if the cells died only by mitotic death, a dose of nearly 4000 rads would be required. At 600–800 rads whole body, sufficient numbers of hematopoietic stem cells are eliminated so that death due to infection allowed by insufficient numbers of phagocytes or to bleeding caused by insufficient numbers of platelets generally occurs in 10–20 days. At 1000–1200 rads whole body, sufficient numbers of intestinal epithelial stem cells are eliminated so that death due to loss of body fluids through the denuded intestines occurs within 5–10 days. Although one may be able to transfuse hematopoietic stem cells, one cannot replace intestinal cells.

Even if the patient survived the irradiation, the lymphocytes from the donor would recognize the host antigens as foreign and initiate a GVHR, which generally leads to the death of the host.

5–11   (a)   Immunity to MS is not effected by the humoral immune system.
(b)   Part A: EMT6 cells grow less well in MS-R hosts. Perhaps there is a low-level antigenic cross-reactivity between these tumors, or perhaps MS activation of the immune system results in a more active host response to EMT6, for example by nonspecific macrophage activation. Part B: MS grows and regresses in normal mice, but does not grow in MS-R hosts (although EMT6 does). Specific cell-mediated immunity to MS tumors is established.

(c)   Killer cells in this system recognize and destroy MS cells. Even though each EMT6 cell is entrapped in a 50-fold excess of MS tumor cells, the killer cell reaction to MS spares EMT6 cells. Thus both recognition and elimination in this reaction are highly specific *in vivo.* If T-cell lymphokines play any role in this reaction, they must act at extremely short range, and cannot act effectively as diffusable nonspecific toxins.

5–12   (a)   Table 5–9 shows that anti-MSV BALB/c strain lymphocytes recognize and react only to BALB/c strain Moloney lymphomas, that C57Bl strain lymphocytes react only to C57Bl strain Moloney lymphomas, that (BALB/c × C57Bl) F$_1$ lymphocytes react to both C57Bl and BALB/c lymphomas, and that the required identity between killer and target is determined by the H-2 locus. Thus associated recognition of H-2 determinants (Essential Concept 1–13) is necessary for interaction of killer cells with target cells in this system. Table 5–10 demonstrates that (BALB/c × C57Bl) F$_1$ lymphocytes may demonstrate this restriction also, if the Moloney tumor antigens that stimulate the appearance of killer cells are presented in the context of one of the parental H-2 types. This result demonstrates the important point that the context of stimulation determines the range of recognition by killer cells, and that not all (BALB/c × C57Bl) F$_1$ anti-Moloney killer cells recognize Moloney target cells in the same way. One could propose that the repertoire of (BALB/c × C57Bl) F$_1$ anti-Moloney prekiller cells is relatively extensive, and that only those subsets recognizing Moloney antigens in the context of a particular H-2 type are stimulated by the cognate immunogen.

(b)   Table 5–11 demonstrates that preincubation of target cells with anti-H-2 serum directed against the H-2 type of the target cells prevents killer cell reactions to that cell, whereas antiserum to another antigen on that cell (Thy 1.2) does not prevent cytotoxicity. Furthermore, the table shows that the inhibitory activity of the H-2 antisera appears to be removed only by absorption with hosts expressing the correct H-2 type. One could propose that H-2 determinants on the target cells are in or close to the sites recognized by T$_c$-cell receptors, and that masking them with antibodies prevents appropriate T$_c$-cell recognition of the target cells.

Index